MW01121826

APLASTIC ANEMIA
Pathophysiology and treatment

This book takes account of the most recent findings in laboratory research and clinical trials to provide a comprehensive and up-to-date reference on the pathophysiology, epidemiology, diagnosis and treatment of acquired and inherited aplastic anemia.

As well as a comprehensive and detailed overview of the pathophysiology of the disease, the international team of authors covers all aspects of management, including the well established approaches of bone marrow transplantation and immunosuppressive treatment, new approaches such as the use of hematopoietic growth factors and escalated immunosuppression, and controversial issues such as stem cell transplantation. The final section concentrates on the inherited syndrome Fanconi's anemia. Much of the recent work in this area has been coordinated by the European Group for Blood and Marrow Transplantation (EBMT). Included here is an important international consensus document with guidelines on treatment of aplastic anemia which combines the results and views of the EBMT with those of the international experts from America and Japan.

Detailed treatment guidelines are given, making this the definitive resource for hematologists and clinicians from other disciplines involved in the management and supportive care of patients with aplastic anemia. Scientists interested in mechanisms of bone marrow failure will also find this an invaluable reference.

Hubert Schrezenmeier is Professor of Medicine in the Free University of Berlin and Chairman of the EBMT Working Party on Severe Aplastic Anemia. **Andrea Bacigalupo** is Director of the Bone Marrow Transplant Centre, Ospedale San Martino, Genoa, and President of the EBMT.

APLASTIC ANEMIA

Pathophysiology and treatment

Edited by

Hubert Schrezenmeier
Free University of Berlin

and Andrea Bacigalupo
Bone Marrow Transplant Centre, Ospedale San Martino, Genoa

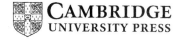

PUBLISHED BY THE PRESS SYNDICATE OF THE UNIVERSITY OF CAMBRIDGE
The Pitt building, Trumpington Street, Cambridge, United Kingdom

CAMBRIDGE UNIVERSITY PRESS
The Edinburgh Building, Cambridge CB2 2RU, UK   www.cup.cam.ac.uk
40 West 20th Street, New York, NY 10011–4211, USA   www.cup.org
10 Stamford Road, Oakleigh, Melbourne 3166, Australia
Ruiz de Alarcón 13, 28014 Madrid, Spain

© Cambridge University Press 2000

This book is in copyright. Subject to statutory exception
and to the provisions of relevant collective licensing agreements,
no reproduction of any part may take place without
the written permission of Cambridge University Press.

First published 2000

Printed in the United Kingdom at the University Press Cambridge

Typeface Utopia (*Adobe*) 9/13pt.   *System* QuarkXPress® [SE]

A catalogue record for this book is available from the British Library

Library of Congress Cataloguing in Publication data
Aplastic anemia : pathophysiology and treatment / edited by Hubert
Schrezenmeier and Andrea Bacigalupo.
p.   cm.
ISBN 0 521 64101 2 (hardback)
I. Schrezenmeier, H. (Hubert)   II. Bacigalupo, A.
[DNLM: 1. Anemia, Aplastic–physiopathology.   2. Anemia, Aplastic–
therapy.   WH 175 A6428 1999]
RC641.7.A6A656   1999
616.1′52–dc21
DNLM/DLC
for Library of Congress   99-10964 CIP

ISBN 0 521 64101 2 hardback

Every effort has been made in preparing this book to provide accurate and up-to-date information
which is in accord with accepted standards and practice at the time of publication. Nevertheless, the
authors, editors and publisher can make no warranties that the information contained herein is totally
free from error, not least because clinical standards are constantly changing through research and
regulation. The authors, editors and publisher therefore disclaim all liability for direct or consequential
damages resulting from the use of material contained in this book. Readers are strongly advised to pay
careful attention to information provided by the manufacturer of any drugs or equipment that they
plan to use.

Contents

Part IV   Fanconi's anemia

Contributors

Blanche P. Alter
Division of Pediatric
  Hematology/Oncology
Children's Hospital C3.270
University of Texas Medical Branch
Galveston, TX 77555-0361
USA

Andrea Bacigalupo
IInd Division of Hematology
Ospedale San Martino
Viale Benedetto XV
I-16132 Genova
Italy

Manuel Buchwald
Department of Molecular and Medical
  Genetics
The Hospital for Sick Children
University of Toronto
Toronto, Ontario
Canada

Bruce M. Camitta
Medical College of Wisconsin
PO Box 26509
8701 Watertown Plank Road
Milwaukee, WI 53226
USA

Madeleine Carreau
Department of Molecular and Medical
  Genetics
The Hospital for Sick Children
University of Toronto
Toronto, Ontario
Canada

H. Joachim Deeg
Clinical Research Division
Fred Hutchinson Cancer Research
  Center
1124 Columbia Street
Seattle, WA 98104
USA

Frances M. Gibson
Department of Haematology
St George's Hospital Medical School
Cranmer Terrace
London SW17 0RE
UK

Eliane Gluckman
Service de Greffe de Moelle Osseuse
Hôpital Saint-Louis
1 Avenue Claude Vellefaux
F-75475 Paris, Cedex 10
France

E. C. Gordon-Smith
Department of Haematology
St George's Hospital Medical School
Cranmer Terrace
London SW17 0RE
UK

Philippe Guardiola
Service de Greffe de Moelle Osseuse
Hôpital Saint-Louis
1 Avenue Claude Vellefaux
F-75475 Paris, Cedex 10
France

Hermann Heimpel
University of Ulm
Robert-Koch-Str aße8
D-89081 Ulm
Germany

Jill M. Hows
Division of Transplant Sciences
Southmead Health Services
Bristol
BS10 5NB
UK

Seiji Kojima
Department of Developmental Paediatrics
Nagoya University School of Medicine
Nagoya 453
Japan

Johnson M. Liu
Hematology Branch
NHLBI, NIH
10/ACRF/7C103
Bethesda, MD 20892
USA

Per Ljungman
Department of Hematology
Karolinska Institute
Huddinge University Hospital
SE-14186 Huddinge
Sweden

Anna Locasciulli
Division of Pediatric Hematology
Ospedale San Gerardo
Via Donizetti 106
I-20052 Monza
Italy

Pedro Marín-Fernandez
Postgraduate School of Hematology
  (EHFC)
Ferreras Valenti Hospital Clinic
C/Villarroel 170
E-08036 Barcelona
Spain

Judith C. W. Marsh
Department of Haematology
St George's Hospital Medical School
Cranmer Terrace
London SW17 0RE
UK

Jean-Yves Mary
Centre de Bioinformatique
INSERM U444
Université Paris VII
Paris
France

Shaun R. McCann
Department of Haematology
St James's Hospital
Dublin 8
Ireland

Shinji Nakao
Third Department of Medicine
Kanazawa University School of Medicine
13-1 Takaramachi, Kanazawa
Ishikawa 920
Japan

Jakob R. Passweg
Department Innere Medizin
Kantonsspital Basel
Petersgraben 4
CH-4031 Basel
Switzerland

N. J. Philpott
Department of Haematology
St George's Hospital Medical School
Cranmer Terrace
London SW17 0RE
UK

Aruna Raghavachar
Dept of Internal Medicine III
University of Ulm
Robert-Koch-Straße8
D-89081 Ulm
Germany

Hubert Schrezenmeier
Benjamin Franklin University Hospital
  Medical Clinic III
Free University of Berlin
Hindenburgdamm 30
D-12200 Berlin
Germany

Gérard Socié
Bone Marrow Transplantation Unit
Hôpital Saint-Louis
1 Avenue Claude Vellefaux
75475 Paris Cedex 10
France

Judith Veum Stone
Statistical Center
Medical College of Wisconsin
PO Box 26509, 8701 Watertown Plank Road
Milwaukee, WI 53226
USA

Rainer Storb
Clinical Research Division
Fred Hutchinson Cancer Research Center
1124 Columbia Street
Seattle, WA 98104
USA

Nydia G. Testa
Department of Experimental Haematology
Paterson Institute for Cancer Research
Wilmslow Road
Manchester M20 9BX
UK

André Tichelli
Hematologie
Kantonsspital Basel
Petersgraben 4-8
CH-4031 Basel
Switzerland

Preface

Recently important progress has been made to improve our understanding of the pathophysiology of aplastic anemia and the clinical management of this rare disease.

For a long time the pathophysiology of aplastic anemia remained a mystery, until a series of new studies provided new insight into this matter. The new information includes demonstration of a defect in bone marrow in those with aplastic anemia at the level of long-term culture-initiating cells; further evidence for the pathophysiological relevance of inhibitory cytokines; the assessment of cytokine action in vitro on bone marrow in aplastic anemia, and the analysis of cytokine expression in aplastic anemia; new results on autoreactive T-cells in aplastic anemia; evidence of roles for Fas-antigen and apoptosis in the pathophysiology of aplastic anemia; the elucidation of the relationship between aplastic anemia and paroxysmal nocturnal hemoglobinuria at the molecular level; and new data on the issue of clonality in bone marrow failure.

The main treatment options for aplastic anemia are bone marrow transplantation and immunosuppressive treatment. Progress in bone marrow transplantation for aplastic anemia includes new conditioning regimens and increasing the number of transplants in aplastic anemia from alternative donors.

During the 1990s a series of clinical studies on treatment with immunosuppression and growth factors were performed. These studies helped to improve standard immunosuppressive treatment. There are, however, still many questions on the place of hemopoietic growth factors in the treatment of aplastic anemia.

Efforts were also focused to analyze late effects of all treatment modalities.

Thus, there is a substantial, recently established body of information on the pathophysiology and treatment of aplastic anemia. This book tries to summarize the established knowledge and the most recent progress in the subject of aplastic anemia.

The idea for this book was generated within the Aplastic Anemia Working Party of the European Group for Blood and Marrow Transplantation (EBMT). However, we tried to avoid restriction to an 'EBMT-view' of the disease and we were fortunate in persuading distinguished experts from many countries to contribute to this volume.

The editors would like to express their appreciation for support of the work of members of the EBMT Aplastic Anemia Working Party by a grant from the European Commission (Biomed-2 programme, contract no. BMH4-CT96-1031).

We are sincerely grateful to all contributors for their excellent work; our thanks to all of them. We hope that this book will be a source of helpful, up-to-date information for students, clinicians, scientists and patients.

Hubert Schrezenmeier
Andrea Bacigalupo

Part I

Pathophysiology of acquired aplastic anemia

Stem cell defect in aplastic anemia

Judith C.W. Marsh

St George's Hospital, London

and

Nydia G. Testa

University of Manchester

Abbreviations

AA	Aplastic anemia
ADA	Adenosine deaminase
BFU-E	Burst-forming unit, erythroid
BL-CFC	Blast-colony forming cells
CAFC	Cobblestone area forming cells
CFU-E	Colony-forming unit, erythroid
CFU-GM	colony-forming unit, granulocyte/macrophage
CSF	Colony-stimulating factor
5-FU	5-Fluorouracil
G-CSF	Granulocyte colony-stimulating factor
GM-CFC	Granulocyte/macrophage colony-forming cells
HPP-CFC	High proliferative potential-colony forming cells
IL-1	Interleukin-1
IFN-γ	Interferon-γ
LTBMC	Long-term bone-marrow culture
LTC-IC	Long-term culture-initiating cell
LTRC	Long-term repopulating cells
M-CSF	Macrophage colony-stimulating factor
MIP1α	Macrophage-inflammatory protein α
Mix-CFC/CFU-Mix	Mixed lineage multipotential colony-forming cells
NOD/SCID	Nonobese diabetic, severe-combined-immunodeficient mice
SCF	Stem cell factor
TGFβ	Transforming growth factor β
TNF-α	Tumor necrosis factor α

Normal stem cells

Definition

The need to continuously replace mature cells in the blood requires the production of about 10^{11} new cells daily in a normal adult, and even more in response to hemopoietic stress. It is known that all these cells are derived from a common ancestor population, the pluripotential stem cells (Lajtha, 1983). The usually accepted definition of stem cells is based on three characteristics: first, their marked capacity for proliferation, as just illustrated, and, second, their potential to undergo differentiation to produce all the lymphohemopoietic mature cell types (Metcalf, 1988). Third, and classically, stem cells are also defined by their reported capacity for self-renewal, i.e., the capacity to generate new stem cells, with the implication that they are able to regenerate their own population (Lajtha, 1983; Metcalf, 1988). As we will discuss later, it is mainly this latter concept that has to be discussed in the context of aplastic anemia (AA).

Regulation

Stem cells comprise only a small minority, between 0.01 and 0.05%, of the total cells found in bone marrow. At least 95% of the hemopoietic cells fall into morphologically recognizable types. The remaining, with nonspecific morphological features, require phenotypic and functional characterization. They encompass not only the stem cells but also their immediate progeny, the progenitor cells which were first characterized by their ability to develop in vitro in response to the colony-stimulating factors (CSF) (Metcalf, 1988). As the hemopoietic tissue is a continuum of differentiating and proliferating cells, the boundaries between different primitive cell populations are ill-defined. However, it is generally agreed that commitment, i.e., a decision to enter a particular differentiation lineage (therefore restricting the multipotentiality of the stem cells), distinguishes between stem and progenitor cell populations. Such commitment appears to be irreversible. For example, macrophage progenitors which are genetically manipulated to present the erythropoietin receptors still develop into macrophages following stimulation with erythropoietin (McArthur et al., 1995). In the converse experiment, erythroid progenitors induced to express the receptor for macrophage colony-stimulating factor (M-CSF) develop into erythroid cells in response to this cytokine (McArthur et al., 1994). In contrast, little is known about the commitment process itself and, at present, the argument rages whether such an event is dictated internally by the cell-driven program, or is the response to external, i.e., environmental, stimuli (Jimenez et al., 1992; Ogawa, 1993). These concepts are important to the understanding of AA, since stem cells, which must supply mature functional cells for a lifetime, must be protected from the competing demands for mature cells in response to physiological or pathological needs. The rapid response of the hemopoietic tissue is met by the more mature, differentiation-restricted progenitors; for example, BFU-E cells (burst-forming unit; erythroid) in response to hypoxia or blood loss, or granulocyte/macrophage colony-forming cells (GM-CFC) in response to infection. These, and equivalent cell populations in the other lineages, are largely controlled by growth factors. However, the steps that *generate* these progenitors from stem cells are, at present, unknown. In the context of AA, it is interesting to speculate whether, in some cases, the 'protection' mechanisms that may act to protect the stem cell population from exhaustion are defective. As stem cells are lodged within bone marrow stroma, it is generally assumed that those stromal cells produce and may present a membrane-bound form, or release a large number of regulatory cytokines, including stimulatory molecules such as interleukin-1 (IL-1), M-CSF, GM-CSF, G-CSF, IL-6 and stem cell factor (SCF), as well as inhibitory cytokines such as transforming growth factor β (TGFβ) and macrophage-inflammatory protein α (MIP1α, for review see Lord et al., 1997). However, whether they have a role in stem cell differentiation is not known. Some do have a role, at least in vitro, in their survival and proliferation (Fairbairn et al., 1993). It may very well be that regulatory factors crucial for the commitment to differentiation are still unknown; such factors may have more in common with those which regulate embryonic and fetal development than with the 20–30 cytokines known to regulate the proliferation, maturation and function of the committed hemopoietic progenitors and their developing progeny (Lord et al., 1997).

The experimental study of primitive hemopoietic cells

While assays for colony-forming cells detect mainly progenitor cells, transplantation experiments define stem cells by their function, i.e., their capacity to repopulate permanently the hemopoietic tissue (Table 1.1). The long-term repopulating cells (LTRC) can, at present, be assayed only in experimental systems.

Currently, the most primitive human cell that can be assayed in vitro is the long-term culture-initiating cell (LTC-IC) (Table 1.1). This cell has certain stem cell characteristics, but it is not yet clear how it is related to the human stem cell. However, Ploemacher (1994) showed that murine LTC-IC (assessed as cobblestone area forming cells or CAFC) were able to repopulate irradiated mice and could, therefore, be regarded as equivalent to the mouse repopulating cell. A number of animal models have been developed for transplantation studies. Sublethally irradiated, severe-combined-immunodeficient, nonobese diabetic (NOD/SCID) mice were used to test the engraftment and repopulating potential

Table 1.1. Assays for primitive stem and progenitor cells

Cells	Assay	Incidence in bone marrow	References*
Long-term repopulating cells (LTRC)	Reconstitution of hemopoietic tissue	$1/(5 \times 10^4 – 10^5)$	Lord et al., 1997; Ploemacher, 1994
Long-term culture initiating cells (LTC-IC)	Generation of progenitor cells (CFC after 5–8 weeks of culture)	$1/(10^4$ to $2 \times 10^4)$	Lord et al., 1997; Ploemacher, 1994; Testa et al., 1996
Also called cobblestone area forming cells (CAFC)	Generation of a cobblestone area of cell proliferation		
Multipotential colony-forming cells (CFC)** HPP-CFC BL-CFC Mix-CFC	Colony formation in vitro	$1/(5 \times 10^4 – 10^5)$	Lord et al., 1997; Metcalf, 1988
Bipotential CFC	Colony formation in vitro	$1–2/10^3$ according to lineage	Lord et al., 1997; Metcalf, 1988

Notes:

* Mostly reviews are quoted.

** Definitions in the text and beginning of chapter.

of putative human stem-cell populations. However, limiting dilution repopulation assays indicate that the frequency of a NOD/SCID mouse repopulating cell is 1 in 10^6 cord blood mononuclear cells, whereas 1 in 3×10^3 to 10^4 mononuclear cells was an LTC-IC (Pettengel et al., 1994). Clearly, the human repopulating cells, as assessed in the NOD/SCID model, appear to be more primitive than the human LTC-IC. Furthermore, a gene-transfer study using a retroviral adenosine deaminase (ADA) vector showed that 30–40% of colony-forming cells and LTC-IC could be transduced with the ADA vector, but, when the cells were transplanted into NOD/SCID mice, none of the colony-forming cells generated were positive for ADA. Although high numbers of colony-forming and mature cells were obtained, it seems that the transfected cells contributed little to the graft, and the cells responsible for repopulation were not transfected. This further indicates that the repopulating cell may be more primitive than the LTC-IC. On the other hand, potentially lethally irradiated mice can be rescued from hemopoietic death by 5×10^4 to 10^5 bone marrow cells (Lord et al., 1997). It is not clear whether the larger numbers of human cells required to rescue the irradiated NOD/SCID mice mean that there are fewer stem cells in humans than in mice. However, there are problems with the maturation of human cells in those mice (Larochell et al., 1996), which suggests that the relatively low incidence of LTRCs in this system may be an assay-driven paradox. The clonogeneic in vitro assays detect mainly the progenitor cells, which are more mature than stem cells. However, because of the continuous spectrum of proliferation and differentiation in the hemopoietic tissue, some of the clonogeneic assays may partially overlap with the stem cell compartment. The blast colony assay (BL-CFC) and the high proliferative potential colony assay (HPP-CFC) are within this category.

Selection of primitive cells by phenotype

It is possible to separate the most primitive cells from their close progeny of progenitor cells. The former have distinct cell membrane markers (Table 1.2) and are also characterized by low metabolic activity. This latter feature allows primitive cells to be isolated by negative selection, using dyes such as rhodamine-123, which concentrates in active mitochondria, or nucleic acid dyes like Hoechst 33342 (Ratajczak and Gerwitz, 1995; Spangrude, 1994).

One of the most useful membrane markers for the selection of primitive cells has been the CD34 antigen, and this feature has been exploited in a number of different positive cell-selection procedures (de Wynter et al., 1995). However, the cells that are CD34+ comprise a wide population, encompassing stem cells, progenitor cells and more differentiated hemopoietic cells. In fact, only 0.1–1% of the CD34+ cells have the most primitive phenotype, while about 10–30% are progenitor cells, and the rest are more differentiated cells (Table 1.3).

Table 1.2. Phenotypic markers of primitive hemopoietic cells

Stem cells	Progenitor cells
CD34+	CD34+
CD38−	CD38+
CD33−	CD33+
Lineage−	Lineage+
HLA-DR− or weakly +	HLA-DR− or weakly +
CD71−	CD71+
Thy 1 *low*	Thy 1+
CD45RA *low*	CD45RA+
c-*kit*+	c-kit *low* or −

Note:

Reviewed in de Wynter et al., 1995; Lord et al., 1997; Spangrude, 1994; Testa et al., 1996.

Table 1.3. Percentage of colony-forming cells (CFC) in the different CD34+ subpopulations expressing stem and progenitor cell phenotype

Phenotype	Percentage of cells	Percentage of CFC
CD34+38+DR+	90	31
CD34+38+DR−	4	N.D.
CD34+38−DR+	6	1.0
CD34+38−DR−	0.3	0.2

Note:

Data calculated from Wynn et al., 1998; N.D. = not determined.

How many stem cells get to express themselves?

Recently, a study demonstrated that one injected cell with a 'stem cell' phenotype is able to reconstitute long-term hemopoiesis in an irradiated mouse (Osawa et al., 1996). The proportion of mice injected with single cells that were reconstituted agrees with the expected proportion (about 20%) of cells seeding in the bone marrow (Testa et al., 1972). Other transplantation studies with marked murine cells have also demonstrated that monoclonal or oligoclonal hemopoiesis may be observed for long periods of time (Capel et al., 1988; Keller and Snodgrass, 1990). Only limited data are available in larger mammals; in experiments with cats, small numbers of syngeneic stem cells are able to maintain hemopoiesis (Abkowitz et al., 1995).

In humans, normal hemopoiesis is polyclonal, and polyclonal hemopoiesis is also usually observed following allogeneic transplantation. Nevertheless, there are anecdotal reports of oligo- or monoclonal hemopoiesis after allogeneic transplantation. This was observed in two out of 12 cases by examining X-chromosome-linked polymorphisms, one of them limited to myeloid cells and the other also comprising lymphoid cells (Turhan et al., 1989). Unfortunately, these observations were made days or weeks after transplant, and the long-term features of hemopoiesis in those patients are not known. However, oligoclonal hemopoiesis, as determined by cytogenetic marks on atomic bomb survivors, may be observed for several years (Amenomori et al., 1988). In one patient, a single identifiable clone provided about 10% of all the lymphohemopoietic cells for an observation period of 10 years, in the absence of any detectable sign of abnormal hemopoiesis (Kusunoki et al., 1995).

Recent studies of normal subjects showed that about 30% of females aged 70 years or older had oligoclonal hemopoiesis in the myeloid, but not the lymphoid lineages (Champion et al., 1997; Gale et al., 1997). It is not clear whether this is caused by altered regulation of cell production or a limited supply of stem cells in the aged. These data, taken together, suggest that only a few stem cells may, under normal steady state, be needed to maintain normal hemopoiesis. They also confirm the early concept that the stem cell population is normally quiescent, and that only a fraction of their vast reserve population needs to express itself, differentiating and giving rise to progeny. In the context of AA, these data also suggest that a mere reduction of stem cell numbers may not be sufficient to cause this syndrome. It is also important to consider how many of the available stem cells are likely to proliferate in AA.

Progressive telomere shortening of CD34+ occurs with age (Vaziri et al., 1994), and we have shown, in paired studies of donors and recipients of allogeneic transplantation, that the telomere length of the recipient's blood cells is significantly shorter than that of their donors. Such shortening is equivalent to that observed during 15 years of normal aging and, in the worst cases, is equivalent to 40 years (Wynn et al., 1998).

Although we do not yet know the molecular mechanisms of this phenomenon, we attribute the accelerated telomere shortening to proliferation stress. If stem cells age, do they conserve their capacity for self-reproduction after the hemopoietic system has reached its adult size? Cultures of human hemopoietic cells have achieved marked expansion of CFC and of LTC-IC (reviewed in Testa et al., 1999), but it is more problematic to assess whether stem cells have increased in number, as assessed by an increase in their capacity to regenerate hemopoiesis. While a primitive phenotype may be conserved, the repopulation capacity may be decreased (Albella et al., 1997). Because of this, it is not known whether the numbers of cells needed for transplantation will be the same when using freshly harvested cells or cells expanded in vitro. Experiments on mice indicate that 6-fold to 50-fold more in-vitro-generated GM-CFC are required to achieve an equivalent number of leukocytes in the blood (Albella et al., 1997). Therefore, it is doubtful that significant expansion of the stem cell population has been achieved. This may not be surprising since the stimulatory cytokines used in those experiments are those known to act on the progenitor cell populations.

Extensive data have also been obtained from experimental systems and patients. Such data indicate that, following serious cytotoxic injury, the stem cell population recovers to a lesser extent than more mature populations, and remains at markedly subnormal levels for the rest of the experimental animal's life, and for several years at least in patients (reviewed in Testa et al., 1996). Progenitor and maturing cell populations have evolved in response to selective pressures that stimulate hemopoiesis, such as infection and blood loss. In contrast, the use of irradiation and the cytotoxic drugs that kill stem cells were developed recently, in the twentieth century; therefore, it is not surprising that they have not developed mechanisms to normalize their numbers after injury. Fortunately, as discussed above, first, their normal numbers far exceed those needed for a normal life span, and second, an adequate output of mature cells may be reached even with a severely restricted stem cell compartment. However, it is apparent that the concept that hemopoietic stem cells in the adult have the capacity to self-reproduce has to be revised. Perhaps it is more realistic to think that while stem cells are characterized by a very extensive proliferation capacity, each cell division results in some stem cell aging. Thus, while operationally the daughter cells may still be defined as stem cells, they are not identical to the parent cell.

Aplastic anemia stem cells

Functional assessment of AA hemopoietic progenitor cells

Early work from the 1970s, with clonogeneic cultures using unpurified bone marrow mononuclear cell preparations and various conditioned media as a source of colony-stimulating activity, demonstrated a reduction or absence of late and early colonies (CFU-GM, CFU-E, BFU-E and CFU-Mix) in patients with AA (Barrett et al., 1979; Hara et al., 1980; Kern et al., 1977). Although variation in colony numbers was seen between individual patients, there was a uniform lack of correlation with disease activity in terms of peripheral blood neutrophil count or marrow granulocytic precursors. Numbers of peripheral blood colonies were at least 10-fold less than bone marrow colonies and more often undetectable. More recent studies using purified (CD34+) hemopoietic cells and recombinant hemopoietic growth factors in clonogeneic culture confirm the reduced numbers of all marrow progenitor cells (Maciejewski et al., 1994; Marsh et al., 1991; Scopes et al., 1996).

The long-term bone-marrow culture (LTBMC) system has been used by several groups to (1) evaluate the earlier stages of hemopoiesis and (2) assess the ability to form a normal stromal layer, the in vitro representation of the marrow micro-environment. All studies of AA patients have demonstrated a marked defect in hemopoiesis, as manifest by a severe reduction in, or cessation of, the generation of hemopoietic progenitor cells within the system (Bacigalupo et al., 1992; Gibson and Gordon–Smith, 1990; Holmberg et al., 1994; Marsh, 1996; Marsh et al., 1990). A similar pattern is seen in untreated patients, whether with severe or nonsevere disease, and treated patients who have responded hematologically to immuno-suppressive therapy (Marsh et al., 1990).

The formation of the stromal layer is normal in most patients with AA (Gibson and Gordon–Smith, 1990; Marsh et al., 1991), although one study reported a lack of stromal confluency in almost half the patients, and that this was associated with a longer duration of disease (Holmberg et al., 1994). Using a different short-term culture system, Nissen and colleagues (1995) reported impairment of stroma formation at 2 weeks but most became confluent at the standard long-term culture time. In contrast, some AA patients form a confluent layer more rapidly than normal (Marsh et al., 1990).

The defect in hemopoiesis seen in LTBMC may reflect either a failing in the stem cell compartment with a deficiency of primitive cells with marrow-repopu-lating ability, or a dysfunctional microenvironment. Cross-over LTBMC experi-ments allow separate examination of these two components. Using AA marrow adherent-cell-depleted mononuclear cells, one group demonstrated defective generation of CFU-GM when the cells were inoculated onto normal irradiated LTBMC stromal layers (Marsh et al., 1990). In contrast, normal stromal function in AA patients was demonstrated by normal numbers of CFU-GM generated from normal marrow mononuclear cells when inoculated onto irradiated stromal layers from AA patients, except in one patient in whom a defective stroma was demonstrated. A second group showed similar results, assessing BL-CFC gener-ation on irradiated stromal layers in AA (Novotski and Jacobs, 1995). Further-more, a similar pattern was seen using purified CD34+ cells as the inoculum, in that the stroma in AA patients supported generation of normal CFU-GM (Marsh et al., 1991) or BL-CFC (Novotski and Jacobs, 1995) from normal marrow CD34+ cells, and purified AA CD34+ cells failed to generate normal numbers of CFU-GM on normal stromas. Hotta and co-workers (1985) had previously demonstrated abnormal stromal function in three out of nine AA patients, although their stem cell function was not examined.

The results of these cross-over experiments indicate a deficiency or defect in primitive cells with marrow-repopulating ability, which in normals had previ-ously been shown to exhibit the CD34+, CD33– phenotype (Andrews et al.,

1989) and within which population LTC-IC are found. Although not all patients form a confluent stroma, in those patients in whom stromal function has been evaluated, in terms of their ability to support the generation of hemopoietic progenitors, the majority function normally. A reported isolated deficiency of a growth factor or increased expression of an inhibitory cytokine (Holmberg et al., 1994) appears not to affect the physiological function of the stroma, as assessed by the long-term marrow-culture system.

Phenotypic quantitation of AA hemopoietic (CD34+) cells

The percentage of bone marrow CD34+ cells is significantly reduced in AA patients compared with normal steady-state bone marrow, with median values of around 0.5%, but with an wide range seen from zero to values falling within the normal range (Maciejewski et al., 1994; Marsh et al., 1991; Scopes et al., 1994). Analysis of the CD34+ subpopulation reveals a significant reduction in the immature CD34+,33– cells, as well as the more mature CD34+,33+ cells (Scopes et al., 1994). A lack of correlation between these compartments and disease severity was reported by one group. Although a second group reported significantly higher percentages of CD34+ and CD33+ cells in patients with recovered AA, almost half the patients had persistently reduced values (Maciejewski et al., 1994). In other words, extreme variability of results was seen among patients who had recovered hematologically after immunosuppressive therapy. It should be remembered that the CD34+ compartment comprises a very heterogeneous collection of cell types in terms of their stage of differentiation, the majority of which comprise the more lineage-restricted progenitors, with the more primitive progenitors comprising only a very small proportion of the CD34+ cells. It appears that, in AA, the CD34+ population contains a much smaller proportion of very primitive cells, with a relative over-representation of more mature progenitors.

AA CD34+ hemopoietic cells have also been shown to be dysfunctional (Scopes et al., 1996). Although marrow mononuclear cells from AA patients consistently produce lower numbers of colonies compared with normal, when the reduced numbers of CD34+ cells in AA bone marrow are considered there is no significant difference in clonogeneic potential. However, when purified AA CD34+ cells cease to be influenced by accessory cells, their clonogeneic potential is significantly reduced, indicating defective function. From the same study, the effects of various hemopoietic growth factors in isolation or in combination on the clonogeneic potential of AA marrow cells was investigated. It was shown that the addition of granulocyte colony-stimulating factor (G-CSF) in vitro was able to correct the dysfunction of AA CD34+ cells to normal in terms of their clonogeneic potential. Thus, in AA there appears to be both a deficiency and a dysfunctionality of marrow CD34+ cells.

Assessment of the long-term marrow-repopulating ability of AA hemopoietic cells

As discussed earlier, the LTC-IC and CAFC assays represent modifications to the LTBMC system to permit quantitation of these primitive hemopoietic cells. Maciejewski and colleagues (1996) demonstrated, by limiting dilution analysis, reduced clonogeneic potential of LTC-IC in two patients; however, for other AA patients examined, limiting dilution analysis was not possible because of low cell numbers. Instead, results of LTC-IC frequency were extrapolated from week-5 clonogeneic cells from bulk cultures and the numbers divided by the average proliferative potential of single AA LTC-IC, based on the small number of formal limiting dilution assays. Using this methodology, the frequency of LTC-IC was reduced compared with normal controls (AA patients had 0.024 colonies/10^5 mononuclear cells compared with 7.8 for normal controls). Furthermore, LTC-IC remained subnormal in those cases, despite achieving normal or near-normal blood counts. LTC-IC were also qualitatively abnormal, demonstrating a markedly reduced clonogeneic potential. Schrezenmeier and colleagues (1996) have also measured the frequency of LTC-IC but used the CAFC as the endpoint for scoring LTC-IC at week 5 instead of the generation of colony-forming cells. They demonstrated a reduction in CAFC in AA patients (mean frequency of CAFC was 6.6/10^5 mononuclear cells (mnc) compared with 84.4 for normal controls). The frequency of LTC-IC is notably higher than reported by Maciejewski et al. (1996), raising questions as to whether the two assay systems are exactly comparable, and whether the CAFC assay detects a somewhat more mature progenitor cell that the LTC-IC (Weaver et al., 1997). In summary, these studies indicate a deficiency in LTC-IC in AA patients, which would account for the deficient marrow-repopulating ability seen in LTBMC.

Podesta and colleagues (1998) have compared the frequency of late hemopoietic progenitors and LTC-IC in AA patients after immunosuppressive therapy with that in AA patients who have undergone successful allogeneic bone marrow transplant (BMT), over a follow-up period of up to 20 years. Although all patients had achieved normal blood counts, bone marrow cellularity and numbers of CFU-GM, BFU-E and CFU-Mix remained subnormal, but there was an even more striking reduction in LTC-IC, equally in transplanted patients and those who had received immunosuppressive therapy (see Figure 1.1). The pattern of recovery of CFU-GM between the two groups was different, with a more rapid normalization of CFU-GM in transplanted patients over a period of 2 years. In contrast, patients treated with immunosuppressive therapy displayed a more prolonged pattern of recovery of CFU-GM over 5–6 years, which may reflect an ongoing process of suppression of hemopoiesis among these patients (see Figure 1.1). From these results, it appears that even a markedly reduced stem cell reservoir (as assessed by LTC-IC frequency) is able to maintain steady-state hemopoiesis, although this

Figure 1.1. Pattern of growth of mixed myeloid cultures (colony-forming unit granulocyte/macrophage or CFU-GM) and long-term culture-initiating cells (LTC-IC) over time following treatment with immunosuppressive therapy (▲) and bone marrow transplantation (■). Numbers are expressed as percentage of expected growth; 100% refers to a median normal of 58/10^5 mononuclear cells (mnc) for CFU-GM and 34/10^6 mnc for LTC-IC; y = years from treatment (reproduced from Podesta et al., 1998, with permission).

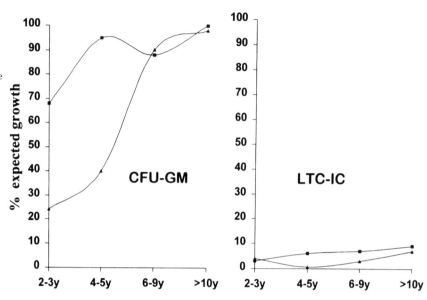

may not be maintained under conditions of hemopoietic stress. In terms of the quality of the LTC-IC, in the transplanted patients LTC-IC generated normal numbers of colony-forming cells at week 5. In contrast, the proliferative potential of LTC-IC was reduced in patients treated with immunosuppressive therapy, compared with normal controls. This would seem to indicate a qualitative abnormality in stem cells derived from patients who recover autologous hemopoiesis after immunosuppressive therapy compared with the normal quality of stem cells (LTC-IC) grown from AA patients receiving an allogeneic stem cell transplant. Persistence of this abnormality may be one explanation for the risk of relapse of AA or later clonal evolution. An alternative explanation for these results is that most stem cells (and LTC-IC) in AA are unable to enter the cell cycle and proliferate normally. This may be compensated for by increased replicative pressure on the more mature hemopoietic progenitor cells (see 'Analysis of telomeric DNA length in AA', p. 16). From a practical viewpoint, the altered cell cycling status of AA stem cells would impact on an attempt to quantitate LTC-IC and make direct comparison of LTC-IC frequency with that of normal controls difficult. Hence LTC-IC assays may not be suitable for the quantitation of very primitive hemopoietic cells in AA.

Very little is known about the kinetics of stem cell proliferation in AA. Maciejewski and colleagues (1994) examined the expression of c-*kit* on AA CD34+ cells, on the basis that in normal marrow CD34+ c-*kit*+ cells contain the highest proportion of cycling cells. Cell cycle analysis was not performed on AA CD34+ cells, but they showed that the percentage of c-*kit*+ cells among the CD34+ cell population was reduced, suggesting that in AA fewer CD34+ progenitors are cycling. Preliminary work by Gibson and colleagues (1996) has demonstrated reduced regeneration of progenitors from 5-fluorouracil-treated (5-FU-treated) AA bone marrow cells inoculated onto irradiated LTBMC stromal layers compared with normal 5-FU-treated cells, and that colonies were produced for only 2–4 weeks. This suggests defective or deficient numbers of primitive noncycling stem cells in AA, and also that the finding of reduced or absent LTC-IC in AA may also reflect abnormal proliferation and differentiation kinetics of the stem cells.

Mobilizing potential of AA progenitor cells

It is well established that primitive hemopoietic progenitor cells (including true stem cells from long-term follow-up of allogeneic peripheral-blood stem-cell transplants) can be mobilized from the bone marrow of normal donors using G-CSF (To et al., 1997). However, it may be possible to mobilize residual stem cells from AA patients. Collection and cryopreservation of mobilized stem cells may allow the subsequent use of intensive immunosuppression followed by reinfusion of the stem cells. One group has attempted to collect mobilized blood progenitor cells in AA patients following treatment with antilymphocyte globulin and cyclosporin and 3 months of daily G-CSF (Bacigalupo et al., 1993). The median number of CD34+ cells collected was 1.8×10^6/kg (range 0.27–3.8) and median CFU-GM 3.9×10^4/kg (range 0–39). Colony growth was only obtained on leukaphereses performed between days +33 and +77. There was marked patient variability in terms of mobilizing ability, but in some cases sufficient CD34+ cells were obtained for potential autologous transplantation. It is not known, however, whether any LTC-IC can be isolated using this procedure, and, so far, we are not aware of any report using this approach to treat AA patients.

Apoptotic properties of AA CD34+ cells

It has recently been demonstrated that AA CD34+ marrow cells are more apoptotic than normal CD34+ marrow cells. In addition, there appears to be a correlation between the percentage that is apoptotic and disease severity, and also between the percentage of CD34+ cells present (Philpott et al., 1995). Increased apoptosis may be an important contributory factor to the stem cell defect in AA. Maciejewski and colleagues (1995a) had shown that AA CD34+ cells show increased expression of Fas-antigen and that tumor necrosis factor-α (TNF-α) and interferon-γ (IFN-γ) upregulate the expression of Fas-antigen on normal CD34+ cells (Maciejewski et al., 1995b). Whether the Fas system is involved in apoptosis in AA remains to be determined. This topic is discussed in detail in Chapter 4. The ability of hemopoietic growth factors such as G-CSF to suppress apoptosis may be an important factor in the effect of G-CSF in vitro and in vivo in AA patients.

Analysis of telomeric DNA length in AA

As discussed earlier, normal hemopoietic stem cells demonstrate progressive telomere shortening with age. A recent study of patients with AA has shown significantly shorter mean telomere length in both granulocytic and mononuclear cell fractions compared with age-matched controls, suggesting some loss at the level of the hemopoietic stem cell (Ball et al., 1998). The degree of telomere loss was proportional to disease duration, and amounted to a loss of 216 base pairs (bp) per year in addition to the normal age-related loss of 36 bp/year. In those patients who had achieved normal blood counts after treatment, the rate of telomere loss had stabilized. It may be that the remaining hemopoietic progenitor cells need to undergo a greater number of cell divisions in order to generate sufficient mature blood cells. This may reflect stem cell loss caused by an increase in apoptosis of stem cells and primitive progenitor cells, or direct immune destruction of these cells. An increase in the replicative capacity of hemopoietic progenitor cells may account for the increased telomere loss in AA patients.

Conclusion

It is now apparent that only a few stem cells are required to maintain normal steady-state hemopoiesis. Normal stem cells exhibit a progressive shortening of telomeric DNA with age, so their self-replicative capacity is not preserved with time. Furthermore, following injury to the stem cells from chemotherapy, for example, the stem cell reservoir does not recover to normal in contrast to the more mature progenitor cells. For these reasons, the classic concept of the hemopoietic stem cell with unlimited self-renewal capacity has been revised, so that with each cell division and after marrow injury, the daughter stem cell is not identical to the parent stem cell in terms of replicative capacity. This concept is important when attempting to define the nature of the hemopoietic defect in AA where there is failure of normal hemopoiesis. Both a deficiency and a dysfunction of hemopoietic progenitor (CD34+) cells occurs, and, with hematological recovery, numbers of mature progenitor cells can return to normal but a deficiency and a dysfunction remains at the level of the primitive progenitor cells (LTC-IC). AA patients also show an exaggeration of the normal pattern of telomere shortening, which may contribute to the markedly reduced replicative capacity of the stem cells. This may occur because of an increased loss of stem cells and committed progenitor cells by apoptosis, or by direct immune destruction. The pattern of recovery of hemopoietic progenitor cell numbers in patients with idiosyncratic AA is similar to that seen following injury to normal bone marrow after chemotherapy, but the exact mechanism behind the injury to the stem cells is poorly understood and likely to be very different.

References

Abkowitz, J. L., Persik, M. T., Shelton, G. H. et al. (1995) Behaviour of haematopoietic stem cells in a large animal. *Proceedings of the National Academy of Sciences of the USA*, **92**, 2031–5.

Albella, B., Segovia, J. C. and Bueren, J. A. (1997) Does the granulocyte-macrophage colony forming unit content in ex-vivo expanded grafts predict the recovery of the recipient leucocytes? *Blood*, **90**, 464–70.

Amenomori, T., Honda, T., Otaka, M. et al. (1988) Growth and differentiation of circulating haemopoietic stem cells with atomic bomb irradiation-induced chromosome abnormalities. *Experimental Hematology*, **16**, 849–53.

Andrews, R. G., Singer, J. W. and Bernstein, I. D. (1989) Precursors of colony forming cells in humans can be distinguished from colony forming cells by expression of the CD33 and CD34 antigens and light scatter properties. *Journal of Experimental Medicine*, **169**, 1721–31.

Bacigalupo, A., Figari, O., Tong, J. et al. (1992) Long term marrow cultures in patients with aplastic anaemia compared with marrow transplant recipients and normal controls. *Experimental Haematology*, **20**, 425–30.

Bacigalupo, A., Piaggio, G., Podesta, M. et al. (1993) Collection of peripheral blood haemopoietic progenitors (PBHP) from patients with severe aplastic anaemia (SAA) after prolonged administration of granulocyte colony stimulating factor. *Blood*, **82**, 1410–14.

Ball, S. E., Gibson, F. M., Rizzo, S. et al. (1998) Progressive telomere shortening in aplastic anemia. *Blood*, **91**, 3582–92.

Barrett, A. J., Faille, A., Balitrand, N. et al. (1979) Bone marrow culture in aplastic anaemia. *Journal of Clinical Pathology*, **32**, 660–5.

Capel, B., Hawley, R., Covarrubias, L. et al. (1988) Clonal contributions of small numbers of retrovirally marked haematopoietic stem cells engrafted in unirradiated neonatal W/W^v mice. *Proceedings of the National Academy of Sciences of the USA*, **86**, 4564–8.

Champion, K. M., Gilbert, J. G. R., Asimakopolos, F. O. et al. (1997) Clonal haemopoiesis in normal elderly women; implications for the myeloproliferative disorders and myelodysplastic syndromes. *British Journal of Haematology*, **97**, 920–6.

de Wynter, E. A., Coutinho, L. H., Pei, X. et al. (1995) Comparison of purity and enrichment of CD34+ cells from bone marrow, umbilical cord and peripheral blood (primed for apheresis) using five different separation systems. *Stem Cells*, **13**, 524–32.

de Wynter, E. A., Nadali, G., Coutinho, L. H. and Testa, N. G. (1996) Extensive amplification of single cells from CD34+ subpopulations in umbilical cord blood and identification of long-term culture initiating cells present in two subsets. *Stem Cells*, **14**, 566–76.

Fairbairn, L. J., Cowling, G. J., Reipert, B. M. and Dexter, T. M. (1993) Suppression of apoptosis allows differentiation and development of a multipotent haemopoietic cell line in the absence of added growth factors. *Cell*, **74**, 823.

Gale, R. E., Fielding, A. K., Harrison, C. N. and Linch, D. C. (1997) Acquired skewing of x-chromosome inactivation patterns in myeloid cells of the elderly suggests stochastic clonal loss with age. *British Journal of Haematology*, **98**, 512–19.

Gibson, F. and Gordon–Smith, E. C. (1990) Long term culture of aplastic anaemia bone marrow. *British Journal of Haematology*, **75**, 421–7.

Gibson, F. M., Scopes, J. and Gordon–Smith, E. C. (1996) Regeneration of aplastic anaemia progenitor cells from 5-fluorouracil treated bone marrow in long term culture. *Experimental Haematology*, **24** [Suppl. 1], 209a.

Hara, H., Kai, S., Fushimi, M. et al. (1980) Pluripotent haemopoietic precursors in vitro (CFU-Mix) in aplastic anaemia. *Experimental Haematology*, **8**, 1165–71.

Holmberg, L. A., Seidel, K., Leisenring, W. et al. (1994) Aplastic anaemia: analysis of stromal cell function in long term marrow cultures. *Blood*, **84**, 3685–90.

Hotta, T., Kato, T., Maeda, H. et al. (1985) Functional changes in marrow stromal cells in aplastic anaemia. *Acta Haematologica*, **74**, 65–9.

Jimenez, G., Griffiths, S. D., Ford, A. M. et al. (1992) Activation of the beta-globulin focus control region precedes commitment to the erythroid lineage. *Proceedings of the National Academy of Sciences of the USA*, **89**, 10618.

Keller, G. and Snodgrass, R. (1990) Life span of multipotential haematopoietic stem cells in vivo. *Journal of Experimental Medicine*, **171**, 1407–18.

Kern, P., Heimpel, H., Heit, W. et al. (1977) Granulocytic progenitor cells in aplastic anaemia. *British Journal of Haematology*, **35**, 613–23.

Kusunoki, Y., Kodama, Y., Hirai, Y. et al. (1995) Cytogenetic and immunologic identification of clonal expansion of stem cells into T and B lymphocytes in one atomic-bomb survivor. *Blood*, **86**, 2106–12.

Lajtha, L. G. (1983) In *Stem cell concepts in stem cells: their identification and characterisation*, ed. C. S. Potten, pp. 1–11. London: Churchill Livingstone.

Larochell, A., Vormoor, J., Hanenberg, M. et al. (1996) Identification of primitive human haematopoietic cells capable of repopulating NOD/SCID mouse bone marrow: implications for gene therapy. *Nature Medicine*, **2**, 1329–37.

Lord, B. I., Heyworth, C. M. and Testa, N. G. (1997) An introduction to primitive haematopoietic cells. In: *Haematopoietic lineages in health and disease*, ed. N. G. Testa, B. I. Lord and T. M. Dexter, pp. 1–27. New York: Marcel Dekker.

Maciejewski, J. P., Anderson, S., Katevas, P. et al. (1994) Phenotypic and functional analysis of bone marrow progenitor cell compartment in bone marrow failure. *British Journal of Haematology*, **87**, 227–34.

Maciejewski, J. P., Selleri, C., Sato, T. et al. (1995*a*) Increased expression of Fas antigen on bone marrow CD34+ cells of patients with aplastic anaemia. *British Journal of Haematology*, **1**, 245–52.

Maciejewski, J., Selleri, C., Anderson, S. et al. (1995*b*) Fas antigen expression on CD34+ human marrow cells is induced by interferon-γ and tumour necrosis factor-α and potentiates cytokine mediated haemopoietic suppression in vitro. *Blood*, **85**, 3183–90.

Maciejewski, J. P., Selleri, C., Sato, T. et al. (1996) A severe and consistent defect in marrow and circulating primitive haemopoietic cells (long term culture initiating cells) in acquired aplastic anaemia. *Blood*, **88**, 1983–91.

Marsh, J. C. W. (1996) Long-term marrow cultures in aplastic anemia. *European Journal of Haematology*, **57** [Suppl. 60], 75–9.

Marsh, J. C. W., Chang, J., Testa, N. G. et al. (1990) The haemopoietic defect in aplastic anaemia assessed by long term marrow culture. *Blood*, **76**, 1748–57.

Marsh, J. C. W., Chang, J., Testa, N. G. et al. (1991) In vitro assessment of marrow 'stem cell' and stromal cell function in aplastic anaemia. *British Journal of Haematology*, **78**, 258–67.

Marsh, J. C. W. (1996) Long-term bone marrow cultures in aplastic anaemia. *European Journal of Haematology*, **57** [Suppl. 60], 75–9.

McArthur, G. A., Rohrschneider, L. R. and Johnson, G. R. (1994) Induced expression of c-fms in normal haematopoietic cells shows evidence for both conservation and lineage restriction of signal transduction in response to macrophage colony-stimulating factor. *Blood*, **83**, 972.

McArthur, G. A., Longmore, G. L., Klingler, K. and Johnson, G. R. (1995) Lineage-restricted recruitment of immature haematopoietic cells in response to erythropoietin after normal haematopoietic cell transfection with erythropoietin receptor. *Experimental Haematology*, **23**, 645.

Metcalf, D. (1988) In *The molecular control of blood cells*. London: Harvard University Press.

Nissen, C., Wodmar-Filipowicz, A., Slanicka-Krieger, M. et al. (1995) Persistent growth impairment of bone marrow stroma after antilymphocyte globulin treatment for severe aplastic anaemia and its association with relapse. *European Journal of Haematology*, **5**, 255–61.

Novotski, N. and Jacobs, P. (1995) Immunosuppressive therapy in bone marrow aplasia: the stroma functions normally to support haemopoiesis. *Experimental Haematology*, **23**, 1472–7.

Ogawa, M. (1993) Differentiation and proliferation in haematopoietic stem cells. *Blood*, **81**, 2844.

Osawa, M., Hanada, K., Hamada, H. and Nakauchi, H. (1996) Long-term lymphohematopoietic reconstitution by a single CD34-low/negative hematopoeitic stem cell. *Science*, **273**, 242–5.

Pettengel, R., Luft, T., Henschler, R. and Testa, N. G. (1994) Direct comparison by limiting dilution analysis of long-term culture initiating cells in human bone marrow, umbilical cord blood and blood stem cells. *Blood*, **84**, 3653–9.

Pflumio, F., Izac, B., Kats, A. et al. (1996) Phenotype and function of human haematopoietic cells engrafting immune-deficient CD17-severe combined immunodeficiency mice and non-obese-diabetic-severe combined immunodeficiency mice after transplant of human cord blood mononuclear cells. *Blood*, **88**, 3731–40.

Philpott, N. J., Scopes, J., Marsh, J. C. W. et al. (1995) Increased apoptosis in aplastic anaemia bone marrow progenitor cells: possible pathophysiological significance. *Experimental Haematology*, **23**, 1642–8.

Ploemacher, R. (1994) Cobblestone area forming cell (CAFC) assay. In *Culture of haematopoietic cells*, ed. R. I. Freshney, I. B. Pragnell and M. G. Freshney, pp. 1–21. New York: Wiley–Liss.

Podesta, M., Piaggio, G., Frassoni, F. et al. (1998) The assessment of the haemopoietic reservoir after immunosuppressive therapy or bone marrow transplantation in severe aplastic anaemia. *Blood*, **91**, 1959–65.

Ratajczak, M. Z. and Gewirtz, A. M. (1995) The biology of haematopoietic stem cells. *Seminars in Oncology*, **22**, 210–17.

Schrezenmeier, H., Jenal, M., Herrmann, F. et al. (1996) Quantitative analysis of cobblestone area forming cells in bone marrow of patients with aplastic anaemia by limiting dilution assay. *Blood*, **88**, 4474–80.

Scopes, J., Bagnara, M., Gordon–Smith, E. C. et al. (1994) Haemopoietic progenitor cells are reduced in aplastic anaemia. *British Journal of Haematology*, **86**, 427–30.

Scopes, J., Daly, S., Atkinson, R. et al. (1996) Aplastic anaemia: evidence for dysfunctional bone marrow progenitor cells and the corrective effect of granulocyte colony stimulating factor. *Blood*, **87**, 3179–85.

Spangrude, G. J. (1994) Biological and clinical aspects of haematopoietic stem cells. *Annual Review of Medicine*, **45**, 93–104.

Testa, N. G., Lord, B. I. and Shore, N. A. (1972) The in vivo seeding of haemopoietic colony forming cells in irradiated mice. *Blood*, **40**, 654–61.

Testa, N. G., de Wynter, E. A. and Weaver, A. (1996) The study of haemopoietic stem cells in patients: concepts, approaches and cautionary tales. *Annals of Oncology*, **7** [Suppl. 2], 5–8.

Testa, N. G., de Wynter, E. and Hows, J. (1999) Haemopoietic stem cells as targets for genetic manipulation: concepts and practical approaches. In: *Haematopoiesis and gene therapy*, ed. L. Fairbairn and N. G. Testa, pp.1–12. London: Plenum Press.

To, L. B., Haylock, D. N., Simmons, P. J. and Juttner, C. A. (1997) The biology and clinical uses of blood stem cells. *Blood*, **89**, 2233–58.

Turhan, A. G., Humphries, R. K., Phillips, G. L., Eaves, A. C. and Eaves, C. J. (1989) Clonal hematopoiesis demonstrated by X-linked DNA polymorphisms after allogeneic bone marrow transplantation. *New England Journal of Medicine*, **320**, 1655–61.

Turner, C. W., Yeager, A. M., Waller, E. K., Wingard, J. R. and Fleming, W. H. (1996) Engraftment potential of different sources of human haematopoietic progenitor cells in BNM mice. *Blood*, **87**, 3237–44.

Vaziri, H., Dragowska, W., Allsopp, et al. (1994) Evidence for a mitotic clock in human haematopoietic stem cells; loss of telomeric DNA with age. *Proceedings of the National Academy of Sciences of the USA*, **91**, 9857–60.

Vormoor, J., Lapidot, T., Pflumio, F. et al. (1994) Immature human cord blood progenitors engraft and proliferate to high levels in severe combined immunodeficiency. *Blood*, **83**, 2489–97.

Weaver, A., Ryder, W. D. J. and Testa, N. G. (1997) Measurement of long term culture initiating cells (LTC-ICs) using limiting dilution: comparison of endpoints and stromal support. *Experimental Haematology*, **25**, 1333–8.

Wynn, R. F., Cross, M. A., Hatton, C. et al. (1998) Accelerated telomere shortening in young recipients of allogeneic bone-marrow transplants. *Lancet*, **351**, 178–81.

2

Cytokine abnormalities in aplastic anemia

Seiji Kojima

Nagoya University School of Medicine, Japan

Introduction

The term aplastic anemia (AA) encompasses a group of stem-cell disorders characterized by peripheral-blood pancytopenia and hypocellular bone marrow. Although the exact mechanisms responsible for its pathogenesis are unknown, possible causes include a primary stem-cell defect, immune-mediated inhibition of hemopoiesis, and an abnormal bone marrow microenvironment (Camitta et al; 1982; Young and Maciejewski, 1997). Normal hemopoiesis is sustained by interactions between hemopoietic stem cells, cells of the bone marrow microenvironment, and cytokines produced by these cells. These cytokines are essential for the viability, proliferation, and differentiation of hemopoietic stem cells. In vitro evidence for the existence of a supporting microenvironment in hemopoiesis comes from the development of a long-term bone marrow culture (LTBMC) system (Dexter et al., 1977; Gartner and Kaplan, 1980). LTBMC is composed of confluent layers of marrow-adherent cells including fibroblasts, endothelial cells, adipocytes, and macrophages. LTBMC forms an in vitro model of the bone marrow microenvironment. Marrow stromal cells are thought to exert their regulatory role in hemopoiesis, at least in part, by the production of certain cytokines. Monolayer cultures of marrow-adherent cells have been shown to produce a variety of cytokines including granulocyte colony-stimulating factor (G-CSF), granulocyte-macrophage colony-stimulating factor (GM-CSF), interleukin-6 (IL-6), and stem cell factor (SCF), either constitutively or after stimulation by interleukin-1 (IL-1) or tumor necrosis factor-α (TNF-α) (Kaushansky et al., 1988; Linenberger et al., 1995; Schadduk et al., 1983).

Several earlier studies showed elevated circulating levels of colony-stimulating activity in patients with AA (Nissen et al., 1985; Yen et al., 1985). These studies employed bioassays to measure colony-stimulating activity and therefore detected the combined stimulatory effects of various cytokines. The recent development of sensitive radioimmunoassays (RIA) and enzyme-linked immunosorbent assays (ELISA) has made it possible to measure specific cytokines even at low levels. To clarify the role of cytokines in the pathophysiology of AA, I will summarize here the circulating levels and production of various cytokines by peripheral mononuclear cells and marrow stromal cells in patients with AA.

Erythropoietin (EPO)

EPO is a glycoprotein produced by cells adjacent to the proximal renal tubules (Erslev, 1991; Kranz, 1991). In the bone marrow, EPO binds to and activates specific receptors on erythroid progenitor cells to regulate the production of red blood cells (RBCs). Under normal steady-state conditions, 10 to 20 mIU/ml of plasma EPO induces the production of enough RBCs to replace senescent cells in the RBC mass, and to maintain a flow of oxygen to the renal oxygen sensor which is sufficient to ensure baseline levels of EPO synthesis. Reduced flow of oxygen to the kidneys increases the rate of EPO synthesis exponentially, such that at a packed cell volume of less than 0.20, the plasma levels of EPO increase 100-fold or more (Erslev et al., 1980).

Several studies have shown highly elevated levels of EPO in patients with AA (Gaines Das et al., 1992; Schrezenmeier et al., 1994; Urabe et al., 1992). We have also measured plasma EPO levels in 75 patients with acquired AA. (Figure 2.1, Kojima et al., 1995). The median hemoglobin concentration was 7.2g/dl with a range of 3.8 to 14.2g/dl, and the median plasma EPO level was 2720 mIU/ml with a range of 103 to 19,800 mIU/ml. The normal range for plasma EPO was 18.3 ± 3.5 mIU/ml. Overall, there was an inverse relationship between the level of plasma EPO and the hemoglobin concentration. Plasma EPO levels varied tremendously among patients with the same degree of anemia. Two factors relevant to this variation were the etiology of AA and the interval between diagnosis and blood sampling. EPO levels in patients with posthepatitis AA were significantly lower than those in patients with idiopathic AA. Higher EPO concentrations were found in patients with a longer duration of disease.

We studied serial changes in plasma EPO levels in patients who showed an erythropoietic response following immunosuppressive therapy or bone marrow transplantation (BMT). A decrease in plasma EPO levels was noted in all erythroid responders. For any given degree of anemia, the plasma EPO level was lower in patients of the BMT group than in patients receiving immunosuppressive therapy. Furthermore, plasma EPO levels were inappropriately decreased in more than half of the patients who received BMT compared with iron-deficient patients. Cyclosporin probably caused the decreased plasma EPO levels in BMT patients.

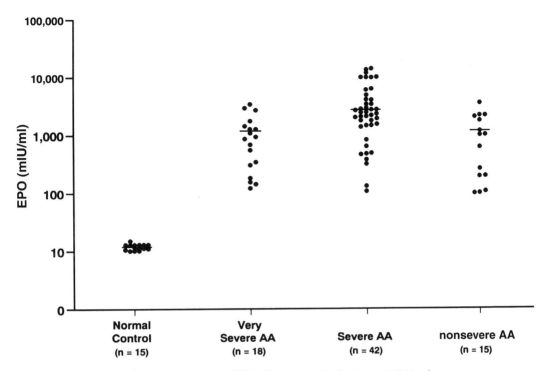

Figure 2.1. Plasma concentrations of erythropoietin (EPO) in 75 patients with aplastic anemia (AA) and 15 normal controls. Each horizontal bar indicates the mean value in the group.

Granulocyte colony-stimulating factor (G-CSF)

G-CSF is a glycoprotein that selectively and specifically stimulates the proliferation and differentiation of neutrophil precursors by binding to a specific cell surface receptor. G-CSF also activates several functions of mature neutrophils, including mobility, adherence, phagocytosis, bacterial killing, and superoxide release. Monocyte/macrophages and bone marrow stromal cells are known to produce G-CSF (Demetri and Griffin, 1991; Lieschke and Burgess, 1992). In recent clinical trials using recombinant human (rh) G-CSF to treat AA, a transient increase in neutrophil counts was induced in the majority of patients (Kojima and Matsuyama, 1994; Kojima et al., 1991).

Although previous studies have shown elevated levels of G-CSF in the sera of some AA patients, serum levels of G-CSF are below the lower limits of detection in a considerable percentage of AA patients or normal controls (Motojima

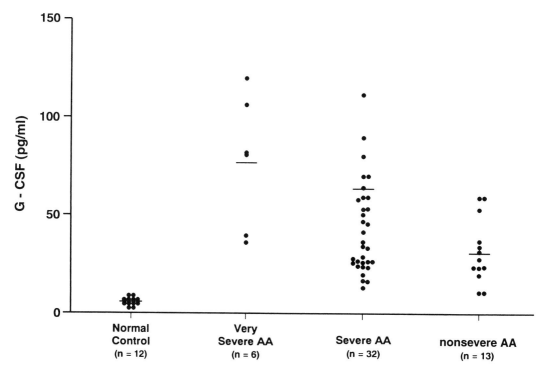

Figure 2.2. Plasma concentrations of granulocyte colony-stimulating factor (G-CSF) in 51 patients with aplastic anemia and no sign of infection and 12 normal controls. Each horizontal bar indicates the mean value in the group.

et al., 1989; Omori et al., 1992; Watari et al., 1989). We measured endogenous plasma G-CSF levels in 68 patients with acquired AA (51 of whom had no sign of infection) by a chemiluminescent immunoassay (Figure 2.2, Kiriyama et al., 1993; Kojima et al., 1996). The minimum detection limit of this assay (0.5 pg/ml) was sufficient to determine G-CSF levels in all AA patients and normal controls. In 51 AA patients who had no signs of infection, plasma G-CSF levels were significantly elevated compared with the normal control group (42.1 ± 23.6 pg/ml versus 6.8 ± 1.7 pg/ml, $P < 0.001$). Plasma G-CSF levels were also significantly higher in the 17 AA patients with signs of infection compared with the 51 AA patients without obvious infection (1211.8 ± 1850.4 pg/ml versus 42.1 ± 23.6 pg/ml, respectively, $P < 0.01$). There was a significant negative correlation between plasma G-CSF levels and absolute neutrophil counts (ANC) in AA patients with no signs of infection. The 51 patients were grouped on the basis of sex, age, interval between diagnosis and time of study entry, and type of therapy at the time of study entry. None of these variables was significantly associated with differences in mean plasma G-CSF levels between subgroups.

Plasma G-CSF levels were determined before and 2–3 months after immuno-suppressive therapy or BMT. In the 13 patients undergoing BMT, the mean ANC increased from $(0.77 \pm 0.48) \times 10^9/l$ to $(1.98 \pm 1.04) \times 10^9/l$ following BMT. The mean ANC also increased from $(0.50 \pm 0.23) \times 10^9/l$ to $(1.64 \pm 1.20) \times 10^9/l$ in ten responders to immunosuppressive therapy. Although a decrease in the plasma G-CSF concentration was observed in all patients who achieved self-sustaining hemopoiesis following BMT or immunosuppressive therapy, it was lower in patients undergoing BMT as compared with those receiving immunosuppressive therapy for any given degree of neutropenia.

Thrombopoietin (TPO)

TPO is a cytokine that supports megakaryocyte colony formation, increases meg-akaryocyte size and ploidy, and is the most important regulator of platelet pro-duction (Kaushansky, 1995). TPO has been identified as a ligand for c-Mpl, and full-length complementary deoxyribonucleic acid sequences (cDNAs) encoding human TPO have been cloned and sequenced (Bartley et al., 1994; Lok et al., 1994; de Sauvage et al., 1994; Sohma et al., 1994; Wendling et al., 1994). The predomi-nant sites of TPO production are the liver and, to a lesser degree, the kidney, although the specific cells responsible for production are not known (Kaushansky, 1995). As TPO is the physiological regulator of platelet production, its circulating levels vary with blood platelet counts.

There are only a few studies that have examined endogenous levels of TPO in patients with AA (Emmons et al., 1996; Marsh et al., 1996). We measured endoge-nous plasma levels of TPO in 76 patients with acquired AA using ELISA (Figure 2.3; Kojima et al., 1997b; Tahara et al., 1996). In patients with AA, the median platelet count was $18 \times 10^9/l$ with a range of $1 \times 10^9/l$ to $110 \times 10^9/l$. The mean plasma TPO level was 29.7 ± 12.9, 21.3 ± 10.6, 16.6 ± 7.4, and 1.3 ± 0.3 fmol/ml in patients with very severe AA, severe AA, nonsevere AA, and normal controls, respectively. The mean plasma TPO level was significantly higher in patients with AA than in normal controls $(P < 0.001)$, and there was a significant negative correlation between plasma TPO levels and platelet counts in 54 AA patients who had not received any platelet transfusions prior to sampling. We did not find any factors responsible for the variation in plasma TPO levels.

We studied serial changes in plasma TPO levels in patients who showed an increase in their platelet counts following immunosuppressive therapy or BMT. In 14 patients undergoing BMT, the mean platelet count increased from $(13 \pm 5) \times 10^9/l$ to $(169 \pm 26) \times 10^9/l$ following BMT. A decrease in TPO level was observed in all patients. However, although the mean platelet count increased from $(13 \pm 6) \times 10^9/l$ to $(55 \pm 35) \times 10^9/l$ in ten responders to immunosuppressive

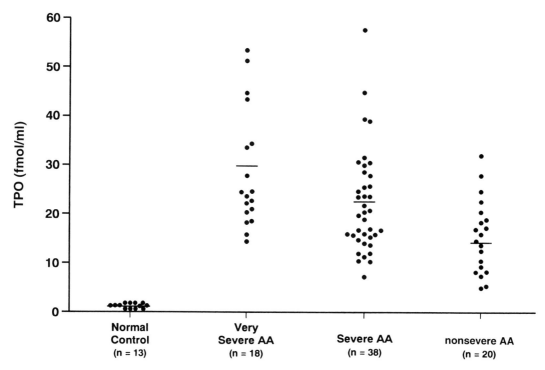

Figure 2.3. Plasma concentrations of thrombopoietin (TPO) in 76 patients with aplastic anemia and 13 normal controls. Each horizontal bar indicates the mean value in the group.

therapy, a decrease in TPO level was observed in only half of them. These findings differed from our previous studies in which decreased plasma EPO and G-CSF levels were observed in all AA patients who achieved self-sustaining hemopoiesis after treatment. Even in patients who respond to immunosuppressive therapy, mild thrombocytopenia and decreased megakaryocyte numbers in the bone marrow are present in the majority. These findings may explain why plasma TPO levels remain high in AA patients who achieved self-sustaining hemopoiesis and further support the model that plasma TPO levels are regulated not only by blood platelet count but also by the number of megakaryocytes or megakaryocyte progenitors in the bone marrow.

Stem cell factor (SCF)

SCF, the ligand for the c-Kit receptor, is produced mainly by marrow stromal cells and has been implicated in the maintenance of an optimal hemopoietic environment (Huang et al., 1990; Martin et al., 1991; Williams et al., 1990; Zsebo et al., 1990). It is biologically active in both a soluble and a membrane-bound

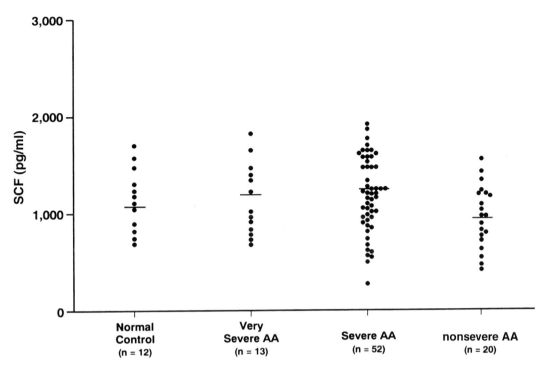

Figure 2.4. Plasma concentrations of soluble stem cell factor (SCF) in 85 patients with aplastic anemia and 12 normal controls. Each horizontal bar indicates the mean value in the group.

form (Anderson et al., 1990). In vitro, SCF alone fails to exhibit any hemopoietic colony-stimulating activity, but it acts synergistically with other more lineage-specific cytokines such as G-CSF, GM-CSF, IL-3, and EPO to augment colony formation by normal human bone marrow cells (McNiece et al., 1991; Tsuji et al., 1991). It can also partially reverse the reduced in vitro colony formation observed in patients with AA (Amano et al., 1993; Bagnara et al., 1992; Wodnar-Filipowicz et al., 1992).

To date, two studies have investigated levels of circulating SCF in patients with AA (Nimer et al., 1994; Wodnar-Filipowicz et al., 1993). Both studies demonstrated that the mean serum levels of SCF in AA patients are significantly lower than those in normal controls. Recently, we studied plasma levels of soluble SCF in 85 patients with AA (Figure 2.4, Kojima et al., 1997a). In contrast to previous studies, the mean SCF level in these 85 patients was 1098 ± 358 pg/ml, which was similar to that of normal controls (1160 ± 316 pg/ml); there was no significant correlation between peripheral blood counts and SCF levels. The mean SCF concentration in patients who received prednisolone with or without anabolic steroids at the time of sampling was significantly lower than in patients who did not receive these agents. We did not find any correlation between changes in SCF levels and the response to immunosuppressive therapy. SCF levels were determined before and 2–3 months after BMT in 21 patients, all of whom achieved self-sustaining hemopoiesis. The mean SCF level was significantly increased after BMT as compared to before BMT (1637 ± 456 pg/ml versus 1052 ± 298 pg/ml, respectively, $P = 0.005$). Although some studies have emphasized the prognostic value of SCF in the treatment of AA (Wodnar-Filipowicz et al., 1993), we did not observe that it had any value in predicting who would and would not respond to immunosuppressive therapy.

Granulocyte-macrophage colony-stimulating factor (GM-CSF)

GM-CSF is a glycoprotein that has the potent effects of stimulating the proliferation, maturation, and function of hemopoietic cells (Metcalf, 1986). GM-CSF can be synthesized by a variety of cell types in response to specific activating signals. T-cells, macrophages, mast cells, endothelial cells, and fibroblasts can be induced to accumulate GM-CSF messenger ribonucleic acid (mRNA) and secrete GM-CSF protein (Gasson, 1991). rhGM-CSF was the first cytokine used in clinical trials for patients with AA, and it has been shown to increase neutrophil counts in some patients with AA (Champlin et al., 1989; Vadhan-Raj et al., 1988). Although it was expected to induce a multilineage response, there is evidence of trilineage recovery following short-term administration of GM-CSF in only a few patients.

Schrezenmeier et al. (1993) measured GM-CSF levels in the sera of 33 patients with AA. In normal controls, GM-CSF does not appear in the circulation at detectable levels. Serum GM-CSF was detected in 25 of 33 untreated AA patients and was significantly higher in AA patients than in normal controls. The median serum GM-CSF level was 45 pg/ml (range: undetectable to 625 pg/ml) in severe AA patients and 24 pg/ml (range: undetectable to 122 pg/ml) in nonsevere AA patients. There was no statistically significant relationship between serum GM-CSF levels and peripheral blood white cell or neutrophil counts.

Several investigators have studied in vitro GM-CSF production by peripheral blood mononuclear cells (PBMNCs) in patients with AA (Kawano et al., 1992; Nimer et al., 1991). We studied the production of GM-CSF by PBMNCs from 48 AA patients using an ELISA (Kojima et al., 1992a). Detectable levels of spontaneous GM-CSF production were observed in 45 of 48 patients; these were not significantly different from levels observed in normal controls. In contrast, phytohemagglutinin-stimulated production of GM-CSF was significantly higher in patients with AA than in normal controls ($P < 0.01$).

Antilymphocyte globulin (ALG) has been used as the first-line therapy for patients with AA. ALG can exert a mitogenic effect on lymphocytes and induce them to produce GM-CSF (Kawano et al., 1988). We found a positive correlation between the clinical response of AA patients to ALG and GM-CSF production by PBMNCs stimulated by ALG (Abe et al., 1991). This finding suggests that an immunostimulatory property of ALG plays an important role in the treatment of AA.

Flt-3 ligand (Flt-3L)

Flt-3L is a novel cytokine that acts as a ligand for the tyrosine kinase receptor flt-3 (Hannum et al., 1994; Lyman et al., 1993; Matthews et al., 1991). While the ligand is expressed by a number of hemopoietic and nonhemopoietic tissues (Hannum et al., 1994), expression of its receptor is restricted to early hemopoietic progenitor cells (Small et al., 1994). The ligand is biologically active in both a soluble and a membrane-bound form (Lyman et al., 1995a). The primary role of flt-3L in the hemopoietic system is the maintenance and proliferation of stem and progenitor cells. By itself, flt-3L does not have strong stimulatory effects on hemopoietic cells, but it synergizes with a number of other cytokines (Hudak et al., 1995; Muench et al., 1995; Rusten et al., 1996). However, Flt-3L has no stimulatory effect on AA bone marrow, either alone or in combination with other cytokines (Scope et al., 1995).

Lyman et al. (1995b) have demonstrated elevated plasma/serum levels of flt-3L in a small number of patients with acquired AA. Recently, Wodnar-Filipowicz et al. (1996) studied circulating levels of flt-3L in 34 patients with AA using ELISA. At diagnosis, flt-3L levels were highly elevated in patients with AA compared with normal controls, 2653 ± 353 pg/ml versus 14 ± 39 pg/ml. Flt-3L levels returned to near normal levels within the first 3 months following BMT or successful immunosuppressive therapy (100 ± 31 and 183 ± 14 pg/ml, respectively). There was a significant negative correlation between serum flt-3L levels and the peripheral-blood neutrophil count.

Interleukin-1 (IL-1)

IL-1 is a polypeptide with an important role in the regulation of the immune system and hemopoiesis. It induces the production of GM-CSF, G-CSF, IL-3, and other cytokines by fibroblasts and endothelial cells. IL-1 also acts synergistically with other cytokines to promote the growth of hemopoietic stem cells. The sources of IL-1 include a variety of cells such as monocytes, tissue macrophages, neutrophils, endothelial cells, fibroblasts, and others (Dinarello, 1991). rhIL-1 has been used in the treatment of AA patients but without an apparent beneficial effect on hemopoiesis (Walsh et al., 1992).

Gascon and Scala (1988) used a bioassay to quantify IL-1 production by monocytes from 15 AA patients prior to immunosuppressive therapy. IL-1 production was markedly diminished in 12 of 15 patients when compared with normal controls ($P < 0.005$). Normalization of IL-1 production was observed in responders to immunosuppressive therapy. Nakao et al. (1989) also found impaired production of IL-1 from PBMNCs in ten of 17 AA patients. Among the cytokines, decreased production has been described only for IL-1 in patients with AA. This finding may reflect defective monocyte–macrophage maturation in patients with AA (Andreesen et al., 1989).

Production of cytokines by marrow stromal cells

A defective marrow microenvironment has been proposed as one possible mechanism of AA (Ershler et al., 1980; Knospe and Crosby, 1971). LTBMC systems have been used to evaluate stromal cell function. These have shown abnormalities in the morphology and function of stromal cells, but the incidence of stromal defects varies widely between individual studies. According to Holmberg et al., (1994), only half of AA patients produce normal-appearing stromal layers with LTBMC. Krieger-Slanicka et al. (1995) have observed defective proliferation of stromal cells in 20 of 30 AA patients. In contrast, we have observed the development of a complete and confluent stromal layer in 29 of 33 patients with AA (Kojima et al., 1992*b*). Other studies have also found that the majority of AA patients are able to form confluent stromal layers within 3–5 weeks of culture (Hotta et al., 1985; Marsh et al., 1990).

Several investigators have studied the role of stroma-derived cytokines to clarify the pathogenesis of AA. Some have measured the concentrations of cytokines in culture supernatants (Gibson et al., 1995; Kojima et al., 1992*b*; Krieger-Slanicka et al., 1995; Tani et al., 1993), while others have analyzed in vitro cytokine mRNA expression using the reverse transcriptase-polymerase chain reaction method (Hirayama et al., 1993; Stark et al., 1993).

In a previous study, we measured production of G-CSF, GM-CSF, and IL-6 by stromal cells from 33 patients with AA (Kojima et al., 1992*b*). The concentration of cytokines in culture media with or without IL-1 stimulation was determined. Spontaneous production of G-CSF, GM-CSF, and IL-6 did not differ significantly between normal controls and AA patients (Figure 2.5). The ability of stromal cells to release these cytokines in response to IL-1 was either normal or elevated in all but one AA patient (Figure 2.6).

SCF is produced mainly by bone marrow stroma (Williams et al., 1990; Zsebo et al., 1990). By itself, it does not have a strong stimulatory effect on hemopoietic cells, but it acts synergistically with a number of other cytokines (McNiece et al., 1991). SCF seems to be the most appropriate cytokine to characterize the hemopoietic function of bone marrow stroma. Recently, we investigated the production of soluble SCF by marrow stromal cells of 46 patients with AA (Kojima et al.,

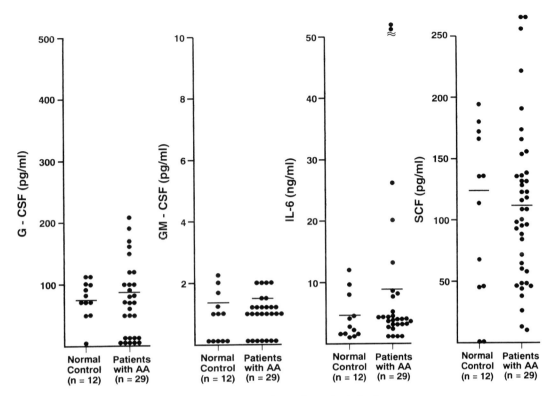

Figure 2.5. Spontaneous release of G-CSF, granulocyte/macrophage colony-stimulating factor (GM-CSF), interleukin-6 (IL-6) and soluble stem cell factor (SCF) by bone marrow stromal cells from patients with aplastic anemia and normal controls. The dots represent the individual values of cytokines for each patient. The mean value is indicated by a horizontal bar.

1997a). The ability of marrow stromal cells to release soluble SCF did not differ significantly between patients with AA and normal controls (Figures 2.5 and 2.6). However, four of 46 patients had SCF levels below the 95% confidence limit of the normal range. Holmberg et al. (1994) have reported on the production of various cytokines from stromal cells in 20 patients with AA using the same method. In agreement with our study, they observed elevated levels of some cytokines, such as macrophage inflammatory protein-1α (MIP-1α) and GM-CSF, and near-normal levels of other cytokines such as IL-6, leukemia-inhibitory factor (LIF) and G-CSF. Increased mRNA expression for cytokines such as G-CSF, GM-CSF and IL-6 was also shown to occur in bone marrow stromal cells derived from patients with AA. However, because the study was based on RNA levels (Hirayama et al., 1993; Stark et al., 1993), it was difficult to quantify the production of cytokines.

Krieger-Slanicka et al. (1995) investigated the in vitro expression of SCF mRNA and protein levels in culture media derived from bone marrow samples of 30 AA patients. Although no deficiencies were found in SCF mRNA expression, they

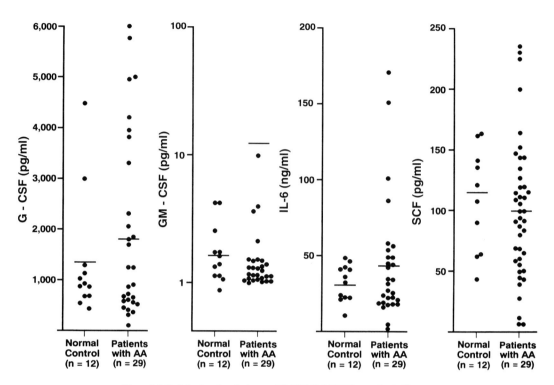

Figure 2.6. IL-1 β-stimulated release of G-CSF, GM-CSF, IL-6 and soluble SCF by bone marrow stromal cells from patients with aplastic anemia and normal controls. The dots represent individual values of cytokines for each patient. The mean value is indicated by a horizontal bar.

found low levels of soluble SCF released from poorly confluent stroma cultures in the majority of AA patients. A significant correlation was found between the concentration of SCF in the culture supernatants and the confluence of stromal growth. The reduced accumulation of SCF was probably related to a reduced cell number and not to any abnormalities in the processes of mRNA translation and/or protein secretion.

Rationale for the therapeutic use of cytokines

Because hemopoietic stem cells will not proliferate or even survive without stimulation by cytokines, a reduction in the rate or cessation of cytokine production might be a cause of AA. As described above, the results of many laboratory studies are against cytokine deficiencies causing AA in most instances. Despite the lack of objective support for their use, several cytokines have been offered to patients with AA to increase the production of mature blood cells from the remaining

Table 2.1. Clinical trials of cytokines in aplastic anemia

		No. of	Hemopoietic response		
Investigator	Cytokines	patients	Neutrophils	Platelets	Red blood cells
Vadhan-Raj et al., 1988	GM-CSF	10	9	0	0
Champlin et al., 1989	GM-CSF	11	10	1	0
Kojima et al., 1991	G-CSF	20	12	0	0
Ganser et al., 1990	IL-3	9	5	1	0
Walsh et al., 1992	IL-1	4	0	0	0
Schrezenmeier et al., 1995	IL-6	6	0	0	0
Urabe et al., 1993	EPO	27	0	0	3

Notes:
EPO = erythropoietin; G-CSF = granulocyte colony-stimulating factor;
GM-CSF = granulocyte-macrophage colony-stimulating factor; IL-1 = interleukin-1;
IL-3 = interleukin-3; IL-6 = interleukin-6.

small pool of precurser cells (Champlin et al., 1989; Ganser et al., 1990; Kojima et al., 1991; Schrezenmeier et al., 1995; Urabe et al., 1993; Walsh et al., 1992; Vadhan-Raj et al., 1988). The results have shown that GM-CSF and G-CSF increase the number of circulating neutrophils in the majority of patients, but other cytokines rarely stimulate hemopoiesis in AA patients (Table 2.1). For example, erythropoietic responses were observed only in patients with mild AA, with lower levels of endogenous EPO (Urabe et al., 1993). The endogenous levels of plasma EPO are so elevated that it seems unlikely that levels of plasma EPO become much higher than endogenous levels after intravenous or subcutaneous injections of rhEPO in patients with severe AA. On the other hand, levels of plasma G-CSF are much higher than endogenous levels after intravenous or subcutaneous injections of rhG-CSF, even in patients with severe AA (Figure 2.7). The ratio of endogenous levels to those after exogenous administration may be useful in predicting AA patients' clinical response to cytokines. Thus, the rationale for treating the cytopenia of AA patients with cytokines is not based on findings of a deficiency of cytokines, but on the expectation that impaired proliferation and differentiation of hemopoietic stem cells may be overcome by pharmacological doses of cytokines.

Conclusion

In patients with AA, the circulating levels and production of various cytokines by peripheral-blood cells or bone marrow stromal cells are usually increased compared to those in healthy controls. Normal or decreased production has been

Figure 2.7. Endogenous levels of plasma G-CSF in patients with aplastic anemia (AA) and assumed plasma levels of G-CSF after intravenous or subcutaneous injection of recombinant G-CSF.

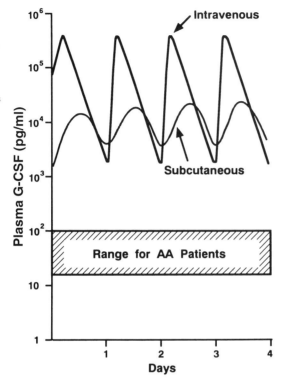

described only for IL-1 and SCF. To date, several cytokines have been used to treat AA patients. G-CSF and GM-CSF have been the most extensively evaluated; they resulted in transient increases in the numbers of myeloid cells in some patients with AA. The use of these cytokines in combination with immunosuppressive agents could reduce early infections and, therefore, increase the number of patients surviving long enough to achieve a hematological response. The European pilot trial has shown very encouraging results (Bacigalupo et al., 1995). Ongoing randomized prospective studies combined with immunosuppression and cytokines will reveal the usefulness of cytokines in the treatment of AA.

References

Abe, T., Matsuoka, H., Kojima, S., Kamachi, Y., Tsuge, I., Kodera, Y. and Matsuyama, T. (1991) Correlation of response of aplastic anemia to antilymphocyte globulin with in vitro lymphocyte stimulatory effect: predictive value of in vitro test for clinical response. *Blood*, **77**, 2225–30.

Amano, Y., Koike, K. and Nakahata, T. (1993) Stem cell factor enhances the growth of primitive erythroid progenitors to a greater exent than interleuin-3 in patients with aplastic anaemia. *British Journal of Haematology*, **85**, 663–9.

Anderson, D. M., Lyman, S. D., Baird, A., Wignall, J. M., Eisenman, J., Rauch, C., March, C. J., Boswell, S., Gimpel, S. D., Cosman, D. and Williams, D. E. (1990) Molecular cloning of mast cell growth factor, a hematopoietin that is active in both membrane bound and soluble forms. *Cell*, **63**, 235–43.

Andreesen, R., Brugger, W., Thomssen, C., Rehm, A., Speck, B. and Lohr, G. (1989) Defective monocyte-to-macrophage maturation in patients with aplastic anemia. *Blood*, **74**, 2150–6.

Bacigalupo, A., Broccia, G., Corda, W., Arcese, W., Carotenuto, A., Coser, P., Lacopino, M. T., van Lint. and Gluckman, E. for the European Group for Blood and Marrow Transplantation (EBMT) Working Party on SAA (1995) Antilymphocyte globulin, cyclosporin, and granulocyte colony-stimulating factor in patients with acquired severe aplastic anemia (SAA): a pilot study of the EBMT SAA Working Party. *Blood*, **85**, 1348–53.

Bagnara, G. P., Strippoli, P., Bonsi, L., Brizzi, M. F., Avanzi, G. C., Timeus, F., Ramenghi, U., Piaggio, G., Tong, J., Podesta, M., Paolucci, G., Pegoraro, L., Gabutti, V. and Bacigalupo, A. (1992) Effect of stem cell factor on colony growth from acquired and constitutional (Fanconi) aplastic anemia. *Blood*, **80**, 382–9.

Bartley, T. D., Bogenberger, J., Hunt, P., Li, Y. S., Lu, H.S., Martin, F., Chang, M. S., Samal, B., Nichol, J. L. and Swift, S. (1994) Identification and cloning of a megakaryocyte growth and development factor that is a ligand for the cytokine receptor Mpl. *Cell*, **77**, 1117–24.

Camitta, B. M., Storb, R. and Thomas, E. D. (1982) Aplastic anemia: pathogenesis, diagnosis, treatment and prognosis. *New England Journal of Medicine*, **306**, 645–50.

Champlin, R. E., Nimer, S. D., Ireland, P., Otte, D. H. and Golde, D. W. (1989) Treatment of refractory aplastic anemia with recombinant human granulocyte-macrophage colony-stimulating factor. *Blood*, **73**, 694–9.

Demetri, G. D. and Griffin, J. D. (1991) Granulocyte colony-stimulating factor and its receptor. *Blood*, **78**, 2791–808.

Dexter, T. M., Allen, T. D. and Lajtha, L. G. (1977) Conditions controlling the proliferation of hemopoietic stem cells in vitro. *Journal of Cell Physiology*, **91**, 335–44.

Dinarello, C. A. (1991) Interleukin-1 and interleukin-1 antagonism. *Blood*, **77**, 1627–52.

Emmons, R. V. B., Reid, D. M., Cohen, R. L., Meng, Y. G., Young, N. S., Dunbar, C. E. and Shulman, N. R. (1996) Human thrombopoietin levels are high when thrombocytopenia is due to megakaryocyte deficiency and low when due to increased platelet destruction. *Blood*, **87**, 4068–71.

Ershler, W. B., Ross, J., Finlay, J. L. and Shahidi, N. T. (1980) Bone marrow microenvironmental defect in congenital hypoplastic anemia. *New England Journal of Medicine*, **302**, 322–7.

Erslev, A. J. (1991) Erythropoietin. *New England Journal of Medicine*, **324**, 1339–44.

Erslev, A. J., Caro, J., Mileer, O. and Silver, R. (1980) Plasma-erythropoietin in health and disease. *Annals of Clinical Laboratory Science*, **10**, 250–7.

Gaines Das, R. E., Milne, A., Rowley, M., Gordon-Smith, E. C. and Cotes, P. M. (1992) Serum immunoreactive erythropoietin in patients with idiopathic aplastic and Fanconi's anaemias. *British Journal of Haematology*, **82**, 601–7.

Ganser, A., Lindemann, A., Seipelt, G., Ottman, O. G., Eder, M., Falk, S., Herrmann, F., Kaltwasser, J. P., Meusers, P., Klausmann, M., Frisch, J., Schulz, G., Mertelsmann, R. and Hoelzer, D. (1990) Effects of recombinant human interleukin-3 in aplastic anemia. *Blood*, **76**, 1287–92.

Gartner, S. and Kaplan, H. S. (1980) Long-term culture of human bone marrow cells. *Proceedings of the National Academy of Sciences of the USA*, **77**, 4756–9.

Gascon, P. and Scala, G. (1988) Decreased interleukin-1 production in aplastic anemia. *American Journal of Medicine*, **85**, 668–74.

Gasson, J. C. (1991) Molecular physiology of granulocyte-macrophage colony-stimulating factor. *Blood*, **77**, 1131–45.

Gibson, F. M., Scopes, J., Daly, S., Ball, S. and Gordon–Smith, E. C. (1995) Haemopoietic growth factor production by normal and aplastic anaemia stroma in long-term bone marrow culture. *British Journal of Haematology*, **91**, 551–61.

Hannum, C., Culpepper, J., Campbell, D., McClanahan, T., Zurawski, S., Bazan, J. F., Kastelein, R., Hudak, S., Wagar, J. and Mattson, J. (1994) Ligand for flt-3/fltk-2 receptor tyrosine kinase regulates growth of haematopoietic stem cells and is encoded by variant RNAs. *Nature*, **368**, 643–8.

Hirayama, Y., Kohgo, Y., Matsunaga, T., Ohi, S., Sakamaki, S. and Niitu, Y. (1993) Cytokine mRNA expression of bone marrow stromal cells from patients with aplastic anemia and myelodysplastic syndrome. British Journal of Haematology, **85**, 676–83.

Holmberg, L. A., Seidel, K., Leisenring, W. and Torok-Storb, B. (1994) Aplastic anemia: analysis of stroma cell function in long-term marrow cultures. *Blood*, **84**, 3685–90.

Hotta, T., Kato, T., Maeda, H., Yamao, H., Yamada, H. and Saito, H. (1985) Functional changes in marrow stromal cells in aplastic anemia. *Acta Haematologica*, **74**, 65–9.

Huang, E., Nocka, K., Beier, D. R., Chu, T. Y., Buck, J., Lahm, H. W., Wellner, D., Leder, P. and Besmer, P. (1990) The hemopoietic growth factor KL is encoded by the Sl locus and it's the ligand of the c-kit receptor, the gene product of the W locus. *Cell*, **63**, 225–33.

Hudak, S., Hunte, B., Culpepper, J., Mennon, S., Hannum, C., Thompson-Snipes, L. and Rennick, D. (1995) Flt-3/flk-2 ligand promotes the growth of murine stem cells and the expansion of colony-forming cells and spleen colony-forming units. *Blood*, **85**, 2747–55.

Kaushansky, K. (1995) Thrombopoietin: the primary regulator of platelet production. *Blood*, **86**, 419–31.

Kaushansky, K., Lin, N. and Adamson, J. W. (1988) Interleukin-1-stimulates fibroblasts to synthesize granulocyte-macrophage and granulocyte colony-stimulating factors. *Journal of Clinical Investigation*, **81**, 92–7.

Kawano, Y., Nissen, C., Gratwohl, A. and Speck, B. (1988) Immuno-stimulatory effects of different antilymphocyte globulin preparations: a possible clue to their clinical effect. *British Journal of Haematology*, **68**, 115–19.

Kawano, Y., Takaue, Y., Hirao, A., Watanabe, T., Abe, T., Shimizu, T., Sato, J., Saito, S., Kitamura, T., Takaku, F. and Kuroda, Y. (1992) Production of interleukin-3 and granulocyte-macrophage colony-stimulating factor from stimulated blood mononuclear cells in patients with aplastic anemia. *Experimental Hematology*, **20**, 1125–8.

Kiriyama, R., Chichibu, K., Matsuno, T. and Ohsawa, N. (1993) Sensitive chemiluminescent immunoassay for human granulocyte colony-stimulating factor (G-CSF) in clinical applications. *Clinica Chimica Acta*, **220**, 201–9.

Knospe, W. H. and Crosby, W. H. (1971) Aplastic anemia: a disorder of the bone marrow sinusoidal microcirculation rather than stem cell failure. *Lancet*, **1**, 20–2.

Kojima, S. and Matsuyama, T. (1994) Stimulation of granulopoiesis by high-dose recombinant human granulocyte colony-stimulating factor in children with aplastic anemia and very severe neutropenia. *Blood*, **83**, 1474–8.

Kojima, S., Fukuda, M., Miyajima, Y., Matsuyama, T. and Horibe, K. (1991) Treatment of aplastic anemia in children with recombinant human granulocyte colony-stimulating factor. *Blood*, **77**, 937–41.

Kojima, S., Matsuyama, T. and Kodera, Y. (1992*a*) In vitro granulocyte-macrophage colony-stimulating factor production by peripheral blood mononuclear cells in aplastic anemia. *Acta Haematologica*, **91**, 175–80.

Kojima, S., Matsuyama, T. and Kodera, Y. (1992*b*) Hematopoietic growth factors released by marrow stromal cells from patients with aplastic anemia. *Blood*, **79**, 2256–61.

Kojima, S., Matsuyama, T. and Kodera, Y. (1995) Circulating erythropoietin in patients with acquired aplastic anaemia. *Acta Haematologica*, **94**, 117–22.

Kojima, S., Matsuyama, T., Kodera, Y., Nishihira, H., Ueda, K., Shimbo, T. and Nakahata, T. (1996) Measurement of endogenous plasma granulocyte colony-stimulating factor in patients with acquired aplastic anemia by a sensitive chemiluminescent immunoassay. *Blood*, **87**, 1303–8.

Kojima, S., Matsuyama, T. and Kodera Y. (1997*a*) Plasma levels and production of soluble stem cell factor by marrow stromal cells in patients with aplastic anemia. *British Journal of Haematology*, **99**, 440–6.

Kojima, S., Matsuyama, T., Kodera, Y., Tahara, T. and Kato, T. (1997*b*) Measurement of endogenous plasma thrombopoietin in patients with acquired aplastic anaemia by a sensitive enzyme-linked immuno-sorbent assay. *British Journal of Haematology*, **97**, 538–43.

Kranz, S.B. (1991). Erythropoietin. *Blood*, **77**, 419–34.

Krieger-Slanicka, M., Nissen, C. and Wodnar-Filipowicz, A. (1995) Stem cell factor in aplastic anaemia: in vitro expression in bone marrow stroma and fibroblast cultures. *European Journal of Haematology*, **54**, 262–9.

Lieschke, G. J. and Burgess, A. W. (1992) Granulocyte colony-stimulating factor and granulocyte-macrophage colony-stimulating factor. *New England Journal of Medicine*, **327**, 28–35.

Linenberger, M. L., Jacobsen, F. W., Bennett, L. G., Broudy, V. C., Martin, F. H. and Abkowitz, J. L. (1995) Stem cell factor production by human marrow stromal fibroblasts. *Experimental Hematology*, **23**, 1104–14.

Lok, S., Kaushansky, K., Holly, R. D., Kuijper, J. F., Lofton-Day, C. E., Oort, P. J., Grant, F. J., Heipel, M. D., Burkhead, S. K., Kramer, J. G., Bell, L. A., Sprecher, C. A., Blumberg, H., Johnson, R., Prunkard, D., Ching, A. F. T., Mathewes, S. L., Bailey, M. C., Forstrom, J. W., Buddle, M. M., Osborn, S. G., Evans, S. J., Sheppard, P. O., Presnell, S. R., O'Hara, P. J., Hagen, F. S., Roth, G. J. and Foster, D. C. (1994) Cloning and expression of murine-thrombopoietin cDNA and stimulation of platelet production in vivo. *Nature*, **369**, 565–8.

Lyman, S. D., James, L., Vanden, B. T., de Vries, P., Brasel, K., Gliniak, B., Hollingsworth, L. T., Picha, K. S., Mckenna, H. J., Splett, R. R., Fletcher, F. F., Maraskovsky, E., Farrach, F., Foxworthe, D., Williams, D. E. and Beckmann, M. P. (1993) Molecular cloning of a ligand for the flt-3/flk-2 tyrosine kinase receptor: a proliferative factor for primitive hematopoietic cells. *Cell*, **75**, 1157–67.

Lyman, S. D., James, L., Escobar, S., Downey, H., de Vries, P., Brasel, K., Stocking, K., Beckman, M. P., Copeland, N. G., Cleveland, L. S., Jenkins, N. A., Belmont, J. W. and Davison, B. L. (1995*a*) Identification of soluble and membrane-bound isoforms of the murine flt-3 ligand generated by alternative splicing of mRNAs. *Oncogene*, **10**, 149–57.

Lyman, S. D., Seaberg, M., Hanna, R., Zappone, J., Brasel, K., Abkowitz, J. L., Prchal, J. T., Schultz, J. C. and Shahidi, N. T. (1995*b*) Plasma/serum-levels of flt-3 ligand are low in normal individuals and are highly elevated in patients with Fanconi anemia and acquired aplastic anemia. *Blood*, **86**, 4091–6.

Marsh, J. C. W., Chang, J., Testa, N. G., Hows, J. M. and Dexter, T. M. (1990) The hematopoietic defect in aplastic anemia assessed by long-term marrow culture. *Blood*, **76**, 1748–57.

Marsh, J. C. W., Gibson, F. M., Prue, R. L., Bowen, A., Dunn, V. T., Hornkohl, A. C., Nichol, J. L. and Gordon-Smith, E. C. (1996) Serum thrombopoietin levels in patients with aplastic anaemia. *British Journal of Haematology*, **95**, 605–10.

Martin, F. H., Suggs, S. V., Langley, K. E., Lu, H. S., Ting, J., Okino, K. H., Morris, C. F., McNiece, I. K., Jacobsen, F. W., Mendiaz, E. A., Birkett, N. C., Smith, K. A., Johnson, M. J., Parker, V. P., Flores, J. C., Patel, A. C., Fisher, E. F., Erjavec, H. O., Herrera, C. J., Wypych, J., Sachdev, R. K., Pope, J. A., Leslie, I., Wen, D., Lin, C-H., Cupples, R. L. and Zsebo, K. M. (1991) Primary structure and functional expression of rat and human stem cell factor DNAs. *Cell*, **63**, 203–12.

Matthews, W., Jordan, C. T., Wiegand, G. W., Pardoll, D. and Lemischka, I. R. (1991) A receptor tyrosine kinase specific to hematopoietic stem and progenitor cell-enriched populations. *Cell*, **65**, 1143–52.

McNiece, I. K., Langley, K. E. and Zsebo, K. M. (1991) Recombinant human stem cell factor synergizes with GM-CSF, G-CSF, IL-3 and Epo to stimulate human progenitor cells of the myeloid and erythroid lineages. *Experimental Hematology*, **19**, 226–31.

Metcalf, D. (1986) The molecular biology and functions of the granulocyte-macrophage colony-stimulating factors. *Blood*, **67**, 257–67.

Motojima, H., Kobayashi, T., Shimane, M., Kamachi, S. and Fukushima, M. (1989) Quantiative enzyme immunoassay for human granulocyte colony-stimulating factor (G-CSF). *Journal of Immunological Methods*, **118**, 187–92.

Muench, M. O., Roncarolo, M. G., Menon, S., Xu, Y., Kastelein, R., Zurawski, S., Hannum, C. H., Culpepper, J., Lee, F. and Namikawa, R. (1995) Flk-2/flt-3 ligand regulates the growth of early myeloid progenitors isolated from human fetal liver. *Blood*, **85**, 963–72.

Nakao, S., Matsushima, K. and Young, N. (1989) Decreased interleukin-1 production in aplastic anaemia. *British Journal of Haematology*, **71**, 431–6.

Nimer, S. D., Golde, D. W., Kwan, K., Lee, K., Clark, S. and Champlin, R. (1991) In vitro production of granulocyte-macrophage colony-stimulating factor in aplastic anemia: possible mechanisms of antithymocyte globulin. *Blood*, **78**, 163–8.

Nimer, S. D., Leung, D. H. Y., Wolin, M. J. and Golde, D. W. (1994) Serum stem cell factor levels in patients with aplastic anemia. *International Journal of Hematology*, **60**, 185–9.

Nissen, C., Moser, Y., Speck, B., Gratwohl, A. and Weis, J. (1985) Stimulatory serum factors in aplastic anaemia. *British Journal of Haematology*, **61**, 499–512.

Omori, F., Okamura, S., Shimoda, K., Otsuka, T., Harada, M. and Niho, Y. (1992) Levels of human serum granulocyte colony-stimulating factor and granulocyte-macrophage colony-stimulating factor under pathological conditions. *Biotherapy*, **4**, 147–53.

Rusten, L. S., Lyman, S. D., Veiby, O. P. and Jacobsen, S. E. W. (1996) The flt-3 ligand is a direct and potent stimulator of the growth of primitive and committed human CD34+ bone marrow progenitor cell in vitro. *Blood*, **87**, 1317–25.

de Sauvage, F. C., Hass, P. E., Spencer, S. D., Malloy, B. E., Gurney, A. L., Spencer, S. A.,

Darbonne, W. C., Henzel, W. J., Wong, S. C., Kuang, W. J., Oles, K. J., Hultgren, B., Solberg, L. A., Jr., Goeddel, D. V. and Eaton, D. L. (1994) Stimulation of megakaryocytopoiesis and thrombopoiesis by the c-Mpl ligand. *Nature*, **369**, 533–8.

Schrezenmeier, H., Raghavachar, A. and Heimpel, H. (1993) Granulocyte-macrophage colony-stimulating factor in the sera of patients with aplastic anemia. *Clinical Investigator*, **71**, 102–8.

Schrezenmeier, H., Noé, G., Raghavachar, A., Rich, I. N., Heimpel, H. and Kubanek, B. (1994) Serum erythropoietin and serum transferrin receptor levels in aplastic anaemia. *British Journal of Haematology*, **88**, 286–94.

Schrezenmeier, H., Marsh, J. C. W., Stromeyer, P., Muller, H., Heimpel, H., Gordon-Smith, E. C. and Raghavachar, A. (1995) A phase I/II trial of recombinant human interleukin-6 in patients with aplastic anaemia. *British Journal of Haematology*, **90**, 283–92.

Scope, J., Daly, S., Ball, S. E., McGuckin, C. P., Gordon–Smith, E. C. and Gibson, F. M. (1995) The effect of human flt-3 ligand on committed progenitor cell production from normal, aplastic anaemia and Diamond–Blackfan anaemia bone marrow. *British Journal of Haematology*, **91**, 544–50.

Shadduck, R. K., Waheed, A., Greenberger, J. S. and Dexter, T. M. (1983) Production of colony-stimulating factor in long-term bone marrow cultures. *Journal of Cell Physiology*, **114**, 88–92.

Small, D., Levenstein, M., Kim, E., Carow, C., Amin, S., Rockwell, P., Witte, L., Burrow, C., Ratajczak, M. Z., Gewirts, A. M. and Civin, C. I. (1994) STK-1, the human homolog of flk-2/flt-3, is selectively expressed in CD34+ human bone marrow cells and is involved in the proliferation of early progenitor/stem cells. *Proceedings of the National Academy of Sciences of the USA*, **91**, 459–63.

Sohma, Y., Akahori, H., Seki, N., Hori, T., Ogami, K., Kato, T., Shimada, Y., Kawamura, K. and Miyazaki, H. (1994) Molecular cloning and chromosomal localization of the human thrombopoietin gene. *FEBS Letters*, **353**, 57–61.

Stark, R., Andre, C., Thierry, D., Cherel, M., Galibert, F. and Gluckman, E. (1993) The expression of cytokine and cytokine receptor genes in long-term bone marrow culture in congenital and acquired marrow hypoplasias. *British Journal of Haematology*, **83**, 560–6.

Tahara, T., Usuki, K., Sato, H., Ohashi, H., Morita, H., Tsumura, H., Matsumoto, A., Miyazaki, H., Urabe, A. and Kato, T. (1996) A sensitive sandwich ELISA for measuring thrombopoietin in human serum: serum thrombopoietin levels in healthy volunteers and in patients with haematopoietic disorders. *British Journal of Haematology*, **93**, 783–8.

Tani, K., Ozawa, K., Ogura, H., Takahashi, S., Takahashi, K., Tsuruta, T., Okano, A., Akiyama, Y., Yoshikubo, T., Shimane, M. and Asano, H. (1993) The production of granulocyte colony-stimulating factor and interleukin-6 by human bone marrow stromal cells in aplastic anemia. *Tohoku Journal of Experimental Medicine*, **169**, 325–32.

Tsuji, K., Zsebo, K. M. and Ogawa, M. (1991) Enhancement of murine blast cell colony formation in culture by recombinant rat stem cell factor, ligand for c-kit. *Blood*, **78**, 1223–9.

Urabe, A., Mitani, K., Yoshinaga, K., Iki, S., Yagisawa, M., Ohbayashi, Y. and Takaku, F. (1992) Serum erythropoietin titers in haematological malignancies and related diseases. *International Journal of Cell Cloning*, **10**, 333–7.

Urabe, A., Mizoguchi, H., Takaku, A., Miyazaki, T., Yachi, A., Niitsu, Y., Miura, Y., Mutoh, Y.,

Fujioka, S., Nomura, T., Toyama, K., Kawato, M. and Kurokawa, K. (1993) Effects of recombinant human erythropoietin on aplastic anemia: Results of a phase II clinical study. *Japanese Journal of Clinical Hematology*, **34**, 1002–10.

Vadhan-Raj, S., Buescher, S., Broxmeyer, H. E., Le Maistre, A., Lepe-Zuniga, J. L., Ventura, G., Jeha, S., Horwitz, L. J., Trujilla, J. M., Gillis, S., Hitterlman, W. N. and Gutterman, J. V. (1988) Stimulation of myelopoiesis in patients with aplastic anemia by recombinant human granulocyte-macrophage colony-stimulating factor. *New England Journal of Medicine*, **139**, 1628–34.

Walsh, C. E., Liu, S. M., Anderson, S. M., Rossio, J. L., Nienhuis, A. W. and Young, N. S. (1992) A trial of recombinant human interleukin-1 in patients with severe refractory aplastic anemia. *British Journal of Haematology*, **80**, 106–10.

Watari, K., Asano, S., Shirafuji, N., Kodo, H., Ozawa, K., Takaku, F. and Kamachi, S. (1989) Serum granulocyte colony-stimulating factor levels in healthy volunteers and patients with various disorders as estimated by enzyme immunoassay. *Blood*, **73**, 117–22.

Wendling, F., Maraskovsky, E., Debili, N., Florindo, C., Teepe, M., Titeux, M., Methia, N., Breton-Gorius, J., Cosman, D. and Vainchenker, W. (1994) c-Mpl ligand is a humoral regulator of megakaryocytopoiesis. *Nature*, **369**, 571–4.

Williams, D. E., Elisenman, J., Baird, A., Rauch, C., van Ness, K., March, C. J., Park, L. S., Martin, U., Mochizuki, D. Y., Boswell, H. S., Burgess, G. S., Cosman, D. and Lyman, S. D. (1990) Identification of a ligand for the c-kit proto-oncogene. *Cell*, **63**, 167–74.

Wodnar-Filipowicz, A., Tichelli, A., Zsebo, K. M., Speck, B. and Nissen, C. (1992) Stem cell factor stimulates the in vitro growth of bone marrow cells from aplastic anemia patients. *Blood*, **79**, 3196–202.

Wodnar-Filipowicz, A., Yancik, S., Moser, Y., dalle Carbonare, V., Gratwohl, A., Tichelli, A., Speck, B. and Nissen, C. (1993) Levels of soluble stem cell factor in serum of patients with aplastic anemia. *Blood*, **81**, 3259–64.

Wodnar-Filipowicz, A., Lyman, S. D., Gratwohl, A., Tichelli, A., Speck, B. and Nissen, C. (1996) Flt-3 ligand level reflects hematopoietic progenitor cell function in aplastic anemia and chemotherapy-induced bone marrow aplasia. *Blood*, **88**, 4493–9.

Young, N. S. and Maciejewski, J. (1997) The pathophysiology of acquired aplastic anemia. *New England Journal of Medicine*, **336**, 1365–72.

Yen, Y. P., Zabala, P., Doney, K., Clemons, G., Gilis, S., Powell, J. S. and Adamson, J. W. (1985) Haematopoietic growth factors in human serum. Erythroid burst-promoting activity in normal subjects and in patients with severe aplastic anaemia. *Journal of Laboratory Clinical Medicine*, **106**, 384–92.

Zsebo, K. M., Williams, D. A., Geissler, E. N., Broudy, V. C., Martin, F. H., Atkins, H. L., Hsu, R-Y., Birkett, N. G., Okino, K. H., Murdock, D. C., Jacobsen, F. W., Langley, K. E., Smith, K. A., Takeishi, T., Cattunach, B. M., Galli, S. J. and Suggs, S. V. (1990) Stem cell factor is encoded at the SI locus of the mouse and is the ligand for the c-kit tryrosine kinase receptor. *Cell*, **63**, 213–24.

3

Role of T-lymphocytes in the pathophysiology of aplastic anemia

Shinji Nakao

Kanazawa University School of Medicine, Japan

Introduction

Although aplastic anemia (AA) is a syndrome of unknown etiology as defined by the clinical picture, a large body of evidence suggests that T-cells have an important role in its development (Nakao, 1997: 127; Young, 1994: 68; 1996: 55). High remission rates in recent clinical trials using a combination of immunosuppressive drugs such as antithymocyte globulin (ATG) and cyclosporin have strengthened the notion that AA is a T-cell disease rather than a stem-cell disease (Bacigalupo et al., 1995: 1348; Frickhofen et al., 1991: 1297; Rosenfeld et al., 1995: 3058). Understanding the immunological abnormalities in individual patients is important in choosing an appropriate therapy; although a >80% rate of response to immunosuppressive therapy is anticipated, some patients may need allogeneic stem-cell transplantation because of nonimmunological pathogenesis, such as drug toxicities or intrinsic stem-cell defects. Moreover, accumulation of patients' data obtained using classic or novel immunological methods would be useful in identifying the inciting events of AA that remain totally unknown.

Immunophenotyping data on T-cells and natural killer cells in bone marrow and peripheral blood

The immune response to foreign antigens or 'self' antigens is usually associated with changes in the T-cell subsets defined by immunophenotype. In AA, where certain antigens probably incite the immune attack against hemopoietic progenitor cells, an imbalance between different T-cell subpopulations in the bone marrow or peripheral blood has been suspected.

Table 3.1. CD4/CD8 ratio in lymphocytes of aplastic anemia patients

Reference	No. of cases	% of patients showing a ratio ≤1.0 in the peripheral blood	Mean ratio in the bone marrow
Zoumbos et al., 1984	28	53	Normal
Ruiz-Arguelles et al., 1984	31	26	Not tested
Falcao et al., 1985	18	17	Normal
Sabbe et al., 1984	53	2	Not tested
Maciejewski et al., 1994	33	Normal	Lower (<0.8) than normals

CD4$^+$ and CD8$^+$ T-cells

Table 3.1 summarizes the results of an investigation into changes in the CD4/CD8 ratio in T-cells of AA patients. Early studies have documented a decreased CD4/CD8 ratio in the peripheral blood of many AA patients (Falcao et al., 1985: 103; Ruiz-Arguelles et al., 1984: 267; Zoumbos et al., 1984: 95). This was mainly because of a reduction of CD4$^+$ cells. In some patients, particularly those with hepatitis-associated AA, virtually all peripheral blood T-cells were CD8$^+$ (Brown et al., 1997: 1059; Kojima et al., 1989: 147). A predominance of CD8$^+$ T-cells in the blood appears to be consistent with results of several studies, indicating that myelosuppressive T-cells generated in vitro or isolated from patients' peripheral blood are CD8$^+$ (Laver et al., 1988: 545; Nakao et al., 1984: 160; Teramura et al., 1997: 80). However, other studies have observed inverted CD4/CD8 ratios only in a minority of AA patients (Maciejewski et al., 1994: 1102; Sabbe et al., 1984: 178). The decrease may be more pronounced in the bone marrow than peripheral blood, although studies of biopsied specimens revealed that the CD4/CD8 ratios were close to 1.0 (Melenhorst et al., 1995: 477a). Since the CD4/CD8 ratios between the two T-cell subsets in AA patients generally vary widely, measuring its value has little role in characterizing the pathophysiology of an AA patient. A marked reduction of the ratio in the peripheral blood may indicate the presence of hepatitis that preceded the development of AA.

Activated T-cell subpopulation

In contrast to the variable nature of the change in the CD4/CD8 ratio in AA, it has repeatedly been shown that the peripheral and bone marrow lymphocytes contain proportionately more activated T-cells than is normal. A National Institutes of Health (NIH) group found for the first time that the ratio between CD4$^+$HLA-DR$^+$ cells and CD8$^+$HLA-DR$^+$ cells of peripheral blood significantly decreased in AA patients as compared with normal individuals (Zoumbos et al.,

1985*a*: 257). The same group recently reevaluated the activated CD8$^+$ T-cells in the peripheral blood and bone marrow, and found that the percentage of CD8$^+$DR$^+$ cells in the bone marrow was a more sensitive marker of the presence of an abnormal cellular immune response (Maciejewski et al., 1994: 1102). An increased proportion of activated CD8$^+$ lymphocytes in the bone marrow has been shown in AA patients responsive to immunosuppressive therapy by the other group (Nakao et al., 1992*a*: 2532). Thus, detection of an increased proportion of activated CD8$^+$ T-cells in the bone marrow appears to be useful in discriminating an immune-mediated marrow failure from a nonimmune-mediated one, as well as in predicting a response to immunosuppressive therapy.

T-cell receptor Vβ subfamily

A few studies have focused on the T-cell repertoire as defined by the expression of T-cell receptors. Melenhorst et al. (1997: 85) studied eight patients with AA for T-cell repertoire in the bone marrow and found no significant change in the usage of the T-cell receptor Vβ gene segment between patients and controls. Manz et al. (1997: 110) found overexpression of certain Vβ families such as Vβ3, Vβ20, Vβ21, and Vβ22 in the bone marrow of five of six AA patients as compared to normal samples. However, the enhanced Vβ species were different for each patient. Reverse dot-blot analysis of the T-cell receptor repertoire in the bone marrow of Japanese patients also failed to reveal biased usage of a certain Vβ gene common to AA patients (Nakao et al., 1996: 647a). It is thus suggested that the involvement of superantigens inducing selective expansion of T-cells that express certain Vβ subfamilies in the pathophysiology is unlikely.

Natural killer cells

The number of cells expressing CD56 with natural killer (NK) cell function in the peripheral blood and their activity are diminished in AA patients (Gascon et al., 1986: 1349). The immaturity of NK cells in AA patients may be related to the marked elevation of serum granulocyte colony-stimulating factor (G-CSF) levels in these patients; a recent study demonstrated that G-CSF inhibits differentiation of NK cells from their progenitor cells (Miller et al., 1997: 3098). However, the percentage of CD8$^-$CD56$^+$ cells in the peripheral blood of AA patients is not different from that of normal controls, while its percentage in the bone marrow of severe AA patients is rather higher than that of normal controls (Maciejewski et al., 1994: 1102). Although the myelosuppressive function of NK cells has been documented by several in vitro studies (Nagler and Greenberg, 1990: 171), the increase in the percentage of CD8$^-$CD56$^+$ cells in the bone marrow does not appear to represent a primary event leading to bone marrow failure, but rather reflects an ongoing autoimmune reaction in the bone marrow, as has been suggested by an increase in activated CD8$^+$ T-cells. Thus, the increased percentage of CD8$^-$CD56$^+$ cells in the bone marrow may be one of the markers of immune-mediated AA.

Markers of T-cell activation

Activation antigens

T-cells express a number of antigens upon activation. Expression of such activation antigens on T-cells of AA patients has been extensively studied since it may correlate with immune-pathophysiology in AA. In AA patients, the percentage of CD3$^+$CD25$^+$ T-cells in the peripheral blood lymphocytes is significantly increased as is that of CD8$^+$HLA-DR$^+$ T-cells (Zoumbos et al., 1985a: 257). The majority of patients with AA have elevated serum levels of the soluble form of the interleukin-2 (IL-2) receptor (Raghavachar et al., 1988: 240).

Cytokine production

Interferon-γ (IFN-γ), IL-2 and tumor necrosis factor (TNF) are overproduced by mononuclear cells from AA patients, both with lectin stimulation and spontaneously (Gascon et al., 1985: 407; Hinterberger et al., 1988: 266; 1989: 2713; Hsu et al., 1996: 31; Schultz and Shahidi, 1994: 32; Zoumbos et al., 1985b: 188). Analysis of T-cell lines or clones from AA patients has also revealed increased secretion of IFN-γ and TNF (Herrmann et al., 1986: 1629; Viale et al., 1991: 1268). To assess the cytokine-producing ability of patients' T-cells, all these studies utilized the culture of mononuclear cells which involves various artifacts; thus, it was difficult to accept that overproduction of cytokines is an unequivocal phenomenon (Schultz and Shahidi, 1994: 32). Detection of cytokine messenger ribonucleic acid (mRNA) using the polymerase chain reaction in freshly obtained bone marrow mononuclear cells resolved this issue. Two studies by different laboratories demonstrated constitutive expression of the IFN-γ gene in bone marrow mononuclear cells of AA patients, particularly of those responsive to immunosuppressive therapy (Figure 3.1) (Nakao et al., 1992a: 2532; Nistico and Young, 1994: 463). The aberrant IFN-γ gene expression of AA patients was not detected after successful immunosuppression. Levels of IFN-γ message were higher in marrow than in blood cells of AA patients, consistent with local activation of T-cells in the bone marrow.

Stress proteins

Lymphocytes of AA patients are presumed to be variously stressed, by exposure to inciting agents and to the resultant inflammatory cytokines. AA patients'

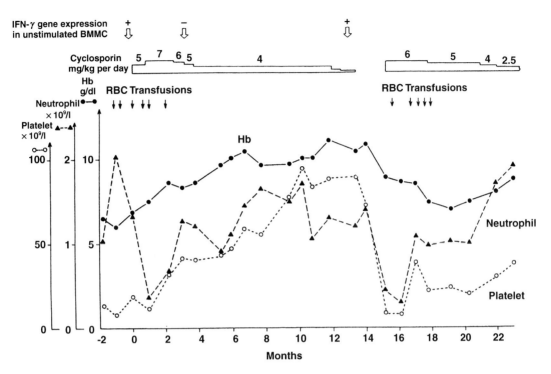

Figure 3.1. Hematological recovery and changes in interferon-γ (IFN-γ) gene expression in bone marrow mononuclear cells (BMMC) of an aplastic anemia (AA) patient following cyclosporin therapy. IFN-γ gene expression was detectable in BMMC of an AA patient before therapy. It was undetectable when the patient obtained remission after cyclosporin therapy and became detectable again in association with the relapse of pancytopenia after the cyclosporin dose was reduced.

lymphocytes express high levels of heat shock protein (HSP) 72 in the cytoplasm when they are incubated at 42°C for 30 min (Figure 3.2) (Takami et al., 1996: 436a). The percentage of HSP72-positive cells after heat treatment in AA patients is particularly high in those responsive to immunosuppressive therapy. Since HSP72 can be induced in the lymphocytes of normal individuals by activation with mitogen, the heat-inducible expression probably reflects an activated state of T-cells (Ferris et al., 1988: 3850).

Production of myelosuppressive cytokines by T-lymphocytes

Secretion of myelosuppressive cytokines by T-cells was first suggested by coculture studies using colony assays. Peripheral-blood and bone-marrow T-cells of AA patients diminish the number of colonies derived from committed hemopoietic progenitor cells when they are cultured with autologous and allogeneic bone marrow cells (Hoffmann et al., 1977: 10; Kagan et al., 1976: 2890; Takaku et al.,

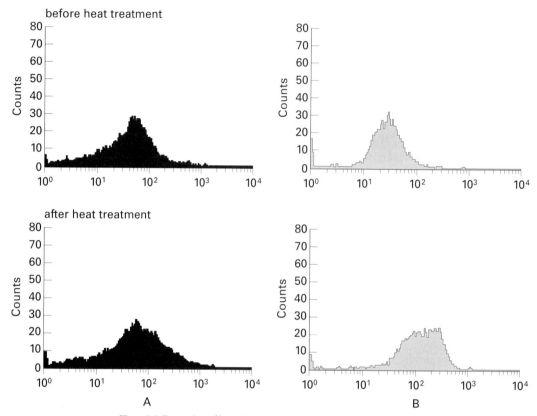

Figure 3.2. Expression of heat shock protein (HSP) 72 in peripheral blood mononuclear cells (PBMC) after heat treatment. PBMC before and after heat treatment were fixed in 4% paraformaldehyde-phosphate-buffered saline, permeabilized in 0.1% Triton X-100, and incubated with monoclonal antibodies to HSP72. A, Normal individual; B, an AA patient who later responded to cyclosporin therapy.

1980: 937). NIH studies identified the molecules responsible for the inhibition of colony formation to be IFN-γ, by demonstrating the abrogation of such inhibition with anti-IFN-γ antibodies (Zoumbos et al., 1985b: 257). This result has been challenged by several studies that failed to reveal a sufficient level of IFN-γ secreted from patients' T-cells for the inhibition of colony formation (Torok-Storb et al., 1987: 629). Growth of hemopoietic progenitor cells in a semisolid medium does not necessarily reflect in vivo hemopoiesis and sufficient levels of IFN-γ are rarely detectable in the bone marrow sera or plasma of AA patients (Schultz and Shahidi 1994: 32; Torok-Storb et al., 1987: 629). Thus, it is reasonable at least to state that IFN-γ is a major soluble factor capable of inhibiting hemopoietic progenitor growth in vitro, but the role of IFN-γ in in vivo myelosuppression of AA is not established.

Recently, the NIH group demonstrated that a very low level of IFN-γ continuously produced by IFN-γ-gene transfected stroma cells can markedly reduce the number of primitive hemopoietic progenitor cells using the long-term marrow culture system (Selleri et al., 1996: 4149). Thus, a low amount of IFN-γ secreted from activated T-cells in the bone marrow may play an active role in the diminution of hemopoietic progenitor cells in AA patients. The results of studies regarding overproduction of myelosuppressive cytokines are summarized in Table 3.2.

Reactivity of T-lymphocytes against hemopoietic progenitor cells

Evidence of the involvement of an antigen-driven response in the development of AA

Hemopoietic progenitor cells as a target of T-cell attack

Although most CD34$^+$ cells express an HLA-DR molecule, little is known about the antigen-presentation capacity of these cells. Recent reports using highly purified CD34$^+$ cells demonstrated that hemopoietic progenitor cells are capable of presenting a purified protein derivative of mycobacterium and alloantigens (van Rhee et al., 1997a: 362a; 1997b: 563a) to T-cells. Harris et al. (1996: 5104) purified peptides bound to HLA-DR of a hemopoietic cell line and identified several peptides derived from endogenous proteins. Thus, it is possible that hemopoietic progenitor cells may stimulate helper T-cells to respond to themselves through the recognition of 'self' peptides. On the other hand, a murine study using a graft-versus-host disease model demonstrated that a small number of CD4$^+$T-cells kill allogeneic hemopoietic stem cells through cell–cell contact, suggesting that hemopoietic progenitor cells expressing HLA-DR can be a target of cytotoxic lymphocytes (Sprent et al., 1994: 307).

Association of certain HLA alleles with a susceptibility to AA

Certain HLA alleles or haplotypes have been implicated in the susceptibility to various autoimmune diseases, such as rheumatoid arthritis and multiple sclerosis (Nishimura et al., 1992: 693). Although the mechanism underlying the association is not fully understood, one possible mechanism is that a human leukocyte antigen (HLA) molecule sensitive to a certain disease may be more likely to bind autoantigens or viral antigens that elicit an autoimmune reaction.

Based on clinical evidence suggesting an immune mechanism for the development of AA, the correlation of a certain type of HLA with the development of AA has been explored. Chapuis et al. (1986: 51) determined the HLA serotypes of 68 patients with AA and revealed an increased frequency of HLA-DR2 compared to a normal population in Switzerland. A survey of Japanese AA patients also

Table 3.2. Evidence of overproduction of myelosuppressive cytokines by lymphocytes of aplastic anemia patients

Assay	Material	Method	Marker	Result
Culture of hemopoietic progenitor cells	Patients' BM	T-cell depletion from BM	No. of colonies	↑
	Patients' BM	Addition of anti-IFN-γ antibodies	No. of colonies	↑*
	PBMC or BM from patients and BM from normal controls	Coculture	No. of colonies from normal BM	↓
Measurement of cytokines	PB or BM serum of patients	Bioassay and RIA	IFN-γ level	↑*
	Patients' PBMC or BMMC	Culture without stimuli	Production of IFN-γ and TNF-α	↑*
	Patients' PBMC	Culture with mitogens	Excessive production of IFN-γ, IL-2, TNF-α, and MIP-1α	↑
	Patients' BMMC	RT-PCR	Amplification of IFN-γ cDNA	+

Notes:

BM = bone marrow; BMMC = bone marrow mononuclear cells; IFN-γ interferon-γ; IL-2 = interleukin-2; MIP-1α = macrophage-inflammatory protein-1α; PB = peripheral blood; PBMC = peripheral-blood mononuclear cells; RIA = radioimmunoassay; RT-PCR = reverse transcriptase-polymerase chain reaction; TNF-α = tumor necrosis factor-α; ↑ = increase; ↓ = decrease; * = findings that cannot be reproduced by different groups.

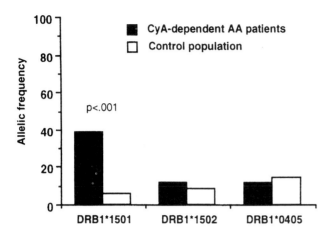

Figure 3.3. Frequency of HLA-DRB1 alleles in patients with cyclosporin-A-dependent AA and a Japanese general population. Frequencies of three HLA-DRB1 alleles that were found frequently in patients with cyclosporin-A-dependent AA were compared to those of a control Japanese population (Nakao, 1997: 127). CyA = cyclosporin.

showed that the frequency of HLA-DR2 (70%) in AA patients was significantly higher than that in the general Japanese population (35%) (Nakao et al., 1994*a*: 108). A recent study of AA patients in North America by Nimer et al. (1994: 923) confirmed the same trend. Thus, it is possible that the hemopoietic system of individuals possessing HLA-DR2 may be vulnerable to primary immune attacks or secondary attacks following exposure to some antigens such as infection. The high rates of response to immunosuppressive therapy shown in the limited numbers of patients with AA are consistent with this hypothesis (Ihan et al., 1997: 291; Nakao et al., 1992*b*: 239; Ragman et al., 1990: 545). However, the study of AA patients in North America failed to reveal a significant correlation between the response to ATG and the presentation of HLA-DR2 (Nimer et al., 1994: 923). Hence, the significance of HLA-DR2 in the immune mechanisms of AA remains unclear.

HLA-DR2 is subdivided into HLA-DR15 and HLA-DR16. These serotypes are further divided into three genotypes including DRB1*1501, DRB1*1502, and DRB1*1602 in the Japanese population. When DRB1 alleles of 13 patients with cyclosporin-A-dependent AA were determined, DRB1*1501, DRB1*1502, and DRB1*0405 were frequently found. Figure 3.3 compares the frequency of these three DRB1 alleles between patients with cyclosporin-A-dependent AA and a general Japanese population. The frequency of DRB1*1501 in the patients was significantly higher than that of the normal control, while those of the other two alleles were comparable between the two groups (Nakao et al., 1994*b*: 4257). Thus, among the alleles that determine HLA-DR2, only DRB1*1501 is thought to be associated with a susceptibility to immune-mediated AA. DRB1*1501 is linked to DQA1*0102-DQB1*0602 in most Japanese because of linkage disequilibrium. It is therefore possible that HLA class II alleles other than DRB1*1501 may actually be responsible for susceptibility to immune-mediated AA.

Table 3.3. Two variants of aplastic anemia (AA)

	HLA allele associated with a susceptibility	T-cell phenotype related to pathophysiology	Clonal predominance in certain Vβ^+ T-cell subfamilies
Cyclosporin-A-dependent AA	HLA-DRB1*1501	Presence of CD4$^+$ T-cells to autologous hemopoietic cells in the bone marrow	+
Hepatitis-associated AA	HLA-B8	Increased percentage of CD8$^+$ T-cells in the peripheral blood	?

Another subgroup of AA, characterized by an HLA antigen and a good response to immunosuppressive therapy, is hepatitis-associated AA. Brown and Young (1997: 439a) found that the presentation of HLA-B8 was much more common in hepatitis-associated AA patients than in the control population in the USA. The association with a certain HLA-B antigen appears to be consistent with the markedly increased percentage of activated CD8$^+$ cells in the peripheral blood of the patients with hepatitis-associated AA (Brown et al., 1997: 1059; Kojima et al., 1989: 147). Table 3.3 summarizes the characteristics of two variants of AA.

Clonal predominance in T-cell subsets defined by T-cell receptor Vβ expression

To clarify the immunological events that precede the destruction of hemopoietic cells, it is important to determine whether an antigen-driven response is involved in the development of bone marrow failure. Several studies explored this point by analyzing clonal rearrangement of the T-cell receptor Vβ gene. Earlier studies demonstrated clonal expansion of a limited number of T-cells with several Vβ families in the bone marrow of AA patients responsive to cyclosporin (Figure 3.4) (Nakao et al., 1996: 647a; Takamatsu et al., 1994: 9a). Melenhorst et al. (1997: 85) also detected clonal predominance in several Vβ families of three out of seven patients with AA, although the presence of clonal predominance did not correlate with the response to immunosuppressive therapy. Manz et al. (1997: 110) determined the complementarity-determining region (CDR3) size variability of T-cells in the bone marrow of five patients and detected subtle abnormalities only in one to two Vβ families of every patient. The discrepancies among these studies may be caused by the heterogeneity of clinical backgrounds of the analyzed patients. Restricting a study population to a subset of patients based on response to immunosuppressive therapy and HLA appears to be important in understanding the role of an antigen-driven T-cell response in the pathophysiology of AA.

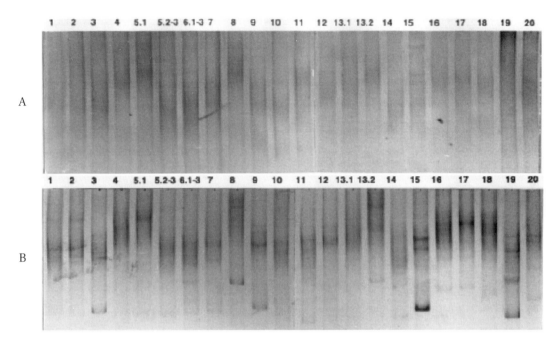

Figure 3.4. Single-strand conformation polymorphism (SSCP) analysis of the amplified products of T-cell receptor (TCR) Vβ cDNA derived from the bone marrow of a normal individual and a patient with CyA-dependent AA. Amplified products of TCRVβ cDNA were denatured in the formamide solution and electrophoresed in 8% polyacrylamide gel. The SSCP of each Vβ cDNA was visualized by silver staining. A, a normal individual; B, a patient with CyA-dependent AA.

Establishment of a T-cell clone reactive to hemopoietic cells from AA patients

Isolating T-cell lines or T-cell clones that specifically recognize autologous hemopoietic progenitor cells would provide direct evidence for the involvement of T-cells in the pathogenesis of AA. Several T-cell clones capable of inhibiting in vitro hemopoiesis have been isolated from patients with AA. Moebius et al. (1991: 1567) found that a CD4$^+$CD8$^+$ T-cell clone isolated from the peripheral blood of a patient with AA lysed autologous and allogeneic lymphoblastic cell lines (LCLs) in an HLA-DP-restricted fashion and inhibited the growth of hemopoietic progenitor cells. In this study, the cytotoxicity of the CD4$^+$CD8$^+$ T-cell clone was not restricted by a certain HLA-DP allele and the inhibition of hemopoietic progenitor cells was nonspecific. A CD4$^+$VB17$^+$ T-cell clone that was isolated from a cyclosporin-A-dependent AA patient with HLA-DRB1*1501 in a previous study secreted IFN-γ in response to autologous CD34$^+$ cells and inhibited the growth of hemopoietic progenitor cells from CD34$^+$ cells (Nakao

Figure 3.5. Effect of NT4.2 on CFU-GM-derived colony formation by allogeneic CD34+ cells. CD34+ cells ($n = 3 \times 10^3$) from three normal individuals (A, B, C) cultured in the presence of colony-stimulating factors were incubated in medium alone with 3×10^4 cloned T-cells for 4 h and then mixed with methylcellulose medium supplemented with growth factors. Some CD34+ cells were mixed with cloned T-cells just before methylcellulose medium was added. HLA-DRB1 alleles of each individual are shown in parentheses (Nakao 1997: 127).

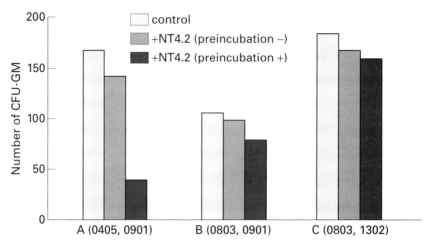

et al., 1995: 433). However, since only a limited number of autologous CD34+ cells were available as target cells, restriction of the inhibition by an HLA allele could not be examined.

A CD4+Vβ21+ T-cell clone (NT4.2) was recently isolated from the bone marrow of an untransfused patient with cyclosporin-A-dependent AA whose HLA-DRB1 alleles included DRB1*1501 and DRB1*0405 (Nakao et al., 1997: 3691). NT4.2 proliferated most dominantly among Vβ21+ T-cells in the bone marrow of the patient as demonstrated by the single-strand conformation polymorphism analysis. This T-cell clone showed potent cytotoxicity against autologous and allogeneic LCL cells as well as against CD34+ cells cultured for 1 week in the presence of colony-stimulating factors in an HLA-DRB1*0405–dependent fashion. Figure 3.5 illustrates the effect of NT4.2 on in vitro growth of allogeneic hemopoietic progenitor cells. Inhibition of myeloid colony formation by allogeneic CD34+ cells by NT4.2 was dependent on cell–cell contact and was restricted to those possessing HLA-DRB1*0405. Thus, these data indicate that the T-cell clone kills autologous hemopoietic cells by recognizing a physiological peptide presented by HLA-DR4. Collectively, there appear to be autoreactive T-cells recognizing antigens on hemopoietic cells in the bone marrow of patients with cyclosporin-A-dependent AA.

Conclusion

Studies on immunological abnormalities in AA that arose from nonspecific findings, such as overproduction of myelosuppressive cytokines by T-cells and T-cell activation, have developed into those involving antigen-specific T-cells that are potentially pathogenic in AA. Further studies on the target molecules of such pathogenic T-cells will help to identify the events that induce AA.

References

Bacigalupo, A., Broccia, G., Corda, G., Arcese, W., Carotenuto, M., Gallamini, A., Locatelli, F., Mori, P. G., Saracco, P., Todeschini, G., Cosar, P., Iacopino, P., van Lint, M. T., Gluckman, E. for the European Group for Blood and Marrow Transplantation (EBMT) Working Party on SAA (1995) Antilymphocyte globulin, cyclosporin, and granulocyte colony-stimulating factor in patients with acquired severe aplastic anemia (SAA): a pilot study of the EBMT SAA Working Party. *Blood*, **85**, 1348–53.

Brown, K. E. and Young, N. S. (1997) HLA antigens in patients with severe aplastic anemia (SAA) and hepatitis associated aplastic anemia. *Blood*, **90**, 439a.

Brown, K. E., Tisdale, J., Barrett, A. J., Dunbar, C. E. and Young, N. S. (1997) Hepatitis-associated aplastic anemia. *New England Journal of Medicine*, **336**, 1059–64.

Chapuis, B., Von Fliedner, V. E., Jeannet, M., Merica, H., Vuagnat, P., Gratwohl, A., Nissen, C. and Speck, B. (1986) Increased frequency of DR2 in patients with aplastic anemia and increased DR sharing in their parents. *British Journal of Hematology*, **63**, 51–7.

Falcao, R. P., Voltarelli, J. C. and Bottura, C. (1985) T-lymphocyte subpopulations in the peripheral blood and bone marrow of patients with aplastic anemia. *British Journal of Hematology*, **50**, 103–7.

Ferris, D. K., Harel Bellan, A., Morimoto, R. I., Welch, W. J. and Farrar, W. L. (1988) Mitogen and lymphokine stimulation of heat shock proteins in T lymphocytes. *Proceedings of the National Academy of Sciences of the USA*, **85**, 3850–4.

Frickhofen, N., Kaltwasser, J. P., Schrezenmeier, H., Raghavachar, A., Vogt, H. G., Herrmann, F., Freund, M., Meusers, P., Salama, A. and Heimpel, H. (1991) Treatment of aplastic anemia with antilymphocyte globulin and methylprednisolone with or without cyclosporine. The German Aplastic Anemia Study Group. *New England Journal of Medicine*, **324**, 1297–304.

Gascon, P., Zoumbos, N. C., Scala, G., Djeu, J. Y., Moore, J. G. and Young, N. S. (1985) Lymphokine abnormalities in aplastic anemia: implications for the mechanism of action of antithymocyte globulin. *Blood*, **65**, 407–13.

Gascon, P., Zoumbos, N. and Young, N. (1986) Analysis of natural killer cells in patients with aplastic anemia. *Blood*, **67**, 1349–55.

Harris, P. E., Maffei, A., Colovai, A. I., Kinne, J., Tugulea, S. and Suciu, F. N. (1996) Predominant HLA-class II bound self-peptides of a hematopoietic progenitor cell line are derived from intracellular proteins. *Blood*, **87**, 5104–12.

Herrmann, F., Griffin, J. D., Meuer, S. G. and Zum Buschenfelde, K. M. (1986) Establishment of an interleukin 2-dependent T cell line derived from a patient with severe aplastic anemia, which inhibits *in vitro* hematopoiesis. *Journal of Immunology*, **136**, 1629–34.

Hinterberger, W., Adolf, G., Huber, C. H., Koller, U., Dudczak, R., Knapp, W., Kalhs, P., Geissler, K., Lechner, K. and Volc-Platzer, B. (1988) Further evidence for lymphokine overproduction in severe aplastic anemia. *Blood*, **72**, 266–72.

Hinterberger, W., Adolf, G., Bettelheim, P., Geissler, K., Huber, C., Irschick, E., Kalhs, P., Koller, U., Lechner, K., Meister, B. and Woloszczuk, W. (1989) Lymphokine overproduction in severe aplastic anemia is not related to blood transfusions. *Blood*, **74**, 2713–17.

Hoffmann, R., Zanjani, E., Lutton, J. D., Zalusky, R. and Wasserman, L. R. (1977) Suppression of erythrocyte-colony formation by lymphocytes from patients with aplastic anemia. *New England Journal of Medicine*, **296**, 10–13.

Hsu, H. C., Tsai, W. H., Chen, L. Y., Hsu, M. L., Ing Tiau, K. B., Ho, C. H., Lin, C. K. and Wang, S. Y. (1996) Production of hematopoietic regulatory cytokines by peripheral blood mononuclear cells in patients with aplastic anemia. *Experimental Hematology*, **24**, 31–6.

Ihan, O., Beksac, M., Arslan, O., Ozcan, M., Koc, H., Akan, H., Gurman, G., Konuk, N. and Uysal, A. (1997) HLA DR2: a predictive marker in response to cyclosporin therapy in aplastic anemia. *International Journal of Hematology*, **66**, 291–5.

Kagan, W. A., Ascensao, J. A., Pahwa, R. N. et al. (1976) Aplastic anemia: presence in human bone marrow of cells that suppress myelopoiesis. *Proceedings of the National Academy of Sciences of the USA*, **73**, 2890–4.

Kojima, S., Matsuyama, K., Kodera, Y. and Okada, J. (1989) Circulating activated suppressor T lymphocytes in hepatitis-associated aplastic anaemia. *British Journal of Hematology*, **71**, 147–51.

Laver, J., Castro, M. H., Kernan, N. A., Levick, J., Evans, R. L., O'Reilly, R. J. and Moore, M. A. (1988) In vitro interferon-gamma production by cultured T-cells in severe aplastic anaemia: correlation with granulomonopoietic inhibition in patients who respond to anti-thymocyte globulin. *British Journal of Hematology*, **69**, 545–50.

Maciejewski, J. P., Hibbs, J. R., Anderson, S., Katevas, P. and Young, N. S. (1994) Bone marrow and peripheral blood lymphocyte phenotype in patients with bone marrow failure. *Experimental Hematology*, **22**, 1102–10.

Manz, C. Y., Dietrich, P. Y., Schnuriger, V., Nissen, C. and Wodnar-Filipowicz, A. (1997) T-cell receptor beta chain variability in bone marrow and peripheral blood in severe acquired aplastic anemia. *Blood Cells, Molecules, and Diseases*, **23**, 110–22.

Melenhorst, I. J., van Kreiken, J. H. J. M., Dreef, E., Landegent, J. E., Willemze, R. and Fibbe, W. E. (1995) T-cell infiltration in bone marrow areas of residual hematopoiesis of patients with aplastic anemia. *Blood*, **86**, 477a.

Melenhorst, J. J., Fibbe, W. E., Struyk, L., van der Elsen, P. J., Willemze, R. and Landegent, J. E. (1997) Analysis of T-cell clonality in bone marrow of patients with acquired aplastic anaemia. *British Journal of Hematology*, **96**, 85–91.

Miller, J. S., Prosper, F. and McCullar, V. (1997) Natural killer (NK) cells are functionally abnormal and NK cell progenitors are diminished in granulocyte colony-stimulating factor-mobilized peripheral blood progenitor cell collections. *Blood*, **90**, 3098–105.

Moebius, U., Herrmann, F., Hercend, T. and Meuer, S. C. (1991) Clonal analysis of CD4+/CD8+ T cells in a patient with aplastic anemia. *Journal of Clinical Investigation*, **87**, 1567–74.

Nagler, A. and Greenberg, P. L. (1990) Bone marrow cell modulation and inhibition of myelopoiesis by large granular lymphocytes and natural killer cells. *International Journal of Cell Cloning*, **8**, 171–83.

Nakao, S. (1997) Immune mechanism of aplastic anemia. *International Journal of Hematology*, **66**, 127–34.

Nakao, S., Harada, M., Kondo, K., Odaka, K., Ueda, M., Matsue, K., Mori, T. and Hattori, K. (1984) Effect of activated lymphocytes on the regulation of hematopoiesis: suppression of *in vitro* granulopoiesis by OKT8+Ia+T cells induced by alloantigen stimulation. *Journal of Immunology*, **132**, 160–4.

Nakao, S., Yamaguchi, M., Shiobara, S., Yokoi, T., Miyawaki, T., Taniguchi, T. and Matsuda, T. (1992*a*) Interferon-gamma gene expression in unstimulated bone marrow mononuclear cells predicts a good response to cyclosporin therapy in aplastic anemia. *Blood*, **79**, 2532–5.

Nakao, S., Yamaguchi, M., Yasue, S., Shiobara, S., Saito, M. and Matsuda, T. (1992*b*) HLA-DR2 predicts a favorable response to cyclosporine therapy in patients with bone marrow failure. *American Journal of Hematology*, **40**, 239–40.

Nakao, S., Takamatsu, H., Chuhjo, T. and Matsuda, T. (1994*a*) HLA-DRB1 alleles of patients with aplastic anemia and response to immunosuppressive therapy. In *Annual Reports by Intractable Hemopoietic Disease Research Group*, pp. 108–9. Tokyo: Ministry of Health and Welfare of Japan.

Nakao, S., Takamatsu, H., Chuhjo, T., Ueda, M., Shiobara, S., Matsuda, T., Kaneshige, T. and Mizoguchi, H. (1994*b*) Identification of a specific HLA class II haplotype strongly associated with susceptibility to cyclosporin-dependent aplastic anemia. *Blood*, **84**, 4257–61.

Nakao, S., Takamatsu, H., Yachie, A., Itoh, T., Yamaguchi, M., Ueda, M., Shiobara, S. and Matsuda, T. (1995) Establishment of a CD4 + T cell clone recognizing autologous hematopoietic progenitor cells from a patient with immune-mediated aplastic anemia. *Experimental Hematology*, **23**, 433–8.

Nakao, S., Zeng, W. H., Takamatsu, H., Takami, A., Kondo, Y., Miura, Y., Yamazaki, H., Chuhjo, T., Shiobara, S., Yoshioka, T., Kaneshige, T. and Matsuda, T. (1996) $V\beta15^+$ T cells with a similar clonotype dominantly proliferate in the bone marrow of aplastic anemia patients with HLA-DRB1*1501 responsive to cyclosporine therapy. *Blood*, **88**, 647a.

Nakao, S., Takami, A., Takamatsu, H., Zeng, W., Sugimori, N., Yamazaki, H., Miura, Y., Ueda, M., Shiobara, S., Yoshioka, T., Kaneshige, T., Yasukawa, M. and Matsuda, T. (1997) Isolation of a T-cell clone showing HLA-DRB1*0405-restricted cytotoxicity for hematopoietic cells in a patient with aplastic anemia. *Blood*, **89**, 3691–9.

Nimer, S. D., Ireland, P., Meshikinpour, A. P. and Frane, M. (1994) An increased HLA DR2 frequency is seen in aplastic anemia patients. *Blood*, **84**, 923–7.

Nishimura, Y., Thorsby, E., Rønningen, K. S., Nelson, L. J., Hansen, J. A., Bias, W. B., Fauchet, R., Dawkins, R. L., TIllikainen, A., Salvaneschi, L., Martinetti, M., Cuccia, M., Vaughan, R. W., Hall, M., Boehm, B. O., Juji, T., Ohno, S., Farid, N. R., Bodmer, J. G., Skamene, E., Marsh, D. G., Svejgaard, A., Thomsen, A. C. and Sasazuki, T. (1992) General organization and overview of the disease component. In *HLA 1991 Proceedings of the 11th International Histocompatibility Workshop*, ed. K. Tsuji, M. Aizawa, T. Sasazuki, pp. 693–700. London: Oxford University Press.

Nistico, A., Young, N. S. (1994) Gamma-interferon gene expression in the bone marrow of patients with aplastic anemia. *Annals of Internal Medicine*, **120**, 463–9.

Raghavachar, A., Frickhofen, N., Taniguchi, Y., Young, N. S. and Heimpel, H. (1988) Soluble interleukin-2 receptors and CD8 like molecules in the sera of patients with aplastic anemia [abstract]. *Blut*, **57**, 240.

Ragman, F. P., Ashby, D. and Davies, J. M. (1990) Does HLA-DR predict response to specific immunosuppressive therapy in aplastic anemia? *British Journal of Hematology*, **74**, 545.

Rosenfeld, S. J., Kimball, J., Vining, D. and Young, N. S. (1995) Intensive immunosuppression with antithymocyte globulin and cyclosporin as treatment for severe acquired aplastic anemia. *Blood*, **85**, 3058–65.

Ruiz-Arguelles. G. J., Katzmann, J. A., Greipp, P. R., Marin, L. A., Gonzalez, L. J. and Cano, C. R. (1984) Lymphocyte subsets in patients with aplastic anemia. *American Journal of Hematology*, **16**, 267–75.

Sabbe, L. J. M., Haak, H. L., Te Velde, J., Bradley, B. A., de Bode, L., Blom, J. and van Rood, J. J. (1984) Immunological investigations in aplastic anemia patients. *Acta Hematologica*, **71**, 178–88.

Schultz, J. C. and Shahidi, N. T. (1994) Detection of tumor necrosis factor-alpha in bone marrow plasma and peripheral blood plasma from patients with aplastic anemia. *American Journal of Hematology*, **45**, 32–8.

Selleri, C., Maciejewski, J. P., Sato, T. and Young, N. S. (1996) Interferon-gamma constitutively expressed in the stromal microenvironment of human marrow cultures mediates potent hematopoietic inhibition. *Blood*, **87**, 4149–57.

Sprent, J., Surh, C. D., Agus, D., Hurd, M., Sutton, S. and Heath, W. R. (1994) Profound atrophy of the bone marrow reflecting major histocompatibility complex class II-restricted destruction of stem cells by CD4+ cells. *Journal of Experimental Medicine*, **180**, 307–17.

Takaku, F., Suda, T., Mizoguchi, H., Miura, Y., Uchino, H., Nagai, K., Kariyone, S., Shibata, A., Akabane, T., Nomura, T. and Maekawa, T. (1980) Effect of peripheral blood mononuclear cells from aplastic anemia patients on the granulocyte-macrophage and erythroid colony formation in samples from normal human bone marrow *in vitro* – a cooperative work. *Blood*, **55**, 937–43.

Takamatsu, H., Nakao, S., Yamaguchi, M., Itoh, T., Chuhjo, T., Shiobara, S. and Matsuda, T. (1994) Analysis of the T-cell clonotype in the bone marrow of immune-mediated aplastic anemia: identification of a T-cell clone that preferentially proliferates in the bone marrow of a cyclosporin-dependent aplastic anemia patient. *Blood (Supplement)*, **84**, 9a.

Takami, A., Nakao, S., Zeng, W., Sugimori, N., Yamazaki, H., Shiobara, S. and Matsuda, T. (1996) Heat shock protein 70 (HSP 70) is inducible in peripheral blood lymphocytes in aplastic anemia patients responsive to cyclosporin therapy. *Blood (Supplement)*, **88**, 436a.

Teramura, M., Kobayashi, S., Iwabe, K., Yoshinaga, K. and Mizoguchi, H. (1997) Mechanism of action of antithymocyte globulin in the treatment of aplastic anaemia: in vitro evidence for the presence of immunosuppressive mechanism. *British Journal of Hematology*, **96**, 80–4.

Torok-Storb, B., Johnson, G. G., Bowden, R. and Storb, R. (1987) Gamma-interferon in aplastic anemia: inability to detect significant levels in sera or demonstrate hematopoietic suppressing activity. *Blood*, **69**, 629–33.

van Rhee, F., Jiang, Y. Z., Vigue, F., Kirby, M., Raptis, A., Hensel, N., Agarwala, V., Read, E. J. and Barrett, A. J. (1997a) Granulocyte colony-stimulating-factor (G-CSF) mobilized CD34+ cells process and present exogenous antigen to T-cells. *Blood (Supplement)*, **90**, 362a.

van Rhee, F., Jiang, Y. Z., Vigue, F., Carter, C., Raptis, A., Read, E. J. and Barrett, A. J. (1997b) Highly purified CD34+ cells induce primary and secondary immune responses despite lack of expression of co-stimulatory molecules on resting cells. *Blood (Supplement)*, **90**, 563a.

Viale, M., Merli, A. and Bacigalupo, A. (1991) Analysis at the clonal level of T-cell phenotype and function in severe aplastic anemia patients. *Blood*, **78**, 1268–74.

Young, N. S. (1994) Pathophysiology II: immune suppression of hematopoiesis. In *Aplastic anemia acquired and inherited*, ed. N. S. Young and B. P. Alter, pp. 68–99. Philadelphia: W. B. Sanders.

Young, N. S. (1996) Immune pathophysiology of acquired aplastic anaemia. *European Journal of Hematology (Supplement)*, **60**, 55–9.

Zoumbos, N. C., Ferris, W. O., Hsu, S. M., Goodman, S., Griffith, P., Sharrow, S. O., Humphries, R. K., Nienhuis, A. W. and Young, N. (1984) Analysis of lymphocyte subsets in patients with aplastic anaemia. *British Journal of Hematology*, **58**, 95–105.

Zoumbos, N. C., Gascon, P., Djeu, J. Y., Trost, S. R. and Young, N. S. (1985*a*) Circulating activated suppressor T lymphocytes in aplastic anemia. *New England Journal of Medicine*, **312**, 257–65.

Zoumbos, N. C., Gascon, P., Djeu, J. Y. and Young, N. S. (1985*b*) Interferon is a mediator of hematopoietic suppression in aplastic anemia *in vitro* and possibly *in vivo*. *Proceedings of the National Academy of Sciences of the USA*, **82**, 188–92.

4

Role of apoptosis in the pathophysiology of aplastic anemia

Frances M. Gibson, N. J. Philpott,
Judith C. W. Marsh and E. C. Gordon-Smith

St George's Hospital Medical School, London

Introduction

Apoptosis is the term coined for the morphologically distinct form of cell death that occurs under primarily physiological conditions (Kerr et al., 1972). Dysregulation of apoptosis (increased or decreased) is believed to be involved in the pathogenesis of a number of diverse disease states, including malignancy (Vaux, 1993; Williams, 1991), acquired immunodeficiency syndrome (AIDS) (Amieson, 1992; Amiesen and Capron, 1991; Martin, 1993) and neurodegenerative disorders, such as Alzheimer's disease and Parkinson's disease (Carson and Ribeiro, 1993; Loo et al., 1993). In multicellular organisms, the rate of cell death must be as tightly controlled as the rate of proliferation and differentiation. Apoptosis is the morphological term to describe cell death as a consequence of a signal from within the cell itself, and is important in embryogenesis (Lockshin et al., 1991), in aging (Newman et al., 1982) and for eliminating cells that are potentially harmful to the whole organism; for example, virally infected, autoreactive or damaged cells (Martin and Green, 1995). In mammalian systems, apoptosis is also readily observed after a number of pathological insults such as cytotoxic drugs or irradiation.

Apoptosis is a critical process in the regulation of cellular proliferation and differentiation. The majority of cells depend on the presence of specific survival factors to inhibit apoptosis; competition for these survival factors ensures a balance between cell division and cell death within a tissue, organ or organism. Apoptosis is particularly important in the hemopoietic system where the extensive cell turnover requires stringent control; expansion and proliferation are continually balanced by apoptosis. Withdrawal of survival factors leads to apoptosis of progenitor cells (Williams et al., 1990).

Features of apoptotic cells

The most striking morphological feature of an apoptotic cell, viewed by light or electron microscopy, is the condensation and aggregation of the nuclear chromatin into dense masses under the nuclear membrane. This must be contrasted with the appearance of necrotic cells, whose hallmarks are swelling of the nucleus and organelles, rupture of the plasma membrane, release of cellular contents, and therefore induction of an inflammatory reaction including chemotaxis of neutrophils. One of the earliest features of apoptosis is the rounding up of the cell, so that it isolates itself from neighboring cells and loses surface projections such as microvilli. The cytoplasm condenses, the cell shrinks and the surface membrane becomes irregular, with the formation of 'blebs'. The nucleus, meanwhile, fragments into several discrete portions and, finally, the whole cell fragments into apoptotic bodies. In vivo, the whole process is rapid and specific membrane changes signal the apoptotic state of the cell, which is then engulfed by phagocytes, without generation of any inflammatory reaction. The chromatin condensation is a consequence of deoxyribonucleic acid (DNA) cleavage, initially into fragments of 300 and/or 50 base pairs (bp) (Brown et al., 1993), followed by more complete digestion to 180- to 200-bp multimers, the hallmark of apoptosis, which can be visualized as the DNA ladder on agarose gel electrophoresis (Cohen and Duke, 1984; Duke et al., 1983; Wyllie, 1980). The identity of the endonucleases responsible for this DNA cleavage remains controversial; however, a number of enzymes are involved and the nature of the enzyme activated probably depends on the cell type undergoing apoptosis.

Control of apoptosis

Apoptosis can be triggered by exogenous factors, such as drugs and irradiation, by intrinsic cellular mechanisms, such as cytotoxic T-cell killing through the Fas system or the granzyme/perforin system, or by changes in the cell's environment, such as growth factor [for example, granulocyte/macrophage colony-stimulating factor (GM-CSF), interleukin-3 (IL-3) or erythropoietin (EPO)] (Koury and Bondurant, 1990; Rodriguez-Tarduchy et al., 1990) or hormone withdrawal. The extent to which such diverse signals share intracellular transduction pathways is unknown. However, certain features are common to many systems and hence are likely to be fundamentally important. Many new genes have been identified that either negatively or positively influence apoptosis.

Alterations in the cell membrane bring new molecules, such as phosphatidylserine (Fadok et al., 1992; Martin et al., 1995), to the cell surface, causing the cell to be phagocytosed by macrophages, without inflammation. Ca^{2+}-dependent enzymes are activated, including endonucleases, calpain (a protease) and transglutaminase. These three act to degrade DNA, disrupt the cytoskeleton and crosslink cytoplasmic proteins, respectively, resulting in DNA fragmentation, cell shrinkage and the formation of apoptotic bodies (Carson and Ribeiro, 1993).

The *bcl-2* oncogene, first identified in the t(14;18) chromosomal translocation characteristic of follicular lymphoma, can be thought of as a generalized cell death suppresser gene, which directly regulates apoptosis in normal cells. All hemopoietic and lymphoid cells, many epithelial cells and neurones contain *bcl-2* protein, localized mainly in the mitochondrial membrane, the nuclear envelope and the endoplasmic reticulum. The mechanism of *bcl-2*-mediated inhibition is unknown. Cells which overexpress *bcl-2* survive longer in culture after growth factor deprivation (Collins et al., 1992; Vaux et al., 1988) and are resistant both to irradiation and to glucocorticoids. High concentrations of *bcl-2* also inhibit apoptosis induced by c-*myc* (Bissonette et al., 1992). The *bcl-2* family is now known to include other proteins which regulate the function of *bcl-2*, such as *bcl-x*$_L$, *bcl-x*$_S$ and *bax*.

Studies of the nematode, *Caenorhabditis elegans*, have identified three intracellular enzymes crucial in apoptosis, Ced-3, Ced-4 and Ced-9. Ced-3 is homologous to the human interleukin-1β converting enzyme (ICE) (Yuan et al., 1993) and Ced-9 to Bcl-2. ICE is probably one representative of a family of proteases, important in transmitting the surface apoptotic signal to the nucleus, by the activation of other enzymes; the process may involve a cascade of enzyme signals within the cell. Several ICE-like proteases have been identified.

Other genes that direct apoptosis include the *p53* tumor suppresser gene which induces apoptosis and mediates the response of hemopoietic cells to survival factors (White, 1996), and c-*myc* which stimulates apoptosis or proliferation if apoptosis is inhibited (Evan et al., 1992).

Apoptosis: role in immune regulation

The most important functions of the mammalian immune system are to eliminate damaged or foreign cells, to reduce the risk of transformation and to rid the system of infected cells. It has now been shown that, in many instances, cytotoxic T-cells accomplish this by stimulating apoptosis in the target cell in two ways. First, in a secretory pathway, granules containing perforin and granzyme are released by the cell and enter the target cell through pores produced by perforin; and, second, in a ligand-induced pathway, by activating a cell surface antigen named Fas (CD95), expressed by the target cell. Fas, also known as Apo-1, is a member of the tumor necrosis factor (TNF) receptor superfamily and can induce apoptosis when crosslinked, either naturally by its ligand (Fas-L) or in vitro by anti-Fas-antibody (Nagata, 1994). Fas is widely expressed; the highest levels are seen in activated T-cells, whilst Fas-L is expressed only by cytotoxic T-cells and in the testes, the small intestine and the lung. Soluble forms of Fas and Fas-L have also been identified. Defective forms of Fas and Fas-L have been identified in two abnormal strains of mice, caused by mutations in the respective genes: *lpr* mice have no functioning Fas and *gld* mice lack Fas-L. These mice suffer massive lymphoproliferation and autoimmune abnormalities, similar to systemic lupus erythematosus, indicating the vital function of the Fas system in eliminating abnormal or autoreactive lymphocytes. Fas-L not only damages Fas-positive cells and tissues, it also plays a role in the concept of immune privilege and protects tissues from immune assault. Conversely, Fas-L has recently been shown to promote inflammation as opposed to apoptosis (Green and Ware, 1997). Although it is not known what determines the choice between the inhibition or promotion of inflammation, other factors such as chemokine or cytokine release are probably involved.

Cells treated with anti-Fas antibody die by apoptosis within 6 h, providing that they express Fas (Itoh et al., 1991). In vivo, anti-Fas antibody kills wild-type but not *lpr* mice within 6 h; the mechanism of death appears to be massive hepatic injury. The speed of cell death implies that the signal mediated by the Fas system is rapidly transduced, although this is variable in nonlymphoid systems. The intracellular portion of Fas has an area of homology with other members of the TNF receptor family, termed the death domain, which is vital in transduction when Fas is crosslinked. ICE-like proteases are involved in downstream transduction of the Fas signal (Enari et al., 1995; Los et al., 1995).

Methods of detecting apoptotic cells

There are many methods of detecting apoptotic cells, but all have disadvantages, particularly in the quantitation of cells. The simplest is light microscopy which can reveal many of the morphological features characteristic of apoptosis as discussed. However, the assessment is, by definition, subjective and may miss a small and transient apoptotic population. Electron microscopy is much more sensitive and readily reveals many of the ultrastructural features of apoptotic cells. However, it is not readily available and is a qualitative assessment of the nature of the cell; apoptotic cells so detected cannot be easily quantitated. Time-lapse photography is believed to be the 'gold standard' for identifying and quantitating apoptotic cells (Evan et al., 1992; Harrington et al., 1994), but the process requires expensive equipment and specific expertise; therefore, it is not widely applicable.

DNA fragmentation has been considered for many years to be the hallmark of apoptosis (Duke et al., 1983; Kerr et al., 1972; Wyllie, 1980; Wyllie et al., 1980). However, the presence of a DNA ladder is purely qualitative. Furthermore, large numbers of apoptotic cells may be required to visualize a DNA ladder, typically

5×10^6 per ladder. It will therefore fail to identify a small apoptotic population, within a larger population of live cells. The amount of fragmented DNA can be quantitated using densitometry (Kawabata et al., 1994) but this gives no information about cell numbers. Also, it is becoming clear that apoptosis can occur (as detected by morphological changes and time-lapse photography) in the absence of a detectable DNA ladder (Cohen, 1994; Cohen et al., 1992; Kulkarni and McCulloch, 1994; Philpott et al., 1996). This may be due in part to technical considerations, to the fact that the formation of a DNA ladder is a very late stage in apoptosis, or that, in some systems, it is not an indispensable feature of the process.

Flow cytometry provides a simple and rapid means of analyzing large numbers of cells and allows easy quantitation of specific populations. Propidium iodide (PI) staining of fixed permeabilized cells has been widely used to detect and quantitate apoptotic cells (Huschtscha et al., 1994; Nicoletti et al., 1992; Pelliciari et al., 1993). PI binds to DNA; since the fragmented DNA of apoptotic cells is able to diffuse more rapidly out of the fixed cell, these cells have a lower DNA content and therefore have lower mean fluorescence than live cells, producing the so-called sub-G1 peak on fluorescence histograms (Telford et al., 1992; Zamai et al., 1993). The method requires permeabilization of the cell membrane and therefore precludes concurrent immunophenotyping, which would allow the nature of the cells undergoing apoptosis to be further defined (Schmid et al., 1994). A sub-G1 peak is not seen in all cell systems where apoptosis is noted to occur by other methods (McConkey et al., 1989). The sub-G1 peak simply represents cells with reduced DNA content and so, in addition to apoptotic cells, may be contaminated with cells whose DNA is nonspecifically degraded during necrosis.

Other DNA-binding agents have been used to detect apoptosis by flow cytometry, but many, such as ethidium bromide, share the disadvantages of PI. Hoechst 33342 binds preferentially to the DNA of apoptotic cells, rather than that of live cells and, in combination with PI for dead-cell discrimination, provides an efficient means of quantitating the three populations (Ormerod et al., 1992). Dual staining for cell surface markers is also possible, as no permeabilization step is necessary if Hoechst 33342 is the only DNA dye used (Hardin et al., 1992). However, this dye requires UV laser excitation, which is not widely available in standard flow cytometers.

Activation of the DNA endonuclease and subsequent DNA cleavage results in free 3'-hydroxyl (3'-OH) groups in apoptotic DNA. These 3'-OH groups can be detected by specific labelling by the enzyme terminal deoxynucleotidyl transferase (TdT), which will add labelled bases to these 3'-ends: TdT-mediated nick end labelling (TUNEL) (Gavrieli et al., 1992; Hotz et al., 1994). Bases can be labelled with fluorescent compounds, e.g., fluorescein isothiocyanate (FITC), and visualized directly by fluorescence microscopy or by flow cytometry, or with biotin or digoxygenin and indirectly identified, using secondary labels such as fluoresceinated avidin, or peroxidase and chromogenic substrate (Gorczyca et al., 1993*a,b*). This method of identifying and quantitating apoptotic cells is both sensitive and specific, but is expensive and, unless performed by flow cytometry, requires manual counting, limiting both the number of cells that can be assessed and the accuracy of the method. Although TUNEL can detect DNA strand breaks before a DNA ladder is detectable, it is still measuring a late stage of apoptosis.

Early changes in the plasma membrane of the apoptotic cell leads to recognition and engulfment of the cell by macrophages (Savill et al., 1993). Studies have demonstrated that, in the early stages of apoptosis, cells lose their plasma membrane phospholipid asymmetry (Martin et al., 1995; Vermes et al., 1995). Phosphatidylserine, normally confined to the inner plasma membrane, becomes externalized during apoptosis. This can be visualized by staining with annexin-V and in conjunction with PI allows discrimination between apoptotic and necrotic cells.

7-Amino actinomycin D (7-AAD) is a fluorescent DNA-binding agent, which intercalates between cytosine and guanine bases (Philpott et al., 1996). The uptake of 7-AAD is associated with the early changes of the plasma membrane and even precedes the translocation of phosphatidylserine as measured by annexin-V binding. It occurs several hours earlier than the loss of membrane integrity or nuclear changes and occurs in the absence of DNA fragmentation. Live, apoptotic and dead-cell populations can be quantitated on the basis of 7-AAD fluorescence intensity, and the method allows concurrent immunophenotyping.

Therefore, it is believed that apoptosis progresses time dependently, and that different stages can be detected using different techniques. That nuclear changes are not essential for detecting apoptosis is highlighted by the fact that apoptosis can occur in cells that do not have nuclei (Nakajima et al., 1995). Initially, plasma membrane changes occur, 7-AAD can enter and annexin-V will bind externalized phosphatidylserine. Hours later, endogenous endonuclease leads to DNA fragments, which can be detected by DNA ladders, PI staining or TUNEL. In vivo, macrophages engulf these cells; whereas, in vitro, in the absence of the phagocytic system, the plasma membrane breaks down and the cell will take up trypan blue.

Apoptosis in progenitor cells in the bone marrow of those with aplastic anemia

Definitive evidence for accelerated apoptosis and its contribution to the stem cell deficiency characteristic of aplastic anemia was provided by our laboratory (Philpott et al., 1995). We quantitated apoptotic cells by flow cytometry in bone marrow and peripheral blood from normal donors and patients with aplastic anemia, using the fluorescent DNA-binding dye 7-AAD, described earlier.

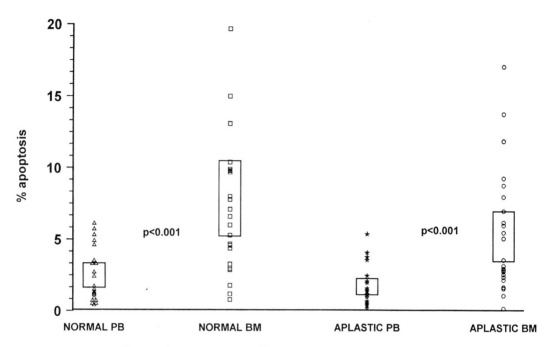

Figure 4.2. Percentage apoptosis of human mononuclear cell samples as defined by 7-AAD staining of normal peripheral blood (PB, △), normal bone marrow (BM, ❑), aplastic peripheral blood (★), aplastic bone marrow (○). Boxes indicate 95% confidence intervals of the mean.

Figure 4.1 shows an example of normal bone marrow. After creating a scattergram combining forward and right-angle light scatter for the whole population, a region (R1) was drawn around mononuclear cells (low forward and low right-angle light scatter), excluding cell debris (Figure 4.1A) and a second scattergram was generated, by combining forward light scatter with 7-AAD fluorescence of those mononuclear cells satisfying R1 (Figure 4.1B). Regions were drawn around clear-cut populations having negative (live cells), dim (apoptotic cells) and bright (dead cells) 7-AAD fluorescence, and the proportion of cells within each region was calculated. When 7-AAD staining was combined with cell surface immunophenotyping for the CD34 antigen, scattergrams were created by combining right-angle light scatter with CD34 fluorescence and a region drawn around a clear-cut population, with low right-angle light scatter and high CD34 fluorescence (R2, Figure 4.1C). A logical gate was then defined to quantitate cells satisfying both CD34+ and 7-AAD-negative, 7-AAD-dim, and 7-AAD-bright regions (Figure 4.1D).

In the mononuclear cell population the proportion of apoptotic cells was significantly reduced in peripheral blood compared to bone marrow, both for normal donors (mean 2.49% versus 7.88%) and patients (mean 1.75% versus 5.24%) (Figure 4.2). This may reflect the greater cell turnover of marrow compared

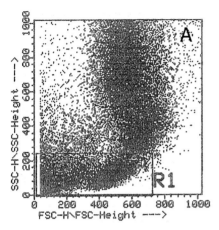
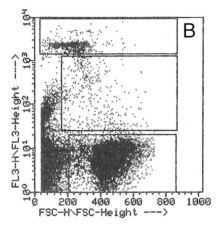
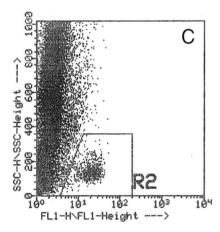
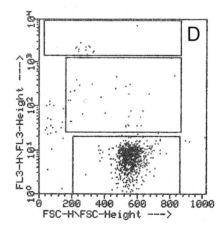

Figure 4.1A–D. Normal bone marrow (BM) stained with 7-amino actinomycin D (7-AAD) and anti-CD34 antibody (anti-HPCA-2). A, Scattergram of FSC versus SSC, to allow gating on mononuclear cells (R1). B, Scattergram of FL3 versus FSC gated on R1, showing 7-AAD-bright cells (dead), 7-AAD-dim cells (apoptotic) and 7-AAD-negative cells (live). C, Scattergram of FL1 versus SSC, to allow gating on CD34$^+$ cells (R2). D, Scattergram of FL3 versus FSC for CD34$^+$ cells (R2) only. FSC = forward light scatter; SSC = right-angle light scatter; FL1 = anti-CD34 fluorescence; FL3 = 7-AAD fluorescence. Similar staining patterns were obtained for peripheral blood and aplastic anemia samples.

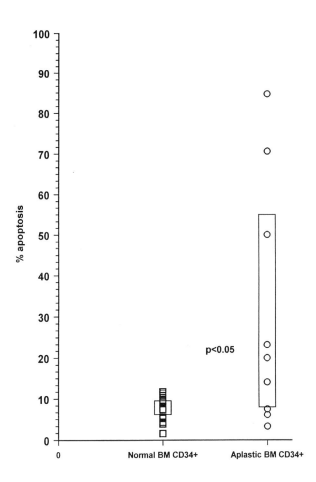

Figure 4.3. Percent apoptosis of CD34+ cells from normal and aplastic bone marrow, defined by 7-AAD staining. Normal bone marrow (BM, □), aplastic marrow (○). Boxes indicate 95% confidence intervals of the mean.

to peripheral blood, where the majority of mononuclear cells are long-lived lymphoid cells. However, there was no significant difference in the proportion of apoptosis between normal donors and aplastic anaemia patients for peripheral blood or marrow mononuclear cells. The process of apoptosis is characterized by the early expression of cell surface antigens which, in vivo, causes rapid phagocytosis by macrophages, so limiting local damage as a result of apoptotic cell death (Fadok et al., 1992). Therefore, even if peripheral blood or marrow mononuclear cells in those with aplastic anemia are dying more rapidly, or in greater numbers than in normal donors, the activity of the reticulo-endothelial system may mask this, before in vitro testing is performed.

CD34+ cells from bone marrow in those with aplastic anemia are significantly more apoptotic (mean 33.44%) than their normal counterparts (mean 7.86%) (Figure 4.3). This is, therefore, preliminary evidence that aplastic CD34+ progenitor cells are more sensitive to apoptosis than their normal bone marrow counterparts. This increase in apoptosis appears to be inversely related to the absolute number of CD34+ cells present (Figure 4.4). Where the percentage of CD34+ cells

Figure 4.4. Percentage apoptosis of CD34$^+$ cells versus percentage CD34$^+$ cells in normal (□) and aplastic marrow [transfusion dependent (●) and transfusion independent (○)].

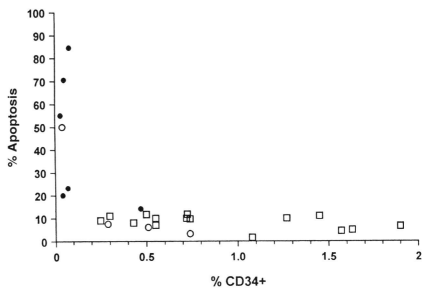

in the bone marrow from aplastic anemia patients is normal, the percentage of apoptotic cells is also within the normal range. In addition, when the proportion of apoptotic CD34$^+$ cells is related to transfusion dependency, as a marker of disease severity at the time of study, it appears that those with the most severe aplasia at the time of study have the highest proportion of apoptotic CD34$^+$ cells, whilst those with milder disease, or recovering marrow, have fewer apoptotic cells. Of the 'low CD34$^+$/high percentage apoptosis' group, five of six were transfusion dependent; the sixth was transfusion independent. Of the 'high CD34$^+$/low percentage apoptosis' group only one of four was transfusion dependent at the time of the study. This difference in the proportion of apoptotic cells between normal and aplastic bone marrow is confined to the early progenitor cell population, since proportions of apoptotic cells within total mononuclear cell populations are not significantly different. We conclude that apoptosis is accelerated in bone marrow progenitor cells in patients with aplastic anemia and that this may contribute to the stem cell deficiency characteristic of this disorder.

Expression of Fas on normal hemopoietic progenitor cells

As well as its expression on lymphoid cells, which increases upon activation, Fas is expressed by many hemopoietic cells (Strahnke et al., 1995). Fas is not expressed on freshly isolated adult bone marrow CD34$^+$ cells, but it is upregulated in these cells by exposure to negative regulators of hemopoiesis, such as interferon-γ (IFN-γ) and tumour necrosis factor α (TNF-α) (Maciejewski et al.,

1995a; Nagafuji et al., 1995). Anti-Fas antibody, which mimics the action of Fas-L, enhances suppression of colony formation by TNF-α and IFN-γ, and this was demonstrated to involve increased apoptosis.

In contrast, Barcena et al. (1996), studying the role of Fas in fetal liver progenitor cells, reported that Fas is expressed on the majority of the earliest, most primitive CD34$^+$ cells (>70% positive) and on a smaller population of less primitive CD34$^+$ cells (>20%). They demonstrated downregulation of Fas during hemopoietic differentiation, which correlated with an increase in the expression of CD38, and a decrease in the expression of CD34. These experiments differ from those cited above (Maciejewski et al., 1995a; Nagafuji et al., 1995), in which freshly isolated adult bone marrow total CD34$^+$ cells displayed negative or low Fas expression. Fas was only expressed after exposure to TNF-α and/or IFN-γ. This discrepancy could be caused by the use of different fluorochromes, resulting in differing sensitivities of the technique, or alternatively may reflect inherent differences between adult marrow and fetal liver CD34$^+$ cells. The functional status of Fas in these fetal liver cells was investigated. Anti-Fas antibody in the presence of TNF-α or IFN-γ had an inhibitory effect on the number of colony-forming units (CFU) generated, which compliments previous reports. However, in contrast, whereas growth factor deprivation induced apoptosis, they were unable to detect DNA fragments (on the basis of Hoechst 33342 staining) in cells treated with TNF-α or IFN-γ in the presence of anti-Fas antibody. This could be because of the different techniques used to detect apoptosis, the previous reports used DNA laddering, or may reflect differences in the susceptibility of fetal liver compared with adult bone marrow progenitor cells to undergo apoptosis. In addition, the hemopoietic suppression after Fas stimulation could be caused by mechanisms other than apoptosis. The demonstration of high expression of *bcl-2* in fetal liver CD34$^+$ cells could explain their protection against Fas-mediated apoptosis.

Expression of Fas on progenitor cells in aplastic anemia

Much evidence suggests that aplastic anemia is an immune-mediated disease; and suppression of hemopoiesis is associated with increased levels of TNF-α (Shinohara et al., 1991), macrophage-inflammatory protein-1α (MIP-1α) (Maciejewski et al., 1992) and IFN-γ (Nakao et al., 1992) as well as increased numbers of cytotoxic T-cells in the marrow (Maciejewski et al., 1994). As these cytokines suppress hemopoiesis, and IFN-γ and TNF-α induce Fas expression on hemopoietic progenitor cells, one may postulate a role for Fas in this function; upregulation of Fas on stem cells will increase their susceptibility to apoptosis. Maciejewski analyzed the expression of Fas on CD34$^+$ cells from patients with acute and recovered aplastic anemia and their results were consistent with this hypothesis (Maciejewski et al., 1995b). The mean percentage of

CD34$^+$ cells expressing Fas was 43% in the acute group and 29% in the recovered group, both levels being significantly greater than the 9% in the normal control group. There was no correlation between expression levels and severity of disease, although patients with acute disease had higher levels than recovered patients.

In addition, the increase in Fas expression correlated with the sensitivity of the cells to the inhibition of colony formation mediated through anti-Fas antibody. Higher levels of inhibition were seen in cultures of CD34$^+$ cells from two patients with aplastic anemia (45% and 63%) than in those from four normal controls (mean of 16%). These results are consistent with the hypothesis that in vivo exposure of CD34$^+$ progenitor cells to inhibitory cytokines leads to increased expression of Fas and greater susceptibility to Fas-mediated killing by cytotoxic T-cells. Although the contribution of autoimmunity to the pathophysiology of aplastic anemia is unproven, increased apoptosis of progenitor cells as a result of upregulated Fas expression may be important in the stem cell depletion that occurs in bone marrow failure.

Modulation of apoptosis by therapeutic intervention

Dysregulation of apoptosis is thought to play an important role in the pathogenesis of aplastic anemia. There are many possible mechanisms by which accelerated apoptosis can explain the hemopoietic stem-cell deficiency in aplastic marrow. An increase in the sensitivity of progenitor cells in aplastic anemia to the induction of apoptosis would result in accelerated cell death; this could explain the reduced numbers of stem cells in this disease (Maciejewski et al., 1996; Scopes et al., 1994) and their dysfunctionality (Scopes et al., 1996). Such an altered sensitivity may be a primary stem-cell defect, or a secondary response to an abnormal environment. Hemopoiesis is a tightly regulated process that requires dynamic changes in the production of soluble factors that stimulate and inhibit the growth and differentiation of progenitor cells. Constitutive release of these factors by various stromal cells is necessary for the maintenance of steady-state hemopoiesis including apoptosis (Koury, 1992; Williams et al., 1990). In vitro, it is known that many cytokines act as survival factors for hemopoietic progenitor cells, by suppressing apoptosis, but it is not clear to what extent this is the case in vivo. One may postulate a deficiency in the local production of survival factors such as granulocyte colony-stimulating factor (G-CSF). The marked increase in response rates in terms of not only neutrophil recovery but also platelet and red cell recoveries seen in patients with aplastic anemia treated with G-CSF after immunosuppressive therapy of antilymphocyte globulin (ALG) and cyclosporin, as opposed to immunosuppressive therapy alone, may be explained by suppression of stem-cell apoptosis in addition to stem-cell proliferation (Bacigalupo et al., 1995). Also, we have shown that only growth factor combinations including G-CSF correct the in vitro defect of purified aplastic CD34$^+$ cells, allowing them to match the growth of normal CD34$^+$ cells in some cases (Scopes et al., 1996). This may be because G-CSF suppresses apoptosis in these cells, because, in addition, G-CSF-mobilized peripheral-blood stem cells are significantly less apoptotic than unmobilized stem cells (Philpott et al., 1997). In light of the success of ALG clinically in combination with cyclosporin and G-CSF at stimulating hemopoiesis to normal levels, ALG may be acting by modulating apoptosis of stem cells or T-cells in aplastic anemia patients.

Alternatively, excess exposure to cytokines such as IFN-γ and TNF-α, which are known to inhibit hemopoiesis and are upregulated in this disease (Nakao et al., 1992, Shinohara et al., 1991), could be responsible for the increased apoptosis. Such negative regulators may exert their effect by increasing apoptosis. There is some evidence that, in normal marrow, IFN-γ and TNF-α upregulate expression of Fas (Maciejewski et al., 1995a). Crosslinking of Fas by Fas-L, expressed on activated T cells, results in apoptotic cell death (Owen-Schaub et al., 1992, 1993). Increased expression of Fas by progenitor cells (Maciejewski et al., 1995b), or excess activity of Fas-L-positive T-cells within the marrow could result in the increased apoptosis of progenitor cells seen in patients with aplastic anemia. Increased Fas-L production by T-cells may provide a link to the abnormalities in immunity noted in some reports to occur in aplastic anemia (Maciejewski et al., 1994). The soluble form of Fas-L could also be present in higher concentrations in the patients' marrow microenvironment. Other apoptosis-inducing stimuli in this disease have not been examined. If the Fas system is shown to be involved in the increased apoptosis that occurs in aplastic anemia, the possibility of blocking this interaction with soluble Fas, or neutralizing antibodies to Fas or Fas-L, should be investigated. In addition, it may be possible to block the action of TNF-α or IFN-γ with neutralizing antibodies to these inhibitory cytokines, or drugs such as pentoxifylline or ciprofloxacin, which have anti-TNF properties, and may reverse apoptosis. These possibilities offer potentially new approaches to the treatment of aplastic anemia.

Conclusion

Having identified an increased proportion of apoptotic progenitor cells in aplastic anemia patients, there is clearly a vast amount of research necessary to delineate the cause of this abnormality. Thus, precise identification of the distinct errors in the complex apoptotic machinery holds great promise for elucidating the pathogenesis of this disease and for devising more specific and effective treatments.

References

Amieson, J. C. (1992) Programmed cell death and AIDS: from hypothesis to experiment. *Immunology Today*, **13**, 388–91.

Amieson, J. C. and Capron, A. (1991) Cell dysfunction and depletion in AIDS: the programmed cell death hypothesis. *Immunology Today*, **12**, 102–5.

Bacigalupo, A., Broccia, G., Corda, G., Arcese, W., Carotenuto, M., Gallamini, A., Locatelli, F., Mori, P. G., Saracco, P., Todeschini, G., Coser, P., Iacopino, P., Van Lint, M. T., Gluckman, E. for the European Group for Blood and Marrow Transplantation (EBMT) Working Party on SAA (1995). Antilymphocyte globulin, cyclosporin and granulocyte colony-stimulating factor in patients with acquired severe aplastic anemia (SAA): a pilot study of the EBMT SAA working party. *Blood*, **85**, 1348–53.

Barcena, A., Park, S. W., Banapour, B., Muench, M. O. and Mechetner, E. (1996) Expression of Fas/CD95 and Bcl-2 by primitive hematopoietic progenitors freshly isolated from human fetal liver. *Blood*, **88**, 2013–25.

Bissonette, R. P., Echerverri, F., Mahboubi, A. and Green, D. R. (1992) Apoptotic cell death induced by c-*myc* is inhibited by *bcl-2*. *Nature*, **359**, 552–4.

Brown, D. G., Sun, X.-M. and Cohen, G. M. (1993) Dexamethasone-induced apoptosis involves cleavage of DNA to large fragments prior to internucleosomal fragmentation. *Journal of Biological Chemistry*, **268**, 3037–9.

Carson, D. A. and Ribeiro, J. M. (1993) Apoptosis and disease. *Lancet*, **341**, 1251–4.

Cohen, G. M., Sun, X.-M., Snowden, R. T., Dinsdale, D. and Skilleter, D. N. (1992) Key morphological features of apoptosis may occur in the absence of internucleosomal DNA fragmentation. *Biochemical Journal*, **286**, 331–4.

Cohen, J. J. (1994) Apoptosis: physiological cell death. *Journal of Laboratory and Clinical Medicine*, **124**, 761–5.

Cohen, J. J. and Duke, R. C. (1984) Glucocorticoid activation of a calcium-dependent endonuclease in thymocyte nuclei leads to cell death. *Journal of Immunology*, **132**, 38–42.

Collins, M. K., Marvel, J., Malde, P. and Lopez-Rivas, A. (1992) Interleukin-3 protects murine bone marrow cells from apoptosis induced by DNA damaging agents. *Journal of Experimental Medicine*, **176**, 1043–51.

Duke, R. C., Chervenak, R. and Cohen, J. J. (1983) Endogenous endonuclease-induced DNA fragmentation: an early event in cell-mediated cytolysis. *Proceedings of the National Academy of Sciences of the USA*, **80**, 6361–5.

Enari, M., Hug, H. and Nagata, S. (1995) Involvement of an ICE-like protease in Fas-mediated apoptosis. *Nature*, **375**, 78–81.

Evan, G. I., Wyllie, A. H., Gilbert, C. S., Littlewood, T. D., Land, H., Brooks, M., Waters, C. M., Penn, L. Z. and Hancock, D. C. (1992) Induction of apoptosis in fibroblasts by c-*myc* protein. *Cell*, **69**, 119–28.

Fadok, V. A., Voelker, D. R., Campbell, P. A., Cohen, J. J., Bratton, D. L. and Henson, P. M. (1992) Exposure of phosphatidylserine on the surface of apoptotic lymphocytes triggers specific recognition and removal by macrophages. *Journal of Immunology*, **148**, 2207–16.

Gavrieli, Y., Sherman, Y. and Ben-Sasson, S. A. (1992) Identification of programmed cell death *in situ* via specific labelling of nuclear DNA fragmentation. *Journal of Cell Biology*, **119**, 493–501.

Gorczyca, W., Gong, J. and Darzynkiewicz, Z. (1993*a*) Detection of DNA strand breaks in individual apoptotic cells by the *in situ* terminal deoxynucleotidyl transferase and nick translation assays. *Cancer Research*, **53**, 1945–51.

Gorczyca, W., Melamed, M. R. and Darzynkiewicz, Z. (1993*b*) Apoptosis of S-phase HL60 cells induced by DNA topoisomerase inhibitors: detection of DNA strand breaks by flow cytometry using the *in situ* nick translation assay. *Toxicology Letters*, **67**, 249–58.

Green, D. R. and Ware, C. F. (1997) Fas-ligand: privilege and peril. *Proceedings of the National Academy of Sciences of the USA*, **94**, 5986–90.

Hardin, J. A., Sherr, D. H., DeMaria, M. and Lopez, P. A. (1992) A simple fluorescence method for surface antigen phenotyping of lymphocytes undergoing DNA fragmentation. *Journal of Immunological Methods*, **154**, 99–107.

Harrington, E. A., Bennett, M. R., Fanidi, A. and Evan, G. I. (1994) c-*myc*-induced apoptosis in fibroblasts is inhibited by specific cytokines. *EMBO Journal*, **13**, 3286–95.

Hotz, M. A., Gong, J., Traganos, F. and Darzynkiewicz, Z. (1994) Flow cytometric detection of apoptosis: comparison of the assays of *in situ* DNA degradation and chromatin changes. *Cytometry*, **15**, 237–44.

Huschtscha, L. I., Jeitner, T. M., Andersson, C. E., Bartier, W. A. and Tattersall, M. H. (1994) Identification of apoptotic and necrotic human leukaemic cells by flow cytometry. *Experimental Cell Research*, **212**, 161–5.

Itoh, N., Yonehara, S., Ishii, A., Yonehara, M., Samashima, M., Hase, A., Seto, Y. and Nagata, S. (1991) The polypeptide encoded by the cDNA for human cell surface antigen Fas can mediate apoptosis. *Cell*, **66**, 233–43.

Kawabata, H., Anzai, N., Yoshida, Y. and Okuma, M. (1994) A new method for quantitative estimation of the degree of DNA fragmentation utilising agarose gel electrophoresis. *International Journal of Hematology*, **59**, 311–16.

Kerr, J. F. R., Wyllie, A. H. and Currie, A. R. (1972) Apoptosis: a basic biological phenomenon with wide-ranging implications in tissue kinetics. *British Journal of Cancer*, **26**, 239–57.

Koury, M. J. (1992) Programmed cell death (apoptosis) in hematopoiesis. *Experimental Hematology*, **20**, 391–4.

Koury, M. J. and Bondurant, M. C. (1990) Erythropoietin retards DNA breakdown and prevents programmed death in erythroid progenitor cells. *Science*, **248**, 378–81.

Kulkarni, G. V. and McCulloch, C. A. G. (1994) Serum deprivation induces apoptotic cell death in a subset of Balb/c 3T3 fibroblasts. *Journal of Cellular Science*, **107**, 1169–79.

Lockshin, R., Alles, A., Kodaman, N. and Zakeri, Z. F. (1991) Programmed cell death and apoptosis: early DNA degradation does not appear to be prominent in either embryonic cell death or metamorphosis of insects. *FASEB Journal*, **5**, A518–A525.

Loo, D. T., Copani, A., Pike, C. J., Whitemore, E. R., Walencewicz, A. J. and Cotman, C. W. (1993) Apoptosis is induced by β-amyloid in cultured central nervous system neurons. *Proceedings of the National Academy of Sciences of the USA*, **90**, 7951–5.

Los, M., Van de Craen, M., Penning, L. C., Schenk, H., Westendorp, M., Baeuerle, P. A., Droge, W., Krammer, P. H., Fiers, W. and Schulzw-Osthoff, K. (1995) Requirement of an ICE/CED-3 protease for Fas/APO-1-mediated apoptosis. *Nature*, **375**, 81–3.

Maciejewski, J., Liu, J., Green, S., Walsh, C., Plump, M. and Young, N. S. (1992) Expression of a stem cell inhibitor (SCI/LD78) gene in patients with bone marrow failure. *Experimental Hematology*, **20**, 1112–17.

Maciejewski, J. P., Hibbs, J., Anderson, S., Prokopis, K. and Young, N. S. (1994) Bone marrow and peripheral blood lymphocyte phenotype in patients with bone marrow failure. *Experimental Hematology*, **22**, 1102–10.

Maciejewski, J., Selleri, C., Anderson, S. and Young, N. S. (1995*a*) Fas antigen expression on CD34+ human marrow cells is induced by interferon-γ and tumour necrosis factor-α and potentiates cytokine-mediated hematopoietic suppression *in vitro*. *Blood*, **85**, 3183–90.

Maciejewski, J. P., Selleri, C., Sato, T., Anderson, S. and Young, N. S. (1995*b*) Increased expression of Fas antigen on bone marrow CD34+ cells of patients with aplastic anaemia. *British Journal of Haematology*, **91**, 245–52.

Maciejewski, J. P., Selleri, C., Sato, T., Anderson, S. and Young, N. S. (1996) A severe and consistent deficit in marrow and circulating primitive heatopoietic cells (long-term culture-initiating cells) in acquired aplastic anemia. *Blood*, **88**, 1983–91.

Martin, S. J. (1993) Programmed cell death and AIDS. *Science*, **262**, 1355–6.

Martin, S. J. and Green, D. R. (1995) Apoptosis and cancer: the failure of controls on cell death and cell survival. *Critical Reviews in Oncology and Haematology*, **18**, 137–53.

Martin, S. J., Reutelingsperger, C. P. M., McGahon, A. J., Rader, J. A., Van Schie, R. C. A. A., Laface, D. M. and Green, D. R. (1995) Early redistribution of plasma membrane phosphatidylserine is ageneral feature of apoptosis regardless of the initiating stimulus: inhibition by overexpression of Bcl-2 and Abl. *Journal of Experimental Medicine*, **182**, 1545–56.

McConkey, D. J., Hartzell, P., Amador-Perez, J. F., Orrenius, S. and Jondal, M. (1989) Calcium-dependent killing of immature thymocytes by stimulation via the CD3/T cell receptor complex. *Journal of Immunology*, **143**, 1801–6.

Nagafuji, K., Shibuya, T., Harada, M., Mizuno, S., Takenaka, K., Miyamoto, T., Okamura, T., Gondo, H. and Niho, Y. (1995) Functional expression of Fas antigen (CD95) on hematopoietic progenitor cells. *Blood*, **86**, 883–9.

Nagata, S. (1994) Apoptosis regulated by a death factor and its receptor: Fas ligand and Fas. *Philosophical Transactions of the Royal Society of London*, **345**, 281–7.

Nakajima, H. P., Golstein, P. and Henkart, P. A. (1995) The target cell nucleus is not required for cell-mediated granzyme- or Fas-based cytotoxicity. *Journal of Experimental Medicine*, **181**, 1905–9.

Nakao, S., Yamaguchi, M., Shiobara, S., Yokoi, T., Miyawaki, T., Taniguchi, T. and Matsuda, T. (1992) Interferon gamma gene expression in unstimulated bone marrow mononuclear cells predicts a response to cyclosporin therapy in aplastic anemia. *Blood*, **79**, 2532–5.

Newman, S. L., Henson, J. E. and Henson, P. M. (1982) Phagocytosis of senescent neutrophils by human monocyte-derived macrophages and rabbit inflammatory macrophages. *Journal of Experimental Medicine*, **156**, 430–42.

Nicoletti, I., Migliorati, G., Pagliacci, M. C., Griganani, F. and Riccardi, C. (1992) A rapid and simple method for measuring thymocyte apoptosis by propidium iodide staining and flow cytometry. *Journal of Immunological Methods*, **139**, 271–9.

Ormerod, M. G., Collins, M. K. L., Rodriguez-Tarduchy, G. and Robertson, D. (1992) Apoptosis in interleukin-3 dependent haemopoietic cells. Quantification by two flow cytometric methods. *Journal of Immunological Methods*, **153**, 57–65.

Owen-Schaub, L. B., Yonehara, S., Crump, W. L. and Grimm, E. A. (1992) DNA fragmentation and cell death is selectively triggered in activated human lymphocytes by Fas antigen engagement. *Cellular Immunology*, **140**, 197–205.

Owen-Schaub, L. B., Meterissian, S. and Ford, R. J. (1993) Fas/APO-1 expression and function on malignant cells of hematologic and non-hematologic origin. *Journal of Immunotherapy*, **14**, 234–41.

Pelliciari, C., Manfredi, A. A., Bottone, M. G., Schaack, V. and Barni, S. (1993) A single-step staining procedure for the detection and sorting of unfixed apoptotic thymocytes. *European Journal of Histochemistry*, **37**, 381–90.

Philpott, N. J., Scopes, J., Marsh, J. C. W., Gordon–Smith, E. C. and Gibson, F. M. (1995) Increased apoptosis in aplastic anemia bone marrow progenitor cells: possible pathophysiologic significance. *Experimental Hematology*, **23**, 1642–8.

Philpott, N. J., Turner, A. J. C., Scopes, J., Westby, M., Marsh, J. C. W., Gordon–Smith, E. C., Dalgleish, A. G. and Gibson, F. M. (1996) The use of 7-amino actinomycin D in identifying apoptosis: simplicity of use and broad spectrum of application compared with other techniques. *Blood*, **87**, 2244–51.

Philpott, N. J., Prue, R. L., Marsh, J. C. W., Gordon–Smith, E. C. and Gibson, F. M. (1997) G-CSF-mobilised CD34+ peripheral blood stem cells are significantly less apoptotic that unstimulated peripheral blood CD34+: role of G-CSF as survival factor. *British Journal of Haematology*, **97**, 146–52.

Rodriguez-Tarduchy, G., Collins, M. and Lopez-Rivas, A. (1990) Regulation of apoptosis in interleukin-3 dependent hematopoietic cells by interleukin-3 and calcium ionophore. *EMBO Journal*, **9**, 2997–3002.

Savill, J. S., Fadok, V., Henson, P. M. and Haslett, C. (1993) Phagocyte recognition of cells undergoing apoptosis. *Immunology Today*, **14**, 131–6.

Schmid, I., Uittenbogaart, C. H., Keld, B. and Giorgi, J. V. (1994) A rapid method for measuring apoptosis and dual-color immunofluorescence by single laser flow cytometry. *Journal of Immunological Methods*, **170**, 145–57.

Scopes, J., Bagnara, M., Gordon–Smith, E. C., Ball, S. E. and Gibson, F. M. (1994) Haemopoietic progenitor cells are reduced in aplastic anaemia. *British Journal of Haematology*, **86**, 427–30.

Scopes, J., Daly, S., Atkinson, R., Ball, S. E., Gordon–Smith, E. C. and Gibson, F. M. (1996) Aplastic anemia: evidence for dysfunctional bone marrow progenitor cells and the corrective effect of granulocyte colony-stimulating factor *in vitro*. *Blood*, **87**, 3179–85.

Shinohara, K., Ayame, H., Tanaka, M., Matsuda, M., Ando, S. and Tajiri, M. (1991) Increased production of tumor necrosis factor-α by peripheral blood mononuclear cells in the patients with aplastic anaemia. *American Journal of Hematology*, **37**, 75–9.

Strahnke, K., Kleihauer, E. and Debatin, K. M. (1995) Differential expression of Apo-1 (Fas/CD95) on human hematopoietic cells. *Experimental Hematology*, **23**, 516.

Telford, W. G., King, L. E. and Fraker, P. J. (1992) Comparative evaluation of several DNA binding dyes in the detection of apoptosis-associated chromatin degradation by flow cytometry. *Cytometry*, **13**, 137–43.

Vaux, D. L. (1993) Toward an understanding of the molecular mechanisms of physiological cell death. *Proceedings of the National Academy of Sciences of the USA*, **90**, 786–9.

Vaux, D. L., Cory, S. and Adams, J. M. (1988) *Bcl-2* gene promotes haemopoietic cell survival and co-operates with *c-myc* to immortalise pre-B cells. *Nature*, **335**, 440–2.

Vermes, I., Haanen, C., Steffens-Nakken, H. and Reutelingsperger, C. (1995) A novel assay for apoptosis. Flow cytometric detection of phosphatidylserine expression on early apoptotic cells using fluorescein labelled Annexin V. *Journal of Immunological Methods,* **184**, 39–51.

White, E. (1996) Life, death and the pursuit of apoptosis. *Genes and Development,* **10**, 1–15.

Williams, G. T. (1991) Programmed cell death: apoptosis and oncogenesis. *Cell,* **65**, 1097–8.

Williams, G. T., Smith, C. A., Spooncer, E., Dexter, T. M. and Taylor, D. R. (1990) Haemopoietic colony stimulating factors promote cell survival by suppressing apoptosis. *Nature,* **343**, 76–9.

Wyllie, A. H. (1980) Glucocorticoid-induced thymocyte apoptosis is associated with endogenous endonuclease activation. *Nature,* **284**, 555–6.

Wyllie, A. H., Kerr, J. F. and Currie, A. R. (1980) Cell death: significance of apoptosis. *International Review of Cytology,* **68**, 251–306.

Yuan, J., Shaham, S., Ledoux, S., Ellis, H. M. and Horvitz, H. R. (1993) The *C. elegans* cell death gene *ced-3* encodes a protein similar to mammalian interleukin-1β-converting enzyme. *Cell,* **75**, 641–52.

Zamai, L., Falcieri, E., Zauli, G., Cataldi, A. and Vitale, M. (1993) Optimal detection of apoptosis by flow cytometry depends on cell morphology. *Cytometry,* **14**, 891–7.

5

The interrelation between aplastic anemia and paroxysmal nocturnal hemoglobinuria

Gérard Socié

Hôpital Saint-Louis, France

Jean-Yves Mary

Université Paris VII

Hubert Schrezenmeier

Free University of Berlin

and Eliane Gluckman

Hôpital Saint-Louis, Paris

Introduction

Since the seminal description of its symptoms by Paul Strübing in 1882 (Strübing, 1882), paroxysmal nocturnal hemoglobinuria (PNH) has captured the attention of physicians and researchers. PNH is an acquired chronic hemolytic anemia, that is classically more frequent at night, and is often associated with neutropenia and/or thrombocytopenia, and episodes of venous thrombosis (Rosse, 1995). From the clinical point of view, the interrelationship between aplastic anemia (AA) and PNH has long been recognized. More than 50 years ago, Dacie and Gilpin (1944) were the first to describe a patient with AA–PNH syndrome and in 1967 Dr Dameshek stated in an editorial that, 'Aplastic anemia, and PNH might have a common denominator in the form of an insult to the marrow' (Dameshek, 1967). Marrow function is frequently found to be impaired in those with PNH, as shown by pancytopenia and a relatively low reticulocyte count in light of the degree of anemia (reviewed by Rosse, 1995). In a number of patients [8-year cumulative incidence rate of 15% (Socié et al., 1996)], moderate to severe marrow failure may occur during the course of the disease. Another group of patients has long been recognized: their first diagnosis is AA, but they go on to develop PNH. Thus, clinically PNH may be considered as a disease that presents in two forms: de novo PNH and the AA–PNH syndrome. In 1967, Lewis and Dacie stated that AA and PNH are associated in two ways:

1. Patients are diagnosed with typical PNH and later develop pancytopenia. This feature was thought to be uncommon (Rosse, 1995). However, in our

experience, this represents an evolution of the disease in 23 of 155 patients with de novo PNH (15%) and the cumulative incidence of this particular complication is 22% at 10 years (Socié et al., 1996).

2. Patients are diagnosed with AA, and the Ham's test becomes positive later. This patient subset, presenting with a so-called AA–PNH syndrome, represents 30% of those studied by Socié et al. (1996). The biological hallmark of PNH is the lack of (or decreased) expression of several proteins that are anchored to the membrane surface by a glycosyl-phosphatidylinositol moiety (GPI) (Yeh and Rosse, 1994). Recently, the *PIG-A* gene was identified using expression cloning (Bessler et al., 1994a; Takeda et al., 1993); its somatic molecular alterations were shown to be responsible for the defect in GPI-anchored protein expression in all PNH patients studied to date (Luzzatto and Bessler, 1996), including patients with the AA–PNH syndrome (Nagarajan et al., 1995). Thus on clinical and cytological grounds, and now at the molecular level, AA and PNH are clearly interrelated.

This chapter, on the inter-relationship between AA and PNH will cover the following:

- Clinical observations, i.e., the evolution of AA to PNH and vice versa.
- The deficiency of GPI-anchored proteins in AA; immunophenotype and clinical implications.
- The mutations of the *PIG-A* gene as a common genetic basis for PNH and the AA–PNH syndrome.

AA–PNH syndrome – clinical observations

A patient diagnosed to have typical PNH may go on to develop pancytopenia. As stated in the Introduction, this feature was thought to be uncommon (Rosse, 1995), but in fact our experience shows that it occurs in 15% of patients with de novo PNH, to give a cumulative incidence of 22% at 10 years (Socié et al., 1996). Other patients are diagnosed with an AA–PNH syndrome. The incidence of this syndrome is not absolutely clear: Socié et al. (1996) measured it as 30% of those with AA, similar to data from Hillmen et al. (1995) and Lewis and Dacie (1967) (29%, 23 out of 80 cases), but less than that reported recently by the Ulm (Späth-Schwalbe et al., 1995) and Japanese (Fujioka and Takayoshi, 1989) groups. This apparent discrepancy may in fact only reflect the bias of referral to centers and/or random fluctuations in sample size. On the other hand, in series involving large numbers of patients with AA, an AA–PNH syndrome is increasingly recognized as a late complication occurring in patients who have been treated with immunosuppressive therapy. Although the exact incidence of PNH in patients with AA is not clearly known (most probably because of changes in basic knowledge and increased recognition of this disease entity), a conservative estimate from large series is that between 15% and 25% of AA patients will eventually develop a PNH clone (Tichelli et al., 1994).

None of the large series of patients with PNH nor those of patients with AA afford direct comparisons between patients with de novo PNH and those with the AA–PNH syndrome. The French study (Socié et al., 1996) of a large group of patients with PNH (either de novo or AA–PNH) allowed for such a comparison. The population of patients included in the French survey has been described previously (Socié et al., 1996). The diagnosis of PNH was based on an unequivocally positive Ham's test. The survey included information on whether PNH was preceded by AA, and, if it was, the date when AA was diagnosed and the treatment subsequently given. At the time of PNH diagnosis, patients with de novo PNH and patients with the AA–PNH syndrome were classified as anemic if their hemoglobin concentration was below 120 g/l, neutropenic if their absolute neutrophil count was below than 1.5×10^9/l and thrombocytopenic if their platelet count was below 150×10^9/l, according to Dacie and Lewis (1972). The entire sample for this study included the 220 patients who were diagnosed with PNH in participating French centers between 1950 and 1995. In this cohort of 220 patients with PNH, AA antedated PNH in 65 patients with a median interval of 3.1 years (0.17–15.0 years). For the purposes of the study, this first group of patients is referred to as the AA–PNH syndrome group, and the remaining 155 patients as the de novo PNH group. Biological and clinical symptoms at diagnosis and initial treatment are summarized in Table 5.1. At diagnosis, age, gender, and symptom (thrombosis, infection and abdominal pain crisis) distributions were similar in both groups. However, when comparing patients with AA–PNH syndrome to patients with de novo PNH at presentation, anemia was less frequently observed (80% versus 93%), while thrombocytopenia and neutropenia were more frequently detected (63% versus 46% and 52% versus 36%, respectively). For patients with anemia, the mean (SD) hemoglobin level was 8.1 (1.8) g/l and 8.0 (1.8) g/l in those with AA–PNH syndrome and de novo PNH, respectively ($P=0.83$). The corresponding figures for neutropenia and thrombocytopenia were 0.8×10^9/l ($\pm 0.4 \times 10^9$/l) versus 0.9×10^9/l ($\pm 0.4 \times 10^9$/l) ($P=0.052$) and 39.9×10^9/l ($\pm 4.0 \times 10^9$/l) versus 48.8×10^9/l ($\pm 30.5 \times 10^9$/l) ($P=0.17$), respectively. Patients with the AA–PNH syndrome were treated initially with androgens (52% versus 18%) or with immunosuppressive therapy (22% versus 5%) more frequently than were patients with de novo PNH. Thus, at diagnosis, presenting symptoms were similar, although patients with de novo PNH tended to be more frequently recognized through the association of abnormal hematological values and abdominal pain crises. Blood examination revealed that patients with the AA–PNH

Table 5.1. Patient characteristics

Variable	Category	Total ($n = 220$)	AA–PNH ($n = 65$)	de novo PNH ($n = 155$)	P* value
Gender (n, %)	Female	120, 55%	37, 57%	83, 54%	0.65
Age (in years, mean $\pm$SD)	NA	37 ± 18	37 ± 18	38 ± 18	0.72
Thrombosis (n, %)	Yes	14, 6%	2, 3%	12, 8%	0.20
Life-threatening thrombosis (n, %)	Yes	9, 4%	1, 2%	8, 5%	0.22
Abdominal pain crisis (n, %)	Yes	28, 13%	4, 6%	24, 15%	0.06
Infection (n, %)	Yes	18, 8%	4, 6%	14, 9%	0.48
Anemia (n, %)	Yes	196, 89%	52, 80%	144, 93%	0.005
Neutropenia (n, %)	Yes	90, 41%	34, 52%	56, 36%	0.03
Thrombocytopenia (n, %)	Yes	112, 51%	41, 63%	71, 46%	0.02
Pancytopenia (n, %)	Yes	70, 32%	26, 60%	44, 72%	0.09
Treatment (n, %)					
Androgens	Yes	62, 28%	34, 52%	28, 18%	<0.0001
Danazole	Yes	11, 5%	4, 6%	7, 5%	0.61
Corticosteroids	Yes	45, 20%	16, 25%	29, 19%	0.32
CSA and/or ATG	Yes	21, 10%	14, 22%	7, 5%	0.0001
BMT	Yes	4, 2%	0, 0%	4, 3%	0.24
Transfusions	Yes	164, 75%	44, 68%	120, 77%	0.13
Others	Yes	13, 6%	1, 2%	12, 8%	0.08

Notes:

ATG = antithymocyte globulin; BMT = bone marrow transplantation; CSA = cyclosporin A.
* Chi-square test, except for age (Mann–Whitney test).

syndrome were more frequently pancytopenic than patients with de novo PNH. However, when comparing patients with the AA–PNH syndrome to those with de novo PNH at presentation, anemia was less frequently observed, while thrombocytopenia and neutropenia were more frequently detected. These blood abnormalities fit with those reported to occur in de novo PNH and in AA patients in 'clinical remission' after immunosuppressive therapy. Treatment options varied with time, but also clearly reflect the physicians' options for both groups, since patients with the AA–PNH syndrome were more frequently treated with immunosuppressive therapy or with androgens than patients with de novo PNH. During follow-up, the prevalence of infections or abdominal pain crises, cumulative incidences of myelodysplastic syndrome or acute leukemia, and the cumulative proportion of patients requiring additional treatment were similar in both groups. The cumulative incidence of thrombosis (or life-threatening thrombosis) was slightly lower in patients with the AA–PNH syndrome as compared to

Table 5.2. Complications occurring overall and in both groups of patients with PNH

Complications	Total (n = 220)	AA–PNH (n = 65)	de novo PNH (n = 155)	P value
MDS or AL				
(n, %)	11 (5%)	4 (6%)	7, (5%)	0.61*
Time (years) since diagnosis (mean ±SD)	1.4 ± 1.8	0.7 ± 0.9	1.7 ± 2.2	
10-year cumulative incidence (%) mean ±SD	6 ± 2	7 ± 3	6 ± 2	
Recurrent abdominal pain crisis (n, %)	41, 19%	12, 18%	29, 19%	0.95**
Recurrent infections (n, %)	41, 19%	10, 15%	31, 20%	0.40**
Pancytopenia	NA	NA		NA
(n, %)			23, 15%	
Time (years) since diagnosis mean +SD			3.4 + 3.8	
10-year cumulative incidence (%) mean ±SD			22 ± 4%	
Any thrombosis				
(n, %)	58, 26%	11, 17%	47, 30%	
Delay (year) since diagnosis (mean ±SD)	4.4 ± 5.1	3.4 ± 3.6	4.7 ± 5.4	
10-year cumulative incidence (%) (mean ±SD)	32 ± 4%	25 ± 8%	34 ± 5%	0.16*
Life-threatening thrombosis				
(n, %)	45, 20%	8, 12%	37, 24%	
Time (year) since diagnosis (mean ±SD)	4.6 ± 5.2	4.2 ± 3.9	4.6 ± 5.5	
10-year cumulative incidence (%) (mean ±SD)	23 ± 4%	20 ± 8%	25 ± 4%	0.16*
Other (n, %)	40, 18%	14, 22%	26, 17%	0.40**
Hemochromatosis (n)	11	3	8	
Hepatitis B or C (n)	11	5	6	
Malignant disorders (n)	9	4	5	
Other (n)	9	2	7	

Notes:
* Log rank test, ** Chi-square test.
Grafted patients are censored at the time of transplantation.

patients with de novo PNH (Table 5.2). Specific causes of death in both groups are summarized in Table 5.3. The data reveal substantial differences in the causes of death in the two groups of patients. Budd–Chiari syndrome was the primary cause of death in 27% of the de novo PNH patients, while none of the six patients with AA–PNH syndrome died of this complication ($P = 0.17$). Similarly, central nervous system (CNS) thrombosis accounted for eight deaths overall (one in the AA–PNH syndrome group and seven in the do novo PNH group, $P = 0.49$). While the cumulative incidence of thrombosis was slightly lower for patients with AA–PNH syndrome than for patients with de novo PNH, and while these latter patients died more frequently of CNS or liver thrombosis, we found in multivariate analyses that patients with AA–PNH syndrome had a fourfold to fivefold

Table 5.3. Primary causes of death in nongrafted patients

Cause of death (excluding patients who underwent BMT)	Total (n = 62) (n, %)	AA–PNH (n = 6) (n, %)	de novo PNH (n = 56) (n, %)
Budd–Chiari syndrome	15, 24%	0, 0%	15, 27%
CNS vascular complications	18, 29%	2, 33%	16, 29%
Thrombosis	8	1	7
Hemorrhage	6	1	5
Unknown	4	0	4
Infectious diseases	12, 19%	2, 33%	10, 18%
Malignancies (including three deaths from MDS/AL)	4, 6%	0, 0%	4, 7%
Other causes	13, 21%	2, 33%	11, 20%
Unknown cause	6	1	5
Disease or treatment related*	6	1	5
Disease or treatment unrelated**	1		1

Notes:

* Three cases of hemorrhage as a consequence of pancytopenia in patients with de novo PNH, two of hemochromatosis (one in each group), one of acute renal insufficiency (hemolysis in a patient with de novo PNH).

** One case of myocardial infarction.

increased risk of dying because of this complication. This apparent discrepancy was solved when we looked at the primary causes of the death of patients with AA–PNH syndrome. These patients died rapidly after having developed life-threatening thrombosis but from causes not directly related to thrombosis (mainly from infection).

The deficiency of GPI-anchored proteins in AA–PNH syndrome

The GPI anchor and its biosynthesis (reviewed in Rosse, 1997; Socié, 1997)

The first identified biochemical defects were the absence of two enzymes: acetylcholinesterase from red blood cells and alkaline phosphatase from leukocytes. However, it was only in the 1980s that the absence of the complement regulatory protein, decay accelerating factor (DAF), now known as CD55, was identified, and its absence did appear to be related to the unusual sensitivity of the red blood cells to the hemolytic action of complement. Since then, at least 30 proteins have been found to be missing from, or only present in markedly diminished numbers on, the abnormal blood cells in those with PNH. This lessened or lack of expression of such a number of proteins in PNH was intriguing, until it was recognized that the missing proteins are tethered to the membrane by a GPI anchor; thus the fundamental defect in PNH was uncovered. Special properties, such as increased translational mobility, phospholipase-mediated shedding, atypical targeting, and transmembrane signal transduction via the caveolae, have been attributed to GPI-anchored proteins.

The most widely studied GPI-anchored proteins (reviewed in Rosse, 1997; Socié, 1997)

- Decay accelerating factor (DAF, CD55). The first protein found to be deficient on red blood cells in those with PNH was identified in the process of analyzing the control of complement activation on the cell surface. This molecule downregulates the activity of the C4b2a complex. This deficiency accounts for the greatly increased deposition of activated C3b on the cells of those with PNH when complement is activated by either the classic or the alternative pathway. It was thus assumed that the deficiency of CD55 accounts for the increased sensitivity of PNH cells to the lytic activity of complement.
- CD59. This is the membrane inhibitor of reactive lysis (MIRL), variably expressed on all types of blood cells. It binds to the C5b–C8 complex.
- CD58 or LFA3. This protein is expressed mostly on the cell surface of lymphocytes and monocytes. It is a ligand for the adhesion molecule CD2. Importantly, it is expressed at the cell surface of lymphocytes as both a GPI-linked and a transmembrane protein.
- CD16 or Fc receptor III (FcγRIII). The CD16 molecule is encoded in a cell-type-restricted manner by two genes, *FcγRIII-A* and *FcγRIII-B*. CD16 exists in two alternative forms, a transmembrane form expressed on natural killer (NK) cells and macrophages and a GPI-anchored form expressed on neutrophils.
- UPAR, or the urokinase plasminogen activator receptor, is a protein of the same superfamily as CD59. Its function is to bind the proteolytic enzyme urokinase, which activates plasminogen to plasmin in the initiation of fibrinolysis.
- CD14 is the endotoxin-binding protein receptor. It is missing from abnormal monocytes in PNH, and this has been shown to affect the responses of these cells to endotoxin.
- CDw52 or Campath-1G. This protein is found on lymphocytes, monocytes and neutrophils. It is capable of activating T-lymphocytes via the CD2 molecule but not the CD3-TCR pathway.
- CD24 is expressed on immature B-cells and to a lesser extent on more mature B-cells.

- CD48 is a pan-leukocyte antigen. Its role as a ligand for the CD2 molecule remains controversial.
- CD66/CD67. This group of proteins is particularly interesting in the study of defects in GPI-anchored proteins on granulocytes. The consequence(s) of this defect for granulocyte function remains unclear.

The GPI-anchored protein deficiency (reviewed in Rosse, 1997; Socié, 1997)

During the past few years a number of papers have been published showing the heterogeneous distribution of GPI-linked proteins on hemopoietic cells and their applicability to the diagnosis of PNH. However, there are a number of potential problems to bear in mind when using cytofluorometry to analyze PNH patients. These problems are even more important now in the late 1990s, as flow cytometry will probably soon become the reference diagnostic tool in clinical practice. These problems can be summarized as follows:

- The number of detectable GPI-linked proteins is large and ever increasing.
- These proteins have various qualitative and quantitative expression patterns in different hemopoietic cell lineages.
- Some molecules (see above) may be GPI-linked *and* transmembrane on the same cell surface.
- Different monoclonal antibodies have different affinities for the pertinent epitopes.
- The lineages towards which the PNH clone(s) differentiate are variable.
- In most patients, both normal residual and mutated hemopoiesis co-exist.

Thus, in practice, diagnosis of PNH using flow cytometry should involve at least two different antibodies (that recognize two different molecules), and two different cytometric gates, on at least two different cell types.

The GPI-anchored protein deficiency in AA–PNH syndrome

The strong clinical links between PNH and AA, and recent advances in flow cytometry in the diagnosis of PNH prompted the search for GPI-anchored protein deficiencies in patients with otherwise typical AA, and for such deficiencies in patients with AA who, after immunosuppressive treatment, had a positive Ham's test. While there are several studies (reviewed in Rosse, 1997; Socié, 1997) of patients with otherwise typical de novo PNH, only four studies to date have focused on the search for a GPI-anchored protein deficiency in patients with AA (Griscelli-Bennaceur et al.,1995; Schrezenmeier et al., 1995; Schubert et al., 1994; Tooze et al., 1995; Yamaguchi et al., 1995). The results of these studies are summarized in Table 5.4: 158 patients have been studied and a GPI-anchored protein defect was found in 62 (40%). However, these studies often mix patients studied at diagnosis and patients studied during follow-up after treatment. Current

Table 5.4. Studies of the GPI-anchored protein deficiency in the AA–PNH syndrome

Number of patients	GPI–n, % in ≤lineage	Red blood cell	PMN	Monocytes	Leukocytes	Response to IST GPI +/− (%)	Author
29	12, 41%	1/12	12/12	11/11	nd	88/58	Schubert et al., 1994
52	27, 52%	7/27	25/27	18/25	7/27	86/30	Schrezenmeier et al., 1995
37	13, 35%	8/14	13/13	8/13	1/12	nd	Griscelli et al., 1995
23	1, 4%	nd	nd	nd	1/23	nd	Yamaguchi et al., 1995
70	16, 23%	?	16/16	16/16	nd	nd	Tooze et al., 1995

Note:
IST = Immunosuppressive therapy.

studies at single centers and an ongoing EBMT prospective study are looking for this deficiency in patients with AA (and a negative Ham's test) at diagnosis. Preliminary data from these ongoing studies suggest that at least 30% of patients with otherwise typical AA have a GPI-anchored protein deficiency at diagnosis (G. Socié, H. Schrezenmeier, and EBMT Severe Aplastic Anemia Working Party; unpublished results). One intriguing clinical result, reported by the Ulm group, is that patients with a GPI-anchored protein deficiency respond less well to immunosuppressive therapy than those without (Schrezenmeier et al., 1995). This preliminary finding requires clarification.

Mutations of the *PIG-A* gene in AA–PNH syndrome

Molecular biology of the *PIG-A* gene

Dr Kinoshita and associates were the first to isolate the gene that is defective in PNH, using expression selection after transduction of defective cells from a patient with PNH. The complementary deoxyribonucleic acid (cDNA) contains 4568 base pairs (bp) and an open reading frame that codes for a protein of 484 amino acids (Iida et al., 1994; Takeda et al., 1993). The protein does not appear to have an N-terminal signal sequence, suggesting that it is external to the endoplasmic reticulum cisterna, but it does have a hydrophobic region suggestive of a transmembrane region. However, to date, the product (protein) of the *PIG-A* gene has not been isolated and its exact role is not known, although the amino acid sequence is strongly homologous to the family of glycotransferases. The genomic structure of the *PIG-A* gene was characterized recently (Bessler et al., 1994; Iida et al., 1994): the gene contains six exons and extends over 17 kilobases (kb). The *PIG-A* gene is located on the short arm of chromosome X at Xp22.1. The same probes as were used to identify *PIG-A* have also been used to identify a pseudogene (Ψ-*PIG-A*) on 12q21. Thus the location of the *PIG-A* gene on the X chromosome explains why there are acquired somatic alterations of this gene in all PNH cases studied to date, since a PNH phenotype caused by alteration of the other genes would require both autosomal gene copies to be altered.

Abnormalities of the *PIG-A* gene in PNH

Since Kinoshita's group first described *PIG-A* gene alteration in PNH patients in 1993 (Takeda et al., 1993), almost 100 PNH cases have been studied at the molecular level (reviewed in Kinoshita et al., 1995; Luzzatto and Bessler, 1996; Luzzatto et al., 1997; Rosse, 1997). The first studies were been done using reverse transcriptase polymerase chain reaction (RT-PCR), cloning, and sequencing. Single-strand conformation polymorphism PCR (SSCP-PCR) is used more widely now the genomic organization of the *PIG-A* gene is known. This latter technique detects most but not all genomic alterations; thus, sequencing is always necessary (either guided by the results of the SSCP analysis, or by sequencing the PCR products of the 6 exons and boundaries). The majority of the alterations are deletions of a few bases, resulting in frameshift abnormalities usually ending with a premature stop codon. A large number of mutations have been located in exon 2 (the largest one). However, more importantly, there is no evidence for recurring genomic alterations in PNH (no 'hot spots'). This latter point leads to the conclusion that it is highly unlikely that a routine molecular method for diagnosing PNH will become available. Thus, as recently stated by Wendel Rosse in a recent review (Rosse, 1997), while it is clear that a defect in the *PIG-A* gene in hemopoietic stem cells is a *necessary* condition for the development of PNH, it is not at all clear if the defect alone is *sufficient* for the manifestation of the disease.

Abnormalities of the *PIG-A* gene in AA–PNH syndrome

Only two studies, of six and five patients respectively, have looked specifically for *PIG-A* gene abnormalities in AA–PNH syndrome (Merk et al., 1997; Nagarajan et al., 1995). To date, there is no clear evidence that the type of mutation determines the clinical phenotype (i.e., there is no evidence yet that the mutations described to occur in de novo PNH are clearly different to those in patients with AA–PNH syndrome).

Conclusion: the mutations of the *PIG-A* gene as a common genetic basis for PNH and AA–PNH syndrome

It has long been demonstrated that the growth of myeloid precursors (CFU-GM, CFU-GEMM, and BFU-E) in semi-solid culture is readily reduced in patients with

PNH. It has also been demonstrated that the growth of these precursors is impaired in unaffected (GPI+) marrow cells. At the present time, we do not have enough data to clearly dissect the mechanism(s) leading to the hemopoietic defect in PNH. Among the theories that have been proposed, the most widely accepted is that of Rotoli and Luzzatto (Luzzatto *et al.*, 1997), which proposes a two-step process. Step 1: the somatic mutation of the *PIG-A* gene occurs commonly but the abnormal clone remains very small. Step 2: a suppressive influence like that seen in AA occurs, but is less effective on the GPI-anchored population. Since over a third of the patients with AA may have *PIG-A* mutation(s), and would probably have been classified as having 'idiopathic' AA some years ago, it is now clear that we have to identify those AA patients who have a GPI-anchored protein defect. However, while it seems clear today that these patients belong to a well-defined biological entity, at both the phenotypic (GPI-anchored protein deficiency) and the molecular (*PIG-A* mutation) levels, it is far from clear whether these patients behave differently to those with other forms of acquired AA. This question will be a major issue in the field of AA research and clinical practice in the forthcoming years.

References

Bessler, M., Hillmen, P., Longo, L., Luzzatto, L. and Mason, P. J. (1994*a*) Genomic organization of the X-linked gene (*PIG-A*) that is mutated in paroxysmal nocturnal haemoglobinuria and of a related autosomal pseudogene mapped to 12q21. *Human Molecular Genetics*, **3**, 751–7.

Bessler, M., Mason, P. J., Hillmen, P., Miyata, T., Yamada N., Takeda, J., Luzzatto, L. and Kinoshita, T. (1994*b*) Paroxysmal nocturnal haemoglobinuria (PNH) is caused by somatic mutations in the PIG-A gene. *EMBO Journal*, **13**, 110–17.

Dacie, J. V. and Gilpin A. (1944) Refractory anaemia (Fanconi type): its incidence in three members of one family, with in one case a relationship to chronic haemolytic anaemia with nocturnal haemoglobinuria. *Archives of Disease in Childhood*, **19**, 155–62.

Dacie, J. V. and Lewis, M. (1972) Paroxysmal nocturnal haemoglobinuria: clinical manifestation, haematology, and nature of the disease. *Series in Haematology*, **3**, 3–23.

Dameshek, W. (1967) What do aplastic anemia, paroxysmal nocturnal hemoglobinuria and 'hypoplastic' leukemia have in common ? *Blood*, **30**, 251–5.

Fujioka, S. and Takayoshi, T. (1989) Prognostic features of paroxysmal nocturnal hemoglobinuria in Japan. *Acta Haematologica Japonica*, **52**, 1386–94.

Griscelli–Bennaceur, A., Gluckman, E., Scrobohaci, M. L., Jonveaux, P., Vu, T., Bazarbachi, A., Carosella, E. D., Sigaux, F. and Socié, G. (1995) Aplastic anemia and paroxysmal nocturnal hemoglobinuria: search for a pathogenetic link. *Blood*, **85**, 1354–63.

Hillmen, P., Lewis, S. M., Bessler, M., Luzzatto, L. and Dacie, J. V. (1995) Natural history of paroxysmal nocturnal hemoglobinuria. *New England Journal of Medicine*, **333**, 1253–8.

Iida, Y., Takeda, J., Miyata, T., Inoue, N., Nishimura, J., Kitani, T., Maeda, K. and Kinoshita, T. (1994) Characterization of genomic PIG-A gene: a gene for glycosylphosphatidylinositol-anchor biosynthesis and paroxysmal nocturnal hemoglobinuria. *Blood*, **83**, 3126–31.

Kinoshita, T., Inoue, N. and Takeda, J. (1995) Defective glycosyl phosphatidylinositol anchor synthesis and paroxysmal nocturnal hemoglobinuria. *Advances in Immunology*, **6**, 60–103.

Lewis, S. M. and Dacie J. V. (1967) The aplastic anaemia–paroxysmal nocturnal hemoglobinuria syndrome. *British Journal of Haematology*, **13**, 236–51.

Luzzatto, L. and Bessler, M. (1996) The dual pathogenesis of paroxysmal nocturnal hemoglobinuria. *Current Opinion in Hematology*, **3**, 101–10.

Luzzatto, L., Bessler, M. and Rotoli, B. (1997) Somatic mutations in paroxysmal nocturnal hemoglobinuria: a blessing in disguise? *Cell*, **88**, 1–4.

Merk, B., Hildebrand, A., Rojewski, M., Raghavachar, A. and Schrezenmeier, H. (1997) Heterogeneous PIG-A mutations in aplastic anemia, paroxysmal nocturnal hemoglobinuria, and non-Hodgkin's lymphoma. *Blood*, **90**, 434a–435a.

Nagarajan, S., Brodsky, R. A., Young N. S. and Medof, M. E. (1995) Genetic defects underlying paroxysmal nocturnal hemoglobinuria that arises out of aplastic anemia. *Blood*, **86**, 4656–61.

Rosse, W. F. (1995) Paroxysmal nocturnal hemoglobinuria. In *Principles and practice of hematology*, ed. T. P. Stossel and S. E. Lux, pp. 367–76. Philadelphia: Lippincott.

Rosse, W. F. (1997) Paroxysmal nocturnal hemoglobinuria as a molecular disease. *Medicine*, **76**, 63–93.

Schrezenmeier, H., Hertenstein, B., Wagner, B., Raghavachar, A. and Heimpel, H. (1995) A pathogenetic link between aplastic anemia and paroxysmal nocturnal hemoglobinuria is suggested by a high frequency of aplastic anemia patients with a deficiency of phosphatidylinositol glycan anchored proteins [Rapid Communication]. *Experimental Hematology*, **23**, 81–7.

Schubert, J., Vogt, H. G., Zielinskaskowronek, M., Freund, M., Kaltwasser, J. P., Hoelzer, D. and Schmidt, R. E. (1994) Development of the glycosylphosphatitylinositol-anchoring defect characteristic for paroxysmal nocturnal hemoglobinuria in patients with aplastic anemia. *Blood*, **83**, 2323–8.

Socié, G. (1997) Recent advances in paroxysmal nocturnal hemoglobinuria. From the biology to the clinic. *Hematology and Cell Therapy*, **39**, 175–87.

Socié, G., Mary, J. Y., De Gramont, A., Rio, B., Leporrier, M., Rose, C., Heudier, P., Rochant, H., Cahn, J. Y. and Gluckman, E. (1996) Paroxysmal nocturnal hemoglobinuria: long-term follow up and prognostic factors. *Lancet*, **348**, 573–7.

Späth-Schwalbe, E., Schrezenmeier, H. and Heimpel, H. (1995) Paroxysmale nächtliche Hämoglobinurie: Klinische Erfahrungen bei 40 Patienten in einem Zentrum über 25 Jahre. *Deutsche Medizinische Wochenschrift*, **120**, 1027–33.

Strübing, P. (1882) Paroxysmale Haemoglobinurie. *Deutsche Medizinische Wochenschrift*, **8**, 1–3.

Takeda, J., Miyata, T., Kawagoe, K., Iida, Y., Endo, Y., Fujita, T., Takahashi, M., Kitani, T. and Kinoshita, T. (1993) Deficiency of the GPI anchor caused by a somatic mutation of the *PIG-A* gene in paroxysmal nocturnal hemoglobinuria. *Cell*, **73**, 703–11.

Tichelli, A., Gratwohl, A., Nissen, C. and Speck, B. (1994) Late clonal complications in severe aplastic anemia. *Leukemia Lymphoma*, **12**, 167–75.

Tooze, J. A., Saso, R., Marsh, J. C. W., Papadopoulos, A., Pulford, K. and Gordon–Smith, E. C. (1995) The novel monoclonal antibody By114 helps detect the early emergence of a paroxysmal nocturnal hemoglobinuria clone in aplastic anemia. *Experimental Hematology*, **23**, 1484–91.

Yamaguchi, M., Nakao, S., Takamatsu, H., Chuhjo, T., Shiobara, S. and Matsuda, T. (1995) Quality of hematologic recovery in patients with aplastic anemia following cyclosporin therapy. *Experimental Hematology*, **23**, 341–6.

Yeh, E. T. H. and Rosse, W. F. (1994) Paroxysmal nocturnal hemoglobinuria and the glycosyl-phosphatidylinositol anchor. *Journal of Clinical Investigation*, **93**, 2305–12.

6

Aplastic anemia and other clonal disorders

Aruna Raghavachar

University of Ulm

Introduction

As the survival of patients with acquired aplastic anemia (AA) improves, patients with autologous marrow recovery have a significant risk of developing malignant disorders of hemopoiesis later in life. The combined cumulative risk of developing myelodysplastic syndrome (MDS), acute myelogenous leukemia (AML) or paroxysmal nocturnal hemoglobinuria (PNH) as a clonal but nonmalignant condition has been calculated to be as high as 40% at 15 years after immunosuppression (Tichelli et al., 1988, 1994). Readers are referred to an excellent review devoted to this issue (Young, 1992) for more details. This chapter focuses on more recent developments, in an attempt to identify patients with AA who are at a high risk of developing MDS or AML as a late clonal complication.

Clinical observations: the evolution of AA to myelodysplastic syndrome and acute myelogenous leukemia

During the past 20 years, treatment of AA has greatly improved, increasing the number of long-term survivors. At the same time, there is mounting evidence that AA is associated with hematological malignancies, as discussed by Dameshek (1967). Table 6.1 summarizes the most meaningful studies which, however, are all retrospective in nature. The evolution of AA to MDS or AML occurs rarely, as compared to transformation to PNH; whilst the exact figure is difficult to establish, it appears to occur in about 10% of cases. The interval between the initial diagnosis of AA and the appearance of MDS or AML is extremely variable and may range from months to more than 10 years (Table 6.1), with a mean onset of about 4 years following treatment.

The relationship between AA, MDS and hypoplastic leukemia is indicated by the difficulty of diagnosing AA reliably. While cytogenetics is not very informative in this respect (Tuzuner et al., 1995), a more recent study recommends immuno-

Table 6.1. Myelodysplastic syndrome (MDS) and acute myelogenous leukemia (AML) as a late clonal complication in acquired aplastic anemia

Patients	No. of patients (n)	Development of MDS/AML		Interval to the onset of MDS/AML (months)*	Reference
		(n)	(%)		
Adults	60	5	8.3	56 (7–142)	De Planque et al., 1988, 1989
Adults	156	5	3.2	? (60–144)	Najean and Haguenauer, 1990
Adults and children	860	43	5	52 (2–122) MDS 47 (7–115) AML	Socié et al., 1993
Adults and children	37	13	35	Not given	Narayanan et al., 1994
Adults	77	5	6.5	49 (30–126)	Paquette et al., 1995
Adults and children	227	20	8.8	Not given	Doney et al., 1997
Children	119	11	9.2	25 (12–74)	Ohara et al., 1997

Note:

* Median, range.

Table 6.2. Primary treatment of acquired aplastic anemia and hematological malignancies

Immunosuppressive therapy	Bone marrow transplant recipients	Reference
43/860*	0/748	Socié et al., 1993
—	0/700	Deeg et al., 1996
20/227	0/168	Doney et al., 1997
—	0/212	Deeg et al., 1998

Note:

* Number of patients developing a hematological malignancy versus the number of patients at risk.

staining of bone marrow biopsies to differentiate between MDS and AA (Orazi et al., 1997). However, in clinical practice and even in randomized trials on the treatment of AA, we continue to observe a significant number of incorrect diagnoses; for example, 6% in the most recent German Multicenter Trial on immunosuppression. From this experience, one might assume that errors in clinical diagnosis partly account for the increased incidence of late clonal disorders.

The most important risk factor for developing a clonal complication in AA is the type of treatment given to the patient (Table 6.2). It is impressive that none of the patients receiving a bone marrow graft in these studies developed MDS or AML. Similarly, treating AA patients with high-dose cyclophosphamide appears to result in recovery of hemopoiesis without evolution to secondary clonal diseases (Brodsky, 1998), although this observation has to be substantiated by clinical trials. Treating AA with androgens (Najean and Haguenauer, 1990) also results in a low frequency of clonal disorders. In addition to immunosuppression with anti-thymocyte globulin with or without cyclosporin, the treatment with hemopoietic growth factors may further increase the AA patients' risk of developing hemo-poietic malignancies (Ohara et al., 1997; Raghavachar et al., 1996). The long-term follow-up of patients treated with immunosuppression and growth factors in several ongoing randomized trials will be of major importance in clarifying this disturbing observation.

The Basel group repeatedly reported that the presence of morphological abnormalities at diagnosis is highly predictive of the development of late clonal disorders (Tichelli et al., 1994). No other clinical parameters, such as age, sex, eti-ology or severity of AA, correlate with an increased risk of developing this com-plication.

A very recent study raised the question of whether accelerated senescence of hematopoietic stem cells underlies the pathophysiology of MDS when it occurs as a late complication of AA (Ball et al., 1998). The authors studied mean telomere length in blood leukocytes from AA patients and were able to show that telomere shortening is associated with the development of cytogenetic abnormalities and MDS, but not with PNH. Further studies are necessary to confirm whether telo-mere loss is an important risk factor in developing MDS as a late complication of AA.

Studies on clonal hemopoiesis in AA patients using X-linked DNA polymorphisms

The clonality of cell populations is significantly important for both the diagnosis and the subsequent studies of the progression of hematological malignancies (Gale and Wainscoat, 1993). When the studies cannot be directed towards the analysis of specific abnormalities, it is necessary to use a more indirect approach based on X-chromosome inactivation. This has been made possible by the obser-vation that in certain genes the active and inactive alleles are differentially methylated at specific cytosine residues. This can be exploited using methyla-tion-sensitive restriction enzymes to determine the X-chromosome inactivation pattern. One of the limiting factors in applying this method is the relatively low frequency of polymorphism – only 40% of females yield information for one of the genes most often used, i.e., those for phosphoglycerate kinase (PGK) and hypox-anthine phosphoribosyl transferase (HPRT). A further problem is that, for a meaningful result, the pattern obtained must be compared with the normal constitutive pattern for that patient in the tissue under investigation. In addition, the X-chromosome inactivation pattern may become more imbalanced with increasing age (Gale et al., 1997). This technique reveals that the T-lymphocytes of AA patients are polyclonal (Melenhorst et al., 1997). As far as hemopoiesis is concerned, the published data are inconsistent. In our own studies of 30 females with AA, and considering the already mentioned limitations of the method, we were able to establish a truly clonal X-chromosome inactivation pattern in only 13% of patients (Raghavachar et al., 1995). In seven patients who later developed clonal disorders of hemopoiesis, X-chromosome inactivation analysis did not predict this event in any case. The method was not sensitive enough to detect clonal populations of less than 5%. However, we showed that cells with a PNH immunophenotype are indeed clonal. We identified patients whose clonal pattern changed over time, indicating transient clones or at least variations in the size of the clones falling below the detection limit. In summary, clonal X-chromosome·inactivation patterns in AA patients are rare. The biological significance of clonal hemopoiesis as defined by this technique remains unclear. The technique's relative lack of sensitivity means that clonal populations may be missed.

Cytogenetic abnormalities in patients with severe aplastic anemia

Cytogenetic investigations in AA patients used to be considered important only for excluding Fanconi's anemia, which is characterized by increased chromosome fragility in the presence of stress from DNA crosslinking agents. However, since the publication of the first large series of cytogenetic studies in AA (Appelbaum et al., 1987), cytogenetic analysis now plays an integral role in the diagnostic work-up of patients with AA. However, difficulties in obtaining sufficient cells for cytogenetics from severely hypoplastic marrows hampers the wider distribution of this technique.

In the cytogenetic sense, a clone is defined by at least two cells having the same additional or structurally rearranged chromosome, or three cells with loss of the same chromosome. Using this definition, Appelbaum et al. (1987) detected chromosomal abnormalities in 4% of 183 patients with AA. The working party on severe aplastic anemia from the European Group for Blood and Marrow Transplantation (EBMT) collected cytogenetic data from 170 patients, treated from 1974 to 1994 within six reporting centers (A. Tichelli, personal communication). An abnormal karyotype was found in 23 cases, with a clonal abnormality observed in 20 cases (11.8%). Numerical aberrations (+8, +6) were the most frequent abnormality. So, from these studies one can conclude that the majority of patients with acquired AA have a normal karyotype at first presentation. Some longitudinal studies from the Geneva group (Mikhailova et al., 1996) add further

Table 6.3. Cytogenetic abnormalities in acquired aplastic anemia longitudinal studies*

Cytogenetic pattern		No. of patients (%)	No. of patients died (%)
At diagnosis	Follow-up		
Normal	Normal	51 (74)	10 (20)
Normal	Abnormal	7 (10)	3 (43)
Abnormal	Abnormal	3 (4)	3 (100)
Abnormal	Normal	8 (12)	1 (13)

Note:

* Adopted from Mikhailova et al., 1996.

information (Table 6.3). The authors showed different patterns of cytogenetic abnormalities during repeated work-up of AA patients over time. This small set of data suggests a correlation between clinical outcome and cytogenetic features, in that patients with persistent abnormalities are at risk of developing MDS or AML, which then negatively affects survival. In addition, these follow-up studies reconfirm the phenomenon of transient clones, as observed in the X-chromosome inactivation studies.

Another critical issue is the question of whether the type of treatment, in particular the use of hemopoietic growth factors in AA, affects the development of MDS/AML in these patients. The clinical data from Ohara et al. (1997), in a trial using granulocyte colony-stimulating factor (G-CSF) to treat children with AA, point to monosomy 7 having a role in this context. Therefore, it is advisable to survey chromosomes for changes at regular intervals, at least for AA patients receiving immunosuppression in combination with hemopoietic growth factors.

Conclusion

The calculated cumulative risk of developing late clonal complications (MDS, AML) is as high as 20% for long-term survivors of AA and autologous bone marrow reconstitution. Studies of clonal hemopoiesis using X-chromosome inactivation analysis demonstrate clonal cell populations in only 13% of patients. Clonal populations may be transient or only occasionally detectable. Karyotype studies show clonal cytogenetic abnormalities in a minority (12%) of AA patients at diagnosis. Patients with a persistent cytogenetic abnormality have a high risk of developing MDS or AML. Telomere shortening may identify a similar-risk population. From the clinical data, the evolution of AA to MDS or AML seems to be influenced by the type of treatment given. Patients treated with immunosuppression have a higher risk of developing late malignant hemopoietic disorders, whereas bone marrow

transplant recipients and perhaps patients treated with high-dose cyclophosphamide do not evolve to such disorders. For further studies, routine cytogenetics
should be included in the diagnostic work-up of AA patients.

References

Appelbaum, F.R., Barall, J., Storb, R., Ramberg, R., Doney, K., Sale, G. E. and Thomas, E. D.
(1987) Clonal cytogenetic abnormalities in patients with otherwise typical aplastic
anemia. *Experimental Hematology*, **15**, 1134–9.

Ball, S. E., Gibson, F. M., Rizzo, S., Tooze, J. A., Marsh, J. C. W. and Gordon–Smith, E. C. (1998)
Progessive telomere shortening in aplastic anemia. *Blood*, **91**, 3582–92.

Brodsky, R. A. (1998) Biology and management of acquired severe aplastic anemia. *Current
Opinion in Oncology*, **10**, 95–9.

Dameshek, W. (1967) Riddle: what do aplastic anemia, paroxysmal nocturnal hemoglobinuria and hypoplastic leukemia have in common? *Blood*, **30**, 251–4.

De Planque, M. M., Kluin–Nelemans, H. C., van Krieken, H. J. M., Kluin, P. M., Brand, A.,
Beverstock, G. C., Willemze, R. and van Rood, J. J. (1988) Evolution of acquired severe
aplastic anemia to myelodysplasia and subsequent leukemia in adults. *British Journal of
Haematology*, **70**, 55–62.

De Planque, M. M., Bacigalupo, A., Würsch, A., Hows, J. M., Devergie, A., Frickhofen, N.,
Brand, A. and Nissen, C. (1989) Long-term follow-up of severe aplastic anemia patients
treated with antithymocyte globulin. *British Journal of Haematology*, **73**, 121–6.

Deeg, H. J., Socié, G., Schoch, G., Henry–Amar, M., Witherspoon, R. P., Devergie, A., Sullivan,
K. M., Gluckman, E. and Storb, R. (1996) Malignancies after marrow transplantation for
aplastic anemia and Fanconi anemia: a joint Seattle and Paris analysis of results in 700
patients. *Blood*, **87**, 386–92.

Deeg, H. J., Leisenring, W., Storb, R., Nims, J., Flowers, M. E. D., Witherspoon, R. P., Sanders,
J. and Sullivan, K. M. (1998) Long-term outcome after marrow transplantation for severe
aplastic anemia. *Blood*,**91**, 3637–45.

Doney, K., Leisenring, W., Storb, R. and Appelbaum, F. R. (1997) Primary treatment of
acquired aplastic anemia: outcomes with bone marrow transplantation and immunosuppressive therapy. *Annals of Internal Medicine*, **126**, 107–15.

Gale, R. E. and Wainscoat, J. S. (1993) Clonal analysis using X-linked DNA polymorphisms.
British Journal of Haematology, **85**, 2–8.

Gale, R. E., Fielding, A. K., Harrison, C. N. and Linch, D. C. (1997) Acquired skewing of X-
chromosome inactivation patterns in myeloid cells of the elderly suggests a stochastic
clonal loss with age. *British Journal of Haematology*, **98**, 512–19.

Melenhorst, J. J., Fibbe, W. E., Struyk, L., van der Elsen, P. J., Willemze, R. and Landegent, J.
E. (1997) Analysis of T-cell clonality in bone marrow of patients with acquired aplastic
anemia. *British Journal of Haematology*, **96**, 85–91.

Mikhailova, N., Sessarego, M., Fugazza, G., Caimo, A., de Filippi, S., van Lint, M. T., Bregante,
S., Valeriani, A., Mordini, N., Lamparelli, T., Gualandi, F., Occhini, D. and Bacigalupo, A.
(1996) Cytogenetic abnormalities in patients with severe aplastic anemia.
Haematologica, **81**, 418–22.

Najean, Y. and Haguenauer, O. (1990) Long-term (5 to 20 years) evolution of nongrafted aplastic anemias. *Blood*, **76**, 2222–8.

Narayanan, M. N., Geary, C. G., Freemont, A. J. and Kendra, J. R. (1994) Long-term follow-up of aplastic anemia. *British Journal of Haematology*, **86**, 837–43.

Ohara, A., Kojima, S., Hamajina, N., Tsuchida, M., Imaskuku, S., Ohta, S., Sasaki, H., Okamura, J., Sugita, K., Kigasawa, H., Kiriyama, Y., Akatsuka, J. and Tsukimotos, I. (1997) Myelodysplastic syndrome and acute myelogenous leukemia as a late clonal complication in children with acquired aplastic anemia. *Blood*, **90**, 1009–13.

Orazi, A., Albitor, M., Heerema, N. A., Haskins, S. and Neiman, R. S. (1997) Hypoplastic myelodysplastic syndromes can be distinguished from acquired aplastic anemia by CD34 and PCNA immunostaining of bone marrow biopsy specimens. *American Journal of Clinical Pathology*, **107**, 268–74.

Paquette, R. L., Tebyani, N., Frane, M., Ireland, P., Ho, W. G., Champlin, R. E. and Nimer, S. D. (1995) Long-term outcome of aplastic anemia in adults treated with antithymocyte globulin: comparison with bone marrow transplantation. *Blood*, **85**, 283–90.

Raghavachar, A., Janssen, J. W. G., Schrezenmeier, H., Wagner, B., Bartram, C. R., Schulz, A. S., Hein, C., Cowling, G., Mubarik, A., Testa, N. G., Dexter, T. M., Hows, J. M. and Marsh, J. C. W. (1995) Clonal hematopoiesis as defined by polymorphic X-linked loci occurs infrequently in aplastic anemia. *Blood*, **86**, 2938–47.

Raghavachar, A., Ganser, A., Freund, M., Heimpel, H., Herrmann, F. and Schrezenmeier, H. (1996) Long-term interleukin-3 and intensive immunosuppression in the treatment of aplastic anemia. *Cytokines and Molecular Therapy*, **2**, 215–23.

Socié, G., Henry–Amar, M., Bacigalupo, A., Hows, J., Tichelli, A., Ljungman, P., McCann, S. R., Frickhofen, N., van't Veer–Korthof, E. and Gluckman, E. (1993) Malignant tumors occuring after treatment of aplastic anemia. *New England Journal of Medicine*, **329**, 1152–7.

Tichelli, A., Gratwohl, A., Würsch, A., Nisse, C. and Speck, B. (1988) Late haematological complications in severe aplastic anemia. *British Journal of Haematology*, **69**, 413–18.

Tichelli, A., Gratwohl, A., Nisse, C. and Speck, B. (1994) Late clonal complications in severe aplastic anemia. *Leukemia and Lymphoma*, **12**, 167–75.

Tuzuner, N., Cox, C., Rowe, J. M., Watrons, D. and Bennett, J. M. (1995) Hypocellular myelodysplastic syndromes (MDS): new proposals. *British Journal of Haematology*, **91**, 612–17.

Young, N. (1992) The problem of clonality in aplastic anemia: Dr. Dameshek's riddle restated. *Blood*, **79**, 1385–92.

Part II

Epidemiology and clinical features of acquired aplastic anemia

7

Epidemiology and etiology of aplastic anemia

Hermann Heimpel

University of Ulm

Introduction

Data on the epidemiology of aplastic anemia predominantly serve several primary purposes: to detect genetic predispositions, to discover external inducing factors, to quantitate the risks of exposure and to generate working hypotheses for the pathophysiology of the disease. There are several specific difficulties of ascertaining and interpreting the data, some of which are discussed in recent reviews (Gordon–Smith and Issaragrisil, 1992; Kaufman et al., 1991; Mary et al., 1996). The most relevant are:

1. The imprecision of diagnostic criteria. Stringent criteria, including adequate bone marrow cytology and histology, are used in collections of cases from single institutions or cooperative therapeutic trials. However, such series include selected cases referred to research institutions. In contrast, stringent criteria have not been applied to older epidemiological studies. As shown by the IAAS (The International Agranulocytosis and Aplastic Anemia Study) and the French registry on aplastic anemia, reviewing notified cases leads to the exclusion of other disorders that involve pancytopenia (Mary et al. 1990; The International Agranulocytosis and Aplastic Anemia Study, 1987), which were most probably included in less well-controlled studies.

2. Differentiating between chronic aplastic anemia and transient pancytopenia. The latter term refers to an entity not generally recognized in the classification of hematological disorders. Cases of pancytopenia with hypo- or normocellular bone marrow and spontaneous recovery within 10–90 days have been described under terms such as transitory bone marrow failure, transient aplastic anemia, bone marrow aplasia or bone marrow suppression, or reversible bone marrow aplasia (for literature see Keisu et al., 1990*a*). In three series defining aplastic anemia according to the criteria proposed by Heimpel and Kubanek (1975) and by Camitta et al. (1982), including bone marrow hypoplasia but not a chronic course, 5% of cases recovered fully within 90 days, and most patients recovered within less than 1 month (Clausen, 1986; Heimpel, 1979; Keisu et al., 1990*a*). In epidemiological

studies, follow-up data are not usually available. Such series may contain cases of transient pancytopenia, particularly if reports on bone marrow biopsy samples are not required. In contrast, series devoted to therapy most probably include none or very few such cases, which often are not referred to specialized research institutions. For drug safety reasons and because of preventive measures in industrial hygiene or environmental policies, chronic aplastic anemia and transient pancytopenia may be grouped together. This does not apply when formulating working hypotheses of pathophysiology and when assessing the efficacy of specific therapy. In chronic aplastic anemia, potential external factors may trigger a self-perpetuating process, whereas in transient pancytopenia one has to assume that they have dose-dependent, reversible effects, modulated by differences in the genetic susceptibility of the hemopoietic tissue.

3. The low incidence of aplastic anemia. This fact leads to the insufficient power of cohort studies in populations of presumed risk. The only solution is to use case–control studies, which have to be based on large populations and are therefore time consuming and expensive to conduct.

4. The difficulty in identifying the onset of the disorder. This is particularly relevant to the role of medical drugs, which may have been given for unspecified symptoms of the disease weeks or months before diagnosis (Heimpel and Heit, 1980).

5. The difficulty of differentiating between socio-economic and genetic factors in comparative epidemiology. The former relates to series of different time periods, while both relate to studies of different ethnic groups, either in the same (Linet et al., 1986; Szklo et al., 1985) or in different (Issaragrisil et al., 1996) geographical areas.

6. Incidence. Reliable data on the overall incidence of aplastic anemia can only be derived from population-based studies. Older estimates based on death certificates or on data from single centers yield much higher numbers than those shown in Table 7.1. These differences can be explained by methodological differences, such as inclusion of states of bone marrow failure that do not fulfil the definition criteria of aplastic anemia (Camitta et al., 1982; Heimpel and Kubanek, 1975), as used by the IAAS and later studies (IAAS, 1987). Szklo et al. (1985) and the IAAS (1987) both demonstrate the need to review and confirm carefully all cases notified to registries before they are used for calculating the incidence of aplastic anemia. In particular, diagnostic confirmation should include bone marrow biopsy (not done in the survey of Szklo et al., 1985) to rule out cases of myelodysplasia and aleukemic myeloid leukemia, and to guarantee that the false-positive rate is as low as possible. Therefore, incidence data shown in Table 7.1, which were obtained before 1980, cannot be compared with later studies, and do not support the hypothesis that aplastic anemia has become less frequent over the last 50 years. Likewise, no secular trends were observed in studies that recorded cases over more than 10 years (Clausen, 1986; Clausen et al., 1996; Szklo et al., 1985; IAAS, 1987).

Table 7.1. Incidence of aplastic anemia

Author	Study period	Area	Age (range)	Population $\times 10^6$	n	Incidence Total	Male	Female
Modan et al., 1975	1961–65	Israel		2.4	93	7.8	7.1	7.8
Wallerstein et al., 1969	1963–64	California		17.5	60	4.8		
Szklo et al., 1985	1970–78	Baltimore	0–60+	1.6	118	4.1	7.1	5.4
IAAS, 1987	1980–84	Europe	0–60+	21.2	208	2.0	1.7	2.3
Carwright et al., 1988	1985	UK	0–80+	21.0	49	2.3	1.4	3.2
Mary et al., 1990	1984–87	France	0–80+		250	1.5	1.6	1.5
Issaragrisil et al., 1991	1989	Thailand	0–60+	8.7	32	3.7	4.8	3.7
Clausen, 1986	1967–82	Scandinavia	0–14		33	2.0		
Clausen et al., 1996	1982 93	Scandinavia	0–14	4.3	101	2.0	2.4	1.5

Note:
Incidence = Cases diagnosed per million per year.

If these factors are considered, the incidence of aplastic anemia, matched for standard age and sex distribution, approximates to two new cases annually per one million inhabitants, without consistent and significant differences between males and females. The true incidence may be moderately higher, because less severe cases may have escaped attention. The overall rate may be higher in Thailand than in European countries, but differences between the Thailand and the IAAS studies, which used identical methodology, are only of borderline significance ($P=0.05$, χ^2). However, the difference in age distribution is striking: whereas the incidence rate is consistently higher in the older age groups in all European and American surveys, the annual probability of 7.2×10^{-6} in 15- to 24-year-olds in Thailand is significantly higher than in all other age groups, in both Thai and European studies. The possible conclusions to be drawn from this difference are discussed below.

There are a few descriptions of clusters of aplastic anemia occurring in circumscribed areas (Linet et al., 1986; Morgan et al., 1988). Unique exposure in these cases could not be detected, and these observations are probably attributable to random distribution.

The role of medical drugs: a good old theory revisited

For many years, aplastic anemia was thought of as a classic example of a drug-induced blood dyscrasia, and was held to be triggered by many medical drugs

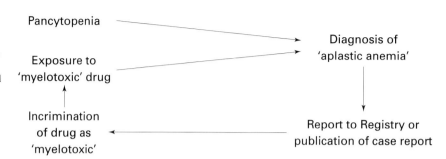

Figure 7.1. Bias circle enhancing the allocation of aplastic anemia or pancytopenia to the group of 'drug-induced aplastic anemia'.

(Girdwood, 1974; Heimpel and Heit, 1980; Williams et al., 1973). After it was reported in 1932 that hemopoietic failure followed the therapy of syphilis with organic arsenical compounds, drugs were suspected as being the single most important etiological factor. This hypothesis was further supported by its apparent similarity with the hemopoietic failure caused by benzene and cytostatic drugs. Fatal hemopoietic aplasia was observed after treating infectious diseases with the antibiotic chloramphenicol. This drug contains a nitrobenzene ring, and induces erythropoietic hypoplasia if given in large doses to dogs and human volunteers. These observations prompted the American Registry of Blood Dyscrasias (Welch et al., 1954) to be set up, which collects data on cases of aplastic anemia following any exposure to drugs within the 6-month interval before the disease (or any of the other blood dyscrasias) is diagnosed. Since exposure to chloramphenicol, the reputed prototype of an inducing agent for aplastic anemia, was frequently recorded within this interval, the hypothesis of a 'lag period' of up to 6 months was established, even though this was not consistent with the kinetics of the hemopoietic cell-renewal system. That hypothesis, although not supported by any epidemiological or experimental evidence, was widely accepted by hematologists, and became a 'self-fulfilling prophecy'. Hematologists recorded all cases of aplastic anemia as 'drug induced' when one of the previously suspected drugs had been taken by the patient up to 6 months before the suspected onset or confirmed diagnosis of the disorder. Such a 'bias circle' (Figure 7.1) may also influence publications: a report on one suspected case may provoke further reports, irrespective of whether the suspected relationship was incidental or not. Such waves of publications were observed for some newly introduced medications, such as chloramphenicol, cimetidine or more recently ticlopidine.

If the subpopulation of transient cases is excluded (Bacigalupo, 1996; Heimpel and Heit, 1980; Tichelli et al., 1994), there is no significant difference in the presentation (except for the drug-associated cases in one study being older) and prognosis between so-called idiopathic and drug-induced aplastic anemia. In studies other than controlled trials, allocation to one of these groups reflects nothing more than the judgment of the individual investigator. The large variation of the ratio between 'idiopathic' and 'drug-induced' cases is shown in Table 7.2. High

Table 7.2. Distribution of 'idiopathic' and 'drug-induced' cases of aplastic anemia selected from the literature

Author	Year	*n*	Drug-induced (%)
Lewis, 1965	1965	60	53
Keiser and Walder, 1970	1965	39	61
Williams et al., 1973	1973	101	86
Camitta et al., 1982	1978	67	10
Abe and Komiya, 1978	1978	396	32
Mir and Geary, 1980	1980	174	23
Heimpel and Heit, 1980	1980	113	35
Doney et al., 1984	1984	54	11
Champlin et al., 1985	1985	121	12
EBMT	1980–86	613	14
EBMT	1987–94	467	7
Issaragrisil, 1997*c*	1989–94	284	5

Notes:
Cases attributed to viral infections not noted. EBMT = EBMT working party on aplastic anemia, courtesy of A. Bacigalupo and H. Schrezenmeier.

proportions of drug-induced aplastic anemia were reported in early studies mainly concerned with etiology, but well-controlled recent series taken from prospective therapeutic trials give much lower values. As already stated, no secular trends in the age-adjusted incidence were observed, and overall drug consumption increased rather than decreased from the 1960s to the present day. Therefore, the large variance demonstrated by the data in Table 7.2 may not reflect true differences between the populations studied. Indeed it may arise because of changing observer-dependent variables, such as stringency of diagnosis and estimations of the strength of the link between exposure to the drug and development of aplastic anemia (Aoki et al., 1978).

The well-known history of chloramphenicol and its association with aplastic anemia is particularly suited to illustrate the methodological problems of establishing a causal link between a drug and the disease (Kaufman et al., 1991). The first four cases reported in 1950, which prompted all subsequent studies, did not describe typical long-lasting aplastic anemia, but rather transient neutropenia and maturation arrest of erythroblasts. In the three nonfatal cases, blood counts returned to normal within 2 weeks after the patients stopped taking the drug. In one fatal case, pancytopenia began during high-dose chloramphenicol therapy, and the patient died soon after the diagnosis was suspected. In these cases the diagnosis ought to be transient pancytopenia (Keisu et al., 1990*a*) rather than aplastic anemia; in a fourth case, it is possible that the drug was given after the onset of neutropenia. Based on the uncontrolled recording of the cases just described, more than 1300 cases of 'chloramphenicol-induced aplastic anemia' were recorded up to 1976 (Swanson and Cook, 1977), and some more series thereafter. Wallerstein's population-based study (Wallerstein et al., 1969), using drug consumption as an estimate of general exposure, suggested that patients treated with chloramphenicol were definitely at an increased risk of developing aplastic anemia. However, since bone marrow diagnostics were not required, and assessment of the temporal relationship between exposure and onset of the disease was inadequate, the study may have been severely biased. An early, though small, epidemiological study comparing chloramphenicol use before development of either aplastic anemia or leukemia showed similar exposure rates for both conditions (Aoki et al., 1978). Also, a recent case–control study from Thailand, where chloramphenicol is still widely used, showed that there was no significant increase in the relative risk of developing aplastic anemia (Issaragrisil et al., 1997c). The overall incidence of aplastic anemia did not change over time, regardless of whether it was measured when chloramphenicol was being commonly used or not. Attempts to detect individual hypersensitivity to chloramphenicol by culture assays with hemopoietic cells from individuals with chloramphenicol-associated aplastic anemia failed (Kern et al., 1975). In conclusion, epidemiological studies have not provided evidence that taking chloramphenicol induces aplastic anemia; indeed it is questionable whether the drug ever induced aplastic anemia as understood in this treatise.

The lesson one learns from the history of chloramphenicol-associated aplastic anemia is that the only instrument capable of revealing distinct associations is the case–control study. There are exceptions for individual drugs, such as remoxipride, which were withdrawn from the market after an unusual cluster of cases was observed in early clinical trials (Philpott et al., 1993). However, aplastic anemia is particularly difficult to study using this method, compared to many other diseases, for a number of reasons. First, experience with other potentially drug-induced blood dyscrasias and from drug-induced hepatitis shows that the most likely candidates are those drugs given shortly before the onset of aplastic anemia. However, the onset of most cases of aplastic anemia is insidious, and one cannot rule out the possibility that the drugs were given for early symptoms of the blood dyscrasias presenting weeks or months before the diagnosis was made. Second, case–control studies rely on the criteria determined at the time of diagnosis, and therefore include both long-lasting aplastic anemia and transient pancytopenia. To group both conditions may be useful in the interests of drug safety, but it does not help to establish working hypotheses for the pathogenesis of either disorder.

Methods established by the IAAS attributed the incidence of drug-induced aplastic anemia as 27%, 17% (Kaufman et al., 1996) and 5% (Issaragrisil et al.,

1997*d*), respectively, of all the cases in three case–control studies. It is not understood whether the differences between these figures reflect differences in the use of potentially harmful drugs, or subtle differences in the stringency of the methods used. Also, the role of single drugs is controversial. Gold and penicillamine may be regarded as exceptions, since case–control and cohort studies both indicate that their use is associated with a greatly increased risk of hemopoietic failure. However, in cases where detailed information is available, the course of the disease is more consistent with transient pancytopenia, with hemopoiesis returning to normal when exposure ends, which in the case of gold salts may be delayed by the substance being retained in the body. The IAAS study in Europe (not including France) identified nonsteroidal anti-inflammatory drugs (NSAIDs) as significant risk factors, but the studies from France (Mary et al., 1996) and Thailand (Issaragrisil et al., 1997*c*) did not show such a link. However, the French study did show that exposure to allopurinol and colchicine increased the risk of developing aplastic anemia. One speculative hypothesis is that regional variations in prescribing practice reflect regional differences in the incidence of diseases that are, themselves, risk factors for aplastic anemia.

Table 7.3 lists the drugs associated with aplastic anemia in case–control studies and case reports (Girdwood, 1974; Goldstein, 1988; Heimpel and Heit, 1980; Kaufman et al., 1991; Swanson and Cook, 1977). The highest reported values are given when there is conflict over the estimated risk. The differences between the controlled studies cited can be explained in many ways. For example, the number of cases for any drug is small, as shown by the large confidence intervals, depending on how much drug is consumed by the population studied. In addition, there are methodological differences, such as matching only for age or for multivariate confounding factors (Kaufman et al., 1991).

Table 7.3 also includes newer drugs, which are not listed in older reviews and were not used when the most recent case–control studies were performed. Remoxipride, a potent antipsychotic agent, was withdrawn after cases of fatal aplasia occurred (Laidlaw et al., 1993; Philpott et al., 1993). Felbamate, an antiepileptic agent, may be associated with both liver and hemopoietic failure in single cases (Blum, 1998; Pennell et al., 1995).

All the methodological problems discussed here can be illustrated by cases involving the drug ticlopidine. Since the first report in 1992 (Troussard et al., 1992), there have been 16 further reported cases, mostly single, of aplastic anemia following ticlopidine administration (Kao et al., 1997). Ticlopidine is used to stop platelet aggregation and has been used instead of acetosalicylic acid to reduce the risk of thromboembolic events in many individuals. The first report of its association with aplastic anemia may have prompted more, and it is not clear whether the association reflects causation. If this drug actually is myelotoxic in predisposed individuals, it may induce transient pancytopenia rather than chronic aplastic anemia: of the 16 reported cases referred to above, four

Table 7.3. Association between aplastic anemia and drug exposure

Author	Method	Drug	RR	95% CI
Custer, 1946	Case–control	Atebrin	12	??
Wallerstein et al., 1969	Drug consumption	Chloramphenicol	13	??
IAAS 91	Case–control	Butazones <4 weeks	12	3.4–42
IAAS 91	Case–control	>4 weeks	33	6.4–173
IAAS 91	Case–control	Indomethacin <4 weeks	10	2.9–36
IAAS 91	Case–control	>4 weeks	17	6.7–46
IAAS 91	Case–control	Gold salts	29	9.7–89
FCGESAA 96	Case–control	Gold salts	12	1.2–109
IAAS 92	Case–control	Penicillamine	49	5.2–464
FCGESAA 96	Case–control	Penicillamine	11	1.2–109
IAAS 91	Case–control	Salicylates >4 weeks	2.7	0.9–7.9
IAAS 91	Case–control	Sulphonamides	2.2	0.6–7.4
IAAS 91	Case–control	Phenothiazines	1.6	0.4–7.4
IAAS 91	Case–control	Antithyroid drugs	11	2.0–16
FCGESAA 96	Case–control	Allopurinol	5.9	1.5–2.4
1992–1996	Case reports	Ticlopidine		
1993	Case reports	Remoxipride		Withdrawn
1995–1996	Case reports	Felbamate*		

Notes:

CI = 95% confidence interval; FCGESAA = French Cooperative Group on Epidemiology of Aplastic Anemia (Baumelou et al., 1993; Mary et al., 1996) (Odds ratio);

IAAS = International Agranulocytosis and Aplastic Anemia Study (Kaufman et al., 1991);

RR = relative risk.

*Kaufman et al., 1997.

died, but all surviving patients recovered between 10 and 60 days after withdrawal of the medication.

There are particular problems in interpreting the data relating to antipsychotic and antiepileptic drugs. Evidence for their role comes from numerous case reports (e.g., Adams et al., 1983; Durrant and Read, 1982; Evreux and Loupi, 1985; Gerson et al., 1983; Hussain et al., 1973; Kanoh et al., 1977; Moore et al., 1985; Pisciotta, 1975; Rapoport and Barratt, 1974; Tomita et al., 1985), but case–control studies either did not calculate the relative risks or estimated them as borderline (Kaufman et al., 1991). This may be because psychiatric institutions, which prescribe larger doses compared with outpatients clinics or nonpsychiatric hospitals, were not included in the IAAS and Thai studies. Acetazolamide (Fraunfelder et al., 1985; Keisu et al., 1990*b*; Shapiro and Fraunfelder, 1992; Wisch et al., 1973), captopril and cimetidine (Iro et al., 1986; Israeli et al., 1985; Kim et al., 1989; Strair et al., 1985) are highlighted by series of case reports but not case–control studies. Again, surviving patients exposed to the latter agents recovered quickly, and can be classified as having suffered from transient pancytopenia.

In conclusion, epidemiological studies are suitable for detecting positive associations between medical drugs and blood dyscrasias, and by exclusion of confounding factors may also suggest etiological relationships between exposure and disease. Well-known examples include the risk of developing myeloid leukemia following radio-chemotherapy treatment for some malignant disorders, and drug-dependent agranulocytosis or hemolytic anemia, where the in vivo interaction can be simulated in vitro. For the case of chronic aplastic anemia, conclusive evidence is still not available except for some drugs listed in Table 7.3 and it is highly questionable whether such evidence will be obtained by further case–control studies. To prevent any misunderstanding, it should be stated that the inverse is not true: actual etiological relationships may be rare enough to reach significance because of the low overall incidence of aplastic anemia. Until the pathogenesis of the disorder is understood, medical drugs should be considered able to trigger downregulation of hemopoiesis at the stem-cell level or immunological events leading to long-lasting hemopoietic aplasia. Physicians should continue to report suggestive temporal associations between new drugs and aplastic anemia (Begaud et al., 1994), but such reports should be interpreted with care in order to prevent misinterpretations which may lead to useful drugs being withdrawn from the market.

Environmental and industrial chemicals

Benzene is very similar to chloramphenicol in its induction of aplastic anemia. Animal studies (Kissling and Speck, 1972) and reports of industrial exposure (Goldstein, 1988; Rothman et al., 1996; Smith, 1996) leave little doubt that benzene is toxic to many organs, in particular to the liver and hemopoietic tissue. Toxicity is attributed to metabolites activated in the bone marrow, for example highly reactive quinones and free radicals (Smith, 1996). This effect depends on the dose, and differences in individual susceptibility are probably caused by the liver's detoxification capacity. In discussing human data, three situations should be distinguished:

1. Changes of the blood count during exposure. Older data obtained from workers in the rubber industry or other plants using benzene are contradictory, with a tendency towards lower white blood cell counts (WBC), lower lymphocyte counts, and a higher mean corpuscular volume (MCV) (macrocytosis) (Goldstein, 1988). These observations were recently confirmed by a study, using modern automated technology, of heavily exposed Chinese workers exposed to an 8-hour daily average (TWA) of up to more than 300 ppm in the air at their workplace (to compare with a permissible TWA of about 1 ppm in western countries). WBC, absolute lymphocyte counts and platelet counts were lower than those of matched controls, and workers exposed to more than 32 ppm had an increased MCV (within the commonly used reference values). Similar trends were seen

when blood counts of workers of the cohort from a plant in Ohio, which was repeatedly analyzed for the incidence of cancer (Rinsky et al., 1987), were correlated with the changing exposure rate between 1940 and 1970 (Ward et al., 1996). These data, though the confidence intervals are very large, suggest that chronic exposure to low benzene levels (less than 5 ppm) leads to a cumulative change in hemopoietic cell production.

2. Benzene intoxication. Exposure to high benzene concentrations leads to severe, life-threatening hemopoietic failure (Goldstein, 1988; Saita, 1974; Wilson, 1942). Dimmel (1933) reported on the largest number of cases with follow-up of blood counts, and showed that regeneration occurred quickly in those who survived the period of profound pancytopenia. There are no data on the delayed effects on individuals surviving transient hemopoietic failure secondary to benzene intoxication.

3. Chronic blood dyscrasias during or after benzene exposure. Workers exposed to more than 20 ppm per year have a definitely increased relative risk of hemopoietic neoplasias (Crump, 1994; Rinsky et al., 1987; Yin et al., 1996a,b). All relevant studies show that this is significant for acute myelogenous leukemia, and some studies reveal significance for the lymphomas. Latency may be as long as 20 years after the initial exposure; however, there are no data on the latency after exposure has ended.

It is not at all clear whether these types of benzene-induced damage to hemopoiesis can serve as a model for the pathogenesis of aplastic anemia as discussed elsewhere in the book. One problem is the fact that estimations of toxicity to hemopoiesis in humans are based on older reports from Europe (Aksoy et al., 1984; Saita, 1974), or on contemporary studies analyzing historical data (Paci et al., 1989), or on studies carried out in regions with lower levels of diagnostic technology, such as Turkey (Aksoy et al., 1984, 1987) and China (Yin et al., 1996a). The cohort and case–control studies just cited do not acknowledge myelodysplastic syndromes as a disease. Since this type of hemopoietic malignancy is over-represented in series of leukemia that develops after exposure to cytostatic drugs, and is associated with benzene in noncontrolled studies (Lowenthal and Marsden, 1997), it may well be that some of the cases of aplastic anemia attributed to benzene exposure are actually cases of myelodysplastic syndrome. Recently, large cohort studies in China (Yin et al., 1996a,b) estimated an increased risk of aplastic anemia after chronic benzene exposure as significant, but again it is uncertain whether stringent diagnostic criteria were fulfilled. Daily and cumulative doses were much higher, with average workplace air concentrations of about 17 ppm. From these data an incidence of 1 $\times 10^{-4}$ was estimated for persons chronically exposed to 10–100 ppm (that is more than 10–100 times the permissible workplace dose) (Smith, 1996). However, this estimate underlies all the possible diagnostic errors in patients with pancytopenia of any cause.

In conclusion, metabolic and epidemiological studies favor the theory that aplastic anemia is induced by exposure to benzene levels greater than those that are currently permissible in Western countries. The magnitude of the risk remains uncertain, and it is rather unlikely that benzene contributes to the incidence of aplastic anemia in areas with modern standards of industrial hygiene.

Even less convincing is the evidence for induction of aplastic anemia by other xenobiotics. Various 'solvents' other than benzene are termed hematotoxic in some textbooks, but single cases of hemopoietic failure and the increased risk in Thailand (Issaragrisil et al., 1996) may be caused by benzene contained in non-volatile solvents and cleaning fluids, as well as in gasoline. Pesticides, for example chlorinated hydrocarbons such as lindane (Morgan et al., 1980; Rugman and Cosstick, 1990) or pentachlorophenol (Roberts, 1990), have been implicated as causing aplastic anemia on the basis of casual observations. However, many of these studies are of low quality and do not provide any evidence for the etiological link. In a few cases, hemopoietic failure after exposure to lindane was associated with raised concentrations in subcutaneous fat (Rauch et al., 1990; Rugman and Cosstick, 1990), but elevated values were not found in bone marrow samples from German patients with aplastic anemia as compared with normal controls (Anselstetter et al., 1985). Common topical applications of lindane as a delousing agent for children and adults did not damage hemopoiesis. Case–control studies from the USA (Linet et al., 1989; Wang and Gruffermann, 1981) and France (Guiget et al., 1995) have not provided any evidence that exposure to pesticides or any other xenobiotic increases the risk of developing aplastic anemia. Occupational exposure to paints and glues moderately increased the chance of developing aplastic anemia in two of these studies (Guiguet et al., 1995; Linet et al., 1989) and in Thailand (Issaragrisil et al., 1996). Dioxins, which are clearly carcinogenic, apparently do not induce aplastic anemia, since no excess was found in the large cohorts followed for many years following the Seveso accident (Bertazzi et al., 1989).

The results of the large case–control study in Thailand are especially interesting, since this is the only work performed with modern epidemiological and hematological methods in a country with standard of industrial hygiene lower than those in middle Europe and the USA. This study shows that, in Thailand, individuals of lower socio-economic status, and those who are younger are at greater risk than their counterparts in other parts of the world following exposure to solvents, glues, and hepatitis A (regarded as a surrogate marker of an undetermined factor). Grain farmers are similarly affected, regardless of whether they use insecticides (Issaragrisil et al., 1996, 1997a,b). It is not fully understood whether these data reflect differences in exposure per se, the confounding effects of an unknown inducer, or a different susceptibility in the Thai population.

The present state of knowledge is summarized in Table 7.4. Aplastic anemia is an unusual consequence of exposure to industrial or environmental xenobiotics, including derivatives that are carcinogenic. This fits with the epidemiological data

Table 7.4. Xenobiotics other than benzene and their association with aplastic anemia

Exposure	Method	Aplastic anemia	Transient pancytopenia	Leukemia
Lindane	Case reports	Yes	Yes	?
PCP	Case reports	Yes		Yes
	Cohort studies	No	No	No
Dioxin	Seveso cohort	No	No	?
Paints and glues	Case–control (Guiguet et al., 1995)	4.0 (0.8–19)		
	Case–control (Linet et al., 1989)	6.1 (1.2–30)		
Pesticides	Case–control (Guiguet et al., 1995)	1.6; 0.4***		
Solvents	Case–control (Guiguet et al., 1995)	0.9 (0.5–1.7)		
Irradiation	Case–control (Guiguet et al., 1995)	1.0 (0.1–11)		
Benzopyrene	Mice	No	Yes	Yes

Notes:
Figures are odds ratio (95% CI).
*** Hospital, neighborhood controls.

from a large number of patients followed for decades after intensive cytoreductive therapy for cancer. As is the case for medical drugs, these epidemiological data do not exclude an etiological relationship in single cases, either by undetected accidents of high-level exposure or infrequent states of individual idiosyncrasy.

Viruses

Hemopoietic damage leading to single or combined hemocytopenias is induced by a variety of viruses, such as parvovirus B19, cytomegalovirus, Dengue, Epstein–Barr virus, or herpes simplex virus-6 (Young and Mortimer, 1984). Individuals with severe preexisting hemopoietic depression seem to be particularly susceptible, as shown by severe and prolonged hemopoietic failure after allogeneic or autologous hemopoietic stem cell or allogeneic liver transplantation (Inoue et al., 1994; Mayer et al., 1997; Singh and Carrigan, 1996). An early onset of aplastic anemia during severe acute, presumably viral, hepatitis is well known, and an etiological relationship is supported by this syndrome's poor prognosis

(Brown et al., 1997*a*; Zeldis, 1989). However, virus was not identified in most cases and, with a few exceptions, the type of hepatitis was nonA, nonB. Recent suspicions that hepatitis virus G is the responsible viral agent could not be confirmed in controlled studies (Brown et al., 1997*b*; Loya, 1996). Since some drugs induce both liver and hemopoietic failure, which may occur simultaneously, it may even be speculated that metabolic changes in liver failure cause hemopoiesis to fail.

There are no quantitative risk estimates for developing aplastic anemia following any specified viral infection, but clinical experience indicates that only a small minority of individuals respond with hemopoietic failure to the viral infections named above. Any genetic or acquired cofactors required are not known, except for severe depression of hemopoiesis, as mentioned. In contrast, there are reliable data on the proportion of cases of aplastic anemia attributable to viruses or hepatitis. It is noteworthy that, in contrast to the fraction of 'drug-induced aplastic anemia' the proportion of cases attributed to viral diseases has remained stable over time. This may be explained by the short time lag between viral disease and the development of aplastic anemia, and also by the inappropriate emphasis placed on casual clinical observations. In Europe and the USA, the percentage of aplastic anemia cases attributable to viral infection, including all incidences of hepatitis, varies between 5% and 8% (Champlin et al., 1985; Doney et al., 1984; Heimpel and Heit, 1980), a value similar to that obtained from case–control studies (Kaufman et al., 1991; Mary et al., 1990).

The case–control study carried out in Thailand (Issaragrisil et al., 1996, 1997*b*) presented no evidence that aplastic anemia is associated with hepatitis B or C. Previous exposure to the hepatitis A virus, as determined by immunoglobulin G (IgG) seropositivity, was significantly associated with aplastic anemia. The relative risk was 2.9 (95% confidence interval 1.2–6.7), similar to the risk for cases of clinical hepatitis within 6 months prior to onset of aplastic anemia in the French study (2.8, 1.2–7) (Guiguet et al., 1995). In Thailand, people under 25 also have the same relative risk, even though the prevalence of hepatitis A IgG in this group is lower than that in the total population. However, no patients showed evidence of recent infection with hepatitis A, as estimated by IgM seropositivity. These results indicate that being exposed to a hepatitis virus places one at risk of developing aplastic anemia in Thailand. Whilst it is unlikely that the hepatitis A virus itself is the etiological agent for aplastic anemia, it may be a surrogate marker for another enteric microbial agent that is more commonly found in young adults of low socio-economic status in Thailand.

Risk factors others than exposure

Risk factors other than age or exposure to chemical agents or viruses may reflect both the tendency to develop aplastic anemia unrelated to external factors – comparable to the association of HLA-B-27 to rheumatic disorders such as ankylosing spondylitis – or increased susceptibility to potentially hematotoxic drugs or viruses. An example of the latter is the strong association between clozapine-induced agranulocytosis (presenting as a transient pancytopenia in severe cases) with subtypes of HLA-DR1. Whereas older studies could not find any significant association between aplastic anemia and HLA class I alleles, more recent ones did report an increased frequency of HLA-DR 2 (Chapuis et al., 1986; Nimer et al., 1994). This may be due to over-representation of its subtype, HLA-DRB1*1501, in patients that respond to cyclosporin (Nakao et al., 1996). It will be interesting to see whether larger immunogenetic studies, including genetic HLA-typing, can identify particular subgroups of aplastic anemia.

Apparently unrelated diseases such as rheumatoid arthritis may be a risk factor, as they select patients for the use of particular medications, and may therefore result in erroneous attribution to drugs used to treat the associated disorder (Mary et al., 1996). This may explain the borderline increased relative risks of taking corticosteroids or peripheral analgesics, as shown in some studies (Kaufman et al., 1996).

Conclusion

Epidemiological data are useful for shedding light on the etiology and pathophysiology of aplastic anemia, but may also result in erroneous hypotheses if the accuracy of diagnostic and epidemiological methods are neglected. Data obtained before the IAAS introduced stringent methodological standards are to be challenged, and future studies must use the critical approach of the IAAS, as has been done in French and Thai studies. Nevertheless, reports of single cases or groups of cases are useful for detecting possible associations, particularly with new drugs or newly identified viral agents.

References

Abe, T. and Komiya, K. (1978) Some clinical aspects of aplastic anemia. In *Aplastic anemia*, ed. S. Hibino, p. 197. Tokyo: University Park Press.

Adams, P. C., Robinson, A., Reid, M. M., Vishu, M. C. and Livingston, M. (1983) Blood dyscrasias and mianserin. *Postgraduate Medical Journal*, **59**, 31–3.

Aksoy, M., Erdem, S., Dincol, G., Bakioglu, I. and Kutlar, A. (1984) Aplastic anemia due to chemicals and drugs: a study of 108 patients. *Sexually Transmitted Diseases*, **11**, 347–50.

Aksoy, M., Ozeris, S., Sabuncu, H., Inanici, Y. and Yanardag, R. (1987) Exposure to benzene in Turkey between 1983 and 1985: a haematological study on 231 workers. *British Journal of Industrial Medicine*, **44**, 785–7.

Anselstetter, V., Balschmiter, K., Dmochewitz, S. and Heimpel, H. (1985) Aplastic anemia: residue analysis of chlorinated hydrocarbons in human bone marrow biopsy specimens by high resolution chromatography. *Acta Haematologica (Basel)*, **73**, 6–10.

Aoki, K., Ohtani, M., and Shimizu, H. (1978) Aplastic anemia. In *Epidemiological approach to the etiology of aplastic anemia*, ed. S. Hibino, F. Takaku and N. T. Shahidi, p. 155–70. Tokyo: University of Tokyo Press.

Bacigalupo, A. (1996) Aetiology of severe aplastic anaemia and outcome after allogeneic bone marrow transplantation or immunosuppression therapy. Working Party on Severe Aplastic Anaemia of the European Blood and Marrow Transplantation Group. *European Journal of Haematology Supplement*, **60**, 16–19.

Baumelou, E., Guiguet, M. and Mary, J. Y. (1993) Epidemiology of aplastic anemia in France: a case–control study. I. Medical history and medication use. The French Cooperative Group for Epidemiological Study of Aplastic Anaemia. *Blood*, **81**, 1471–8.

Begaud, B., Moride, Y., Tubert, Bitter, P., Chaslerie, A. and Haramburu, F. (1994) False-positives in spontaneous reporting: should we worry about them? *British Journal of Clinical Pharmacology*, **38**, 401–4.

Bertazzi, P. A., Zocchetti, C., Pesatori, A. C., Guercilena, S., Sanarico, M. and Radice, L. (1989) Ten-year mortality study of the population involved in the Seveso incident in 1976. *American Journal of Epidemiology*, **129**, 1187–200.

Blum, D. E. (1998) New drugs for persons with epilepsy. *Advances in Neurology*, **76**, 57–87.

Brown, K. E., Tisdale, J., Barrett, A. J., Dunbar, C. E and Young, N. S. (1997*a*) Hepatitis associated aplastic anemia. *New England Journal of Medicine*, **336**, 1059–64.

Brown, K. E., Wong, S. and Young, N. S. (1997*b*) Prevalence of GBV-C/HGV, a novel 'hepatitis' virus, in patients with aplastic anaemia. *British Journal of Haematology*, **97**, 492–6.

Camitta, B. M., Storb, R. and Thomas, E. D. (1982) Aplastic anemia. II. Pathogenesis, diagnosis, treatment, and prognosis. *New England Journal of Medicine*, **306**, 712–18.

Cartwright, R. A., McKinney, P. A., Williams, L., Miller, J. G., Evans, D. I., Bentley, D. P and Bhavnani, M. (1988) Aplastic anaemia incidence in parts of the United Kingdom in 1985. *Leukaemia Research*, **12**, 459–63.

Champlin, R. E., Ho, W. G., Feig, S. A., Winston, D. J., Lenarsky, C and Gale, R. P. (1985) Do androgens enhance the response to antithymocyte globulin in patients with aplastic anemia? A prospective randomized trial. *Blood*, **66**, 184–8.

Chapuis, B., Von Fliedner, V. E., Jeannet, M., Merica, H., Vuagnat, P., Gratwohl, A., Nissen, C. and Speck, B. (1986) Increased frequency of DR2 in patients with aplastic anaemia and increased DR sharing in their parents. *British Journal of Haematology*, **63**, 51–7.

Clausen, N. (1986) A population study of severe aplastic anemia in children. Incidence, etiology and course. *Acta Paediatrica Scandinavica*, **75**, 58–63.

Clausen, N., Kreuger, A., Salmi, T., Storm Mathisen, I. and Johannesson, G. (1996) Severe aplastic anaemia in the Nordic countries: a population based study of incidence, presentation, course, and outcome. *Archives of Disease in Childhood*, **74**, 319–22.

Crump, K. S. (1994) Risk of benzene-induced leukemia: a sensitivity analysis of the pliofilm cohort with additional follow-up and new exposure estimates. *Journal of Toxicology and Environmental Health*, **42**, 219–42.

Custer, R. P. (1946) Aplastic anemia in soldiers treated with Atebrin (Quinacrine). *American Journal of Medical Science*, **212**, 211–24.

Dimmel, H. (1933) Zur Klinik der chronischen Benzolvergiftung. *Archiv der Gewerbehygiene und Gewerbepathologie*, **4**, 414–64.

Doney, K., Dahlberg, S. J., Monroe, D., Storb, R., Buckner, C. D. and Thomas, E. D. (1984) Therapy of severe aplastic anemia with anti-human thymocyte globulin and androgens: the effect of HLA-haploidentical marrow infusion. *Blood*, **63**, 342–8.

Durrant, S. and Read, D. (1982) Fatal aplastic anaemia associated with mianserin [Letter]. *British Medical Journal [Clinical Research]*, **285**, 437.

Evreux, J. C. and Loupi, E. (1985) Responsibility of meprobamate in bone marrow aplasia [Letter]. *Presse Medicale (Paris)*, **14**, 793.

Fraunfelder, F. T., Meyer, S. M., Bagby, G. C. Jr. and Dreis, M. W. (1985) Hematologic reactions to carbonic anhydrase inhibitors. *American Journal of Ophthalmology*, **100**, 79–81.

Gerson, W. T., Fine, D. G., Spielberg, S. P. and Sensenbrenner, L. L. (1983) Anticonvulsant-induced aplastic anemia: increased susceptibility for toxic drug metabolites in vitro. *Blood*, **61**, 889–93.

Girdwood, R. H. (1974) *Blood disorders due to drugs and other agents*. Amsterdam: Excerpta Medica.

Goldstein, B. D. (1988) Benzene toxicity. *State of the Art Review of Occupational Medicine*, **3**, 541–54.

Gordon–Smith, E. C. and Issaragrisil, S. (1992) Epidemiology of aplastic anemia. *Baillieres Clinical Haematology*, **5**, 475–92.

Guiguet, M., Baumelou, E. and Mary, J. Y. (1995) A case–control study of aplastic anaemia: occupational exposures. The French Cooperative Group for Epidemiological Study of Aplastic Anaemia. *International Journal of Epidemiology*, **24**, 993–9.

Heimpel, H. (1979) Laboratory aspects of aplastic anemia. In *Aplastic anemia*, ed. C. G. Geary, p. 63–81. London: Balliere Tindall.

Heimpel, H. and Heit, W. (1980) Drug-induced aplastic anaemia: clinical aspects. *Clinical Haematology*, **9**, 641–62.

Heimpel, H. and Kubanek, B. (1975) Pathophysiology of Aplastic Anaemia. *British Journal of Haematology Supplement*, **31**, 57–68.

Hussain, M. Z., Khan, A. G and Chaudhry, Z. A. (1973) Aplastic anemia associated with lithium therapy. *Canadian Medical Association Journal*, **108**, 724–5.

Inoue, H., Shinohara, K., Nomiyama, J. and Oeda, E. (1994) Fatal aplastic anemia caused by Epstein–Barr virus infection after autologous bone marrow transplantation for non-Hodgkin malignant lymphoma. *Internal Medicine*, **33**, 303–7.

Iro, H., Henschke, F. and Koenig, H. J. (1986) Reversible Panmyelopathie nach Captopril-Medikation. (Reversible panmyelopathy following captopril treatment). *Deutsche Medizinische Wochenschrift*, **111**, 139–41.

Israeli, A., Or, R. and Leitersdorf, E. (1985) Captopril-associated transient aplastic anemia. *Acta Haematologica (Basel)*, **73**, 106–7.

Issaragrisil, S., Sriratanasatavorn, C., Piankijagum, A., Vannasaeng, S., Porapakkham, Y., Leaverton, P. E., Kaufman, D. W., Anderson, T. E., Shapiro, S. and Young, N. S. (1991) Incidence of aplastic anemia in Bangkok. The Aplastic Anemia Study Group. *Blood*, **77**, 2166–8.

Issaragrisil, S., Kaufman, D. W and Anderson, T. (1996) Incidence and non-drug aetiologies of aplastic anaemia in Thailand. The Thai Aplastic Anaemia Study Group. *European Journal of Haematology Supplement*, **60**, 31–4.

Issaragrisil, S., Chansung, K., Kaufman, D. W., Sirijirachai, J., Thamprasit, T. and Young, N. S. (1997a) Aplastic anemia in rural Thailand: its association with grain farming and agricultural pesticide exposure. Aplastic Anemia Study Group. *American Journal of Public Health*, **87**, 1551–4.

Issaragrisil, S., Kaufman, D., Thongput, A., Chansung, K., Thamprasit, T., Piankijagum, A., Anderson, T., Shapiro, S., Leaverton, P. and Young, N. S. (1997b) Association of seropositivity for hepatitis viruses and aplastic anemia in Thailand. *Hepatology*, **25**, 1255–7.

Issaragrisil, S., Kaufman, D. W., Anderson, T., Chansung, K., Thamprasit, T., Sirijirachai, J., Piankijagum, A., Porapakkham, Y., Vannasaeng, S., Leaverton, P. E. et al. (1997c) Low drug attributability of aplastic anemia in Thailand. The Aplastic Anemia Study Group. *Blood*, **89**, 4034–9.

Kanoh, T., Jingami, H. and Uchino, H. (1977) Aplastic anaemia after prolonged treatment with chlorpheniramine [Letter]. *Lancet*, **1**, 546–7.

Kao, T. W., Hung, C. C., Chen, Y. C. and Tien, H. F. (1997) Ticlopidine-induced aplastic anemia: report of three Chinese patients and review of the literature. *Acta Haematologica (Basel)*, **98**, 211–13.

Kaufman, D. W., Kelly, J. P., Anderson, T., Harmon, D. C. and Shapiro, S. (1997) Evaluation of case reports of aplastic anemia among patients treated with felbamate. *Epilepsia*, **38**, 1265–9.

Kaufman, D. W., Kelly, J. P., Levy, M. et al. (1991) *The drug etiology of agranulocytosis and aplastic anemia.* New York: Oxford University Press.

Kaufman, D. W., Kelly, J. P., Jurgelon, J. M., Anderson, T., Issaragrisil, S., Wiholm, B. E., Young, N. S., Leaverton, P., Levy, M. and Shapiro, S. (1996) Drugs in the aetiology of agranulocytosis and aplastic anaemia. *European Journal of Haematology Supplement*, **60**, 23–30.

Keiser, G. and Walder, H. R. (1970) Die idiopathischen und die medikamentös erworbenen aplastischen Anämien. *Schweizerische Medizinische Wochenschrift*, **100**, 697.

Keisu, M., Heit, W., Lambertenghi Deliliers, G., Parcells Kelly, J., Polliack, A. and Heimpel, H. (1990a) Transient pancytopenia. A report from the International Agranulocytosis and Aplastic Anemia Study. *Blut*, **61**, 240–4.

Keisu, M., Wiholm, B. E., Ost, A. and Mortimer, O. (1990b) Acetazolamide-associated aplastic anaemia. *Journal of Internal Medicine*, **228**, 627–32.

Kern, P., Heimpel, H., Heit, W. and Kubanek, B. (1975) Bone-marrow cells resistant to chloramphenicol in chloramphenicol-induced aplastic anaemia [Letter]. *Lancet*, **1**, 1190.

Kim, C. R., Maley, M. B. and Mohler, E. R. Jr. (1989) Captopril and aplastic anemia [Letter]. *Annals of Internal Medicine*, **111**, 187–8.

Kissling, M. and Speck, B. (1972) Further studies on experimental benzene induced aplastic anemia. *Blut*, **25**, 97–103.

Laidlaw, S. T., Snowden, J. A. and Brown, M. J. (1993) Aplastic anaemia and remoxipride [Letter]. *Lancet*, **342**, 1245.

Lewis, S. M. (1965) Course and prognosis in aplastic anemia. *British Medical Journal*, **I**, 1027–31.

Linet, M. S., McCaffrey, L. D., Morgan, W. F., Bearden, J. D. III, Szklo, M., Sensenbrenner, L. L., Markowitz, J. A., Tielsch, J. M. and Warm, S. G. (1986) Incidence of aplastic anemia in a three county area in South Carolina. *Cancer Research*, **46**, 426–9.

Linet, M. S., Markowitz, J. A., Sensenbrenner, L. L., Warm, S. G., Weida, S., Van Natta, M. L. and Szklo, M. (1989) A case–control study of aplastic anemia. *Leukaemia Research*, **13**, 3–11.

Lowenthal, R. M. and Marsden, K. A. (1997) Myelodysplastic syndromes. *International Journal of Hematology*, **65**, 319–38.

Loya, F. (1996) Does the hepatitis G virus cause hepatitis? *Texas Medicine*, **92**, 68–73.

Mary, J. C., Baumelou, E. and Guiguet, M. (1990) Epidemiology of aplastic anemia in France: a prospective multicentric study. *Blood*, **75**, 1646–53.

Mary, J. Y., Guiguet, M. and Baumelou, E. (1996) Drug use and aplastic anaemia: the French experience. French Cooperative Group for the Epidemiological Study of Aplastic Anaemia. *European Journal of Haematology Supplement*, **60**, 35–41.

Mayer, A., Podlech, J., Kurz, S., Steffens, H. P., Maiberger, S., Thalmeier, K., Angele, P., Dreher, L. and Reddehase, M. J. (1997) Bone marrow failure by cytomegalovirus is associated with an in vivo deficiency in the expression of essential stromal hemopoietin genes. *Journal of Virology*, **71**, 4589–98.

Mir, M. A. and Geary, C. G. (1980) Aplastic anemia:an analysis of 174 patients. *Postgraduate Medical Journal*, **56**, 322–6.

Modan, B., Segal, S., Shani, M. and Sheba, C. (1975) Aplastic anemia in Israel: evaluation of the etiological role of chloramphenicol on a community wide basis. *American Journal of Medical Science*, **270**, 441–45.

Moore, N. C., Lerer, B., Meyendorff, E. and Gershon, S. (1985) Three cases of carbamazepine toxicity. *American Journal of Psychiatry*, **142**, 974–5.

Morgan, D. P., Roberts, R. J., Walter, A. W. and Stockdale, E. M. (1980) Anemia associated with exposure to lindane. *Archives of Environmental Health*, **35**, 307–10.

Morgan, G. J., Palmer, S. R., Onions, D., Anderson, M., Cartwright, R. A. and Bentley, D. P. (1988) A cluster of three cases of aplastic anaemia in children. *Clinical and Laboratory Haematology*, **10**, 29–32.

Nakao, S., Takami, A., Sugimori, N., Ueda, M., Shiobara, S., Matsuda, T. and Mizoguchi, H. (1996) Response to immunosuppressive therapy and an HLA-DRB1 allele in patients with aplastic anaemia: HLA-DRB1*1501 does not predict response to antithymocyte globulin. *British Journal of Haematology*, **92**, 155–8.

Nimer, S. D., Ireland, P., Meshkinpour, A. and Frane, M. (1994) An increased HLA DR2 frequency is seen in aplastic anemia patients. *Blood*, **84**, 923–7.

Paci, E., Buiatti, E., Seniori Costantini, A. S., Miligi, L., Pucci, N., Scarpelli, A., Petrioli, G., Simonato, L., Winkelmann, R. and Kaldor, J. M. (1989) Aplastic anemia, leukemia and other cancer mortality in a cohort of shoe workers exposed to benzene. *Scandinavian Journal of Work, Environment and Health*, **15**, 313–18.

Pennell, P. B., Ogaily, M. S. and Macdonald, R. L. (1995) Aplastic anemia in a patient receiving felbamate for complex partial seizures. *Neurology*, **45**, 456–60.

Philpott, N. J., Marsh, J. C., Gordon–Smith, E. C. and Bolton, J. S. (1993) Aplastic anaemia and remoxipride [Letter] [see Comments]. *Lancet*, **342**, 1244–5.

Pisciotta, A. V. (1975) Hematologic toxicity of carbamazepine. *Advances in Neurology*, **11**, 355–68.

Rapoport, J. and Barratt, J. (1974) Idiosyncrasy to phenothiazines in phenylbutazone-associated aplastic anaemia [Letter]. *British Medical Journal*, **4**, 48.

Rauch, A. E., Kowalsky, S. F., Lesar, T. S., Sauerbier, G. A., Burkart, P. T. and Scharfman, W. B. (1990) Lindane (Kwell)-induced aplastic anemia. *Archives of Internal Medicine*, **150**, 2393–5.

Rinsky, R. A., Smith, A. B., Hornung, R. et al. (1987) Benzene and leukemia: an epidemiologic risk assessment. *New England Journal of Medicine*, **316**, 1044–50.

Roberts, H. J. (1990) Pentachlorophenol-associated aplastic anemia, red cell aplasia, leukemia and other blood disorders. *Journal of the Florida Medical Association*, **77**, 86–90.

Rothman, N., Li, G. L., Dosemeci, M., Bechtold, W. E., Marti, G. E., Wang, Y. Z., Linet, M., Xi, L. Q., Lu, W., Smith, M. T. et al. (1996) Hematotoxocity among Chinese workers heavily exposed to benzene [see Comments]. *American Journal of Industrial Medicine*, **29**, 236–46.

Rugman, F. P. and Cosstick, R. (1990) Aplastic anaemia associated with organochlorine pesticide: case reports and review of evidence. *Journal of Clinical Pathology*, **43**, 98–101.

Saita, G. (1974) Benzene induced hypoplastic anemias and leukemias. In *Blood disorders due to drugs and other agents*, ed. R. H. Girdwood, pp. 127–46. Amsterdam: Excerpta Medica.

Shapiro, S. and Fraunfelder, F. T. (1992) Acetazolamide and aplastic anemia. *American Journal of Ophthalmology*, **113**, 328–30.

Singh, N. and Carrigan, D. R. (1996) Human herpesvirus-6 in transplantation: an emerging pathogen. *Annals of Internal Medicine*, **124**, 1065–71.

Smith, M. T. (1996) Overview of benzene-induced aplastic anaemia. *European Journal of Haematology Supplement*, **60**, 107–10.

Strair, R. K., Mitch, W. E., Faller, D. V. and Skorecki, K. L. (1985) Reversible captopril-associated bone marrow aplasia [Letter]. *Canadian Medical Association Journal*, **132**, 320–2.

Swanson, M. and Cook, R. (1977) *Drugs, chemicals and blood dyscrasias*. Hamilton, IL: Drug Intelligence Publications.

Szklo, M., Sensenbrenner, L., Markowitz, J., Weida, S., Warm, S. and Linet, M. (1985) Incidence of aplastic anemia in metropolitan Baltimore: a population-based study. *Blood*, **66**, 115–19.

The International Agranulocytosis and Aplastic Anemia Study (1987) Incidence of aplastic anemia: the relevance of diagnostic criteria. *Blood*, **70**, 1718–821.

Tichelli, A., Gratwohl, A., Nissen, C. and Speck, B. (1994) Late clonal complications in severe aplastic anemia. *Leukemia and Lymphoma*, **12**, 167–75.

Tomita, S., Kurokawa, T., Ueda, K. and Higuchi, S. (1985) Aplastic anaemia induced by intravenous phenytoin and lidocaine administration [Letter]. *European Journal of Pediatrics*, **144**, 207–8.

Troussard, X., Mayo, P., Mosquet, B., Reman, O. and Leporrier, M. (1992) Ticlopidine and severe aplastic anaemia. *British Journal of Haematology*, **82**, 779–80.

Wallerstein, R. O., Condit, P. K., Casper, C. K. et al. (1969) State wide study of chloramphenicol therapy and aplastic anemia. *Journal of the American Medical Association*, **208**, 2045–50.

Wang, H. H. and Gruffermann, S. (1981) Aplastic anemia and occupational pesticide exposure: a case–control study. *Journal of Occupationl Medicine*, **23**, 365–6.

Ward, E., Hornung, R., Morris, J., Rinsky, R. A., Wild, D., Halperin, W. and Guthrie, W. (1996) Risk of low red or white blood cell count related to estimated benzene exposure in a rubberworker cohort (1940–1975). *American Journal of Industrial Medicine*, **29**, 247–57.

Welch, H., Lewis, C. N. and Kerlan, I. (1954) Blood dyscrasias, a nationwide survey. *Antibiotics and Chemotherapy*, **4**, 607.

Williams, D. M., Lynch, R. E. and Cartwright, G. E. (1973) Drug-induced aplastic anemia. *Seminars in Hematology*, **10**, 195–223.

Wilson, R. H. (1942) Benzene poisoning in industry. *Journal of Laboratory and Clinical Medicine*, **27**, 1517–21.

Wisch, N., Fischbein, F. I., Siegel, R., Glass, J. L. and Leopold, I. (1973) Aplastic anemia resulting from the use of carbonic anhydrase inhibitors. *American Journal of Ophthalmology*, **75**, 130–2.

Yin, S. N., Hayes, R. B., Linet, M. S., Li, G. L., Dosemeci, M., Travis, L. B., Li, C. Y., Zhang, Z. N., Li, D. G., Chow, W. H. et al. (1996*a*) A cohort study of cancer among benzene-exposed workers in China: overall results. *American Journal of Industrial Medicine*, **29**, 227–35.

Yin, S. N., Hayes, R. B., Linet, M. S., Li, G. L., Dosemeci, M., Travis, L. B., Zhang, Z. N., Li, D. G., Chow, W. H., Wacholder, S. et al. (1996*b*) An expanded cohort study of cancer among benzene-exposed workers in China. Benzene Study Group. *Environmental Health Perspectives*, **104** [Suppl. 6], 1339–41.

Young, N. S. and Mortimer, P. (1984) Viruses and bone marrow failure. *Blood*, **63**, 729–37.

Zeldis, J. B. (1989) Aplastic anemia after liver transplantation for fulminant viral hepatitis: black box or bag of worms. *Hepatology*, **10**, 520–1.

8

Clinical presentation, natural course, and prognostic factors

Pedro Marín-Fernandez

Farreras Valenti Hospital Clinic, Barcelona

Clinical manifestations

Medullary aplasia does not have specific signs and symptoms, and its clinical manifestations are similar to those observed in other oncohematological diseases such as acute leukemia, some types of lymphomas, myelosclerosis, myelodysplasia, and following chemotherapy or radiotherapy treatment. They are caused by hemopoietic failure and the intensity of expression is directly related to the degree of pancytopenia.

The patient usually consults with an anemic syndrome together with skin or mucosal hemorrhages (Marín, 1981:114; Rozman et al., 1981:321; Scott et al.,1959:119; Williams et al., 1973:195). Patients present less frequently with an isolated infection or anemic syndrome as the initial manifestation of the disease (Marín, 1981:116; Rozman et al., 1981:321). Disease perception may vary considerably. While some patients are diagnosed during a routine health check-up and are practically asymptomatic, others present an acute clinical situation. This explains why the time that elapses between the initial presentation of symptoms and medical attention varies considerably, from days to years, reflecting the behavior and severity of the disease (Lynch, 1975:517; Marín, 1981:115; Rozman et al., 1981:321; Williams et al., 1973:195). The anemic syndrome, together with hemorrhages, is the most frequently described clinical presentation, which in half of the cases is accompanied by hemodynamic symptoms that may disclose prior cardiovascular abnormalities (Marín, 1981:114). Hemorrhagic symptoms are usually slight and easily controlled, and manifest as ecchymoses, petechiae, epistaxis or visual field defects. However, in 20% of cases they can be severe and cause death. Fever occurs in 30–40% of cases and is responsible for 6% of deaths at presentation (Marín, 1981:116; Rozman et al., 1981:321; Williams et al., 1973:195). Only physical examination can confirm the presence of anemia, infections or hemorrhages. Splenomegaly or lymph node enlargement can only be explained in the context of an infection (Williams et al., 1973:195).

Complementary investigations

Peripheral blood cell counts

All patients present a low count of all three blood elements during the course of the disease, but in only 83% of cases are they all present at diagnosis (Li et al., 1972:153; Marín, 1981:117; Rozman et al., 1981:321). In the remaining cases, one or two cell lines are initially affected and the complete picture appears during follow-up. Decreased cell production of neutrophils and platelets rather than erythrocytes is observed because of their different cell kinetics (Dreyfus, 1959:62; Heimpel et al., 1975:235; Huhn et al., 1975:7; Van der Weyden and Firkin, 1972:1; Williams, 1973:195).

The most frequent cytopenia at diagnosis is thrombocytopenia (Li et al., 1972:153; Williams et al., 1973:195). Seventy per cent of patients present counts below $30 \times 10^9/l$ (Marín, 1981:115). Platelet size and half-life are normal and no data are available on their functional state (Adam et al., 1973:9; Marín, 1981:118; Najean et al., 1966:1071,1973:529).

Although in less aggressive presentations neutrophil counts may be normal, neutropenia is generally the rule. Differential analysis may disclose a small percentage of myelocytes and metamyelocytes (Scott et al., 1959:119). A decrease in the number of monocytes, in proportion to the number of neutrophils, may be observed (Twomey et al., 1973:187; Williams et al., 1973:195), although the count may be normal or even show a relative monocytosis (Marín, 1981:116; Rozman et al., 1981:321). There is little information on changes in basophil and eosinophil counts in this disease. Studies of the abnormalities of granulocyte function are inconclusive (Clark et al., 1976:22; Territo et al., 1977:245).

Neutropenia is more frequent than leukopenia, since the total number of lymphocytes may be normal or even increased. During follow-up lymphopenia may appear in 40% of cases (Heimpel et al. 1975:235; Huhn et al., 1975:7; Rozman et al., 1981:321; Scott et al., 1959:119; Williams et al., 1973:195). Lymphocyte morphology is normal and a small proportion of stimulating elements may be detected (Bacon et al., 1975:201). No disproportion of the different lymphoid populations has been detected by flow cytometry analysis (Torok-Storb et al., 1985:1015).

Anemia is accompanied by reticulopenia which may be absolute (Heimpel and Kubanek, 1975:57; Hellriegel et al., 1977:11; Huhn et al., 1975:7; Lewis, 1965:1027; Lohrman et al., 1976a:647, 1976b:599; Marín, 1981:118; Rozman et al., 1987:955; Vincent and De Gruchi, 1967:977; Williams et al., 1973:195). The total number of erythrocytes and the hemoglobin value depend on the transfusion requirements. The most reliable parameter for monitoring the red cell series is the number of reticulocytes. Its count may vary depending on the method used. It is preferable to obtain the percentage of reticulocytes corrected for the packed cell volume, than to use the absolute value. In some patients, transfused or not, an increase in the mean corpuscular volume may be detected (Baldridge, 1935:759; Marín, 1981:118; Rozman et al., 1981:321, 1985:982, 1987:955; Scott et al., 1959:119). Erythrocyte morphology is characterized by anisopoichilocytosis. The presence of a small percentage of erythroblasts is not incompatible with the diagnosis (Hasselbach and Thomas, 1960:1253; Scott et al., 1959:119). Increases in the concentrations of fetal hemoglobin (Alter et al., 1976:843; Bloom and Diamond, 1968:304; Marín, 1981:117; Shahidi et al., 1962:117) and some erythrocyte enzymes may also be observed (Boivin, 1977:221; Kleeberg et al., 1971:557). Most of these elements reflect dyserythropoiesis, which may accompany hemopoietic insufficiency and should be considered in the differential diagnosis of medullary aplasia (Alter et al., 1976:843; Lewis, 1969:49; Lewis and Verwilghem, 1973:99, 1977:3).

Other analytical data

The abnormal proliferation and maturation of the red cells induce secondary modifications in iron metabolism with a final positive balance, and a tendency towards liver hemosiderosis, an increase in medullary and macrophagic iron, and an increase in serum iron and ferritinemia (Marín, 1981:120). The transfusion requirements and the presence of severe hemorrhages may alter or increase these abnormalities. No abnormalities in the intestinal absorption of iron have been detected.

No abnormalities in the serum levels of coagulation factors have been detected (Rasche, 1975:1137). Erythrocyte sedimentation rate is increased due either to the anemia and/or the accompanying complications (Heimpel et al., 1975:235; Marín, 1981:119; Vincent and De Gruchy, 1967:977).

Some authors have detected up to 15% of patients with a deficit in their immunoglobulins (Huhn et al., 1975:7). A polyclonal hypergammaglobulinemia may appear during follow-up in relation to the associated complications. Increases in the circulating levels of unconjugated bilirubin, lactodehydrogenase and aldolase are evidence of inefficiencies in erythropoiesis related to the presence of dyserythropoiesis.

The cytology and histopathology of medullary aplasia

A myelogram is not a diagnostic test for medullary aplasia, but it is useful in the differential diagnosis since it may disclose neoplastic cells or the presence of qualitative abnormalities of hemopoiesis. The distribution of the aplastic lesion is heterogeneous, with empty medullary areas coexisting with others of normal aspect. Hypocellularity with decreased numbers or the absence of one or all blood series is usually detected (Gruppo et al., 1977:29; Lewis, 1965:1027; Marín 1981:125). This hypocellularity is accompanied by increased numbers of adipose, stromal, lymphocyte, plasma and macrophage cells. Some of these cells, histori- cally considered as unimportant, are now known to be involved in the patho- physiology of the disease. The decrease in hemopoiesis can be quantified as the percentage of nonmyeloid cellularity. For this, all types of hemopoietic and stromal cellularity are counted in 500–1000 cells: red series elements except erythrocytes, the granulopoietic series, lymphocytes, monocytes, megakaryocy- tes, mast, plasma, and reticular cells. Myeloid cellularity (MC) is considered to be formed by any cell in any maturation stage of the red series, the white series up to the maturation stage of metamyelocytes, and megakaryocytes (Lynch et al., 1975:517). The percentage of nonmyeloid cellularity (%NMC) is obtained from the following calculation:

$$\% \, NMC = [(TC–MC)/TC] \times 100$$

Where TC is total cellularity. Aplastic anemia may be accompanied by dyserythro- poiesis (Frisch et al., 1975:545; Geary et al., 1974:337; Lewis, 1969:49; Lewis and Verwilghem, 1973:99, 1977:3; Lewis et al., 1961:64; McGibbon and Mollin, 1965:59). The visual diagnosis of this entity is based on the bi- or multinuclearity of erythro- blasts, the presence of internuclear bridges, megaloblastosis, nucleocytoplasmatic maturation asynchrony, nuclear degenerative signs, and mitotic abnormalities, cytoplasmatic abnormalities such as vacuolization and an increase in siderotic granulation, intercytoplasmatic bridges, and occasionally ring sideroblasts. Ultra- structural analysis may help by revealing numerous and complex abnormalities such as bi- or multinuclearity with intranuclear chromatinic bridges and microtu- bules, variable mitochondrial size, changes in the quantity and distribution of ribosomes, irregular nuclei with euchromatin and heterochromatin clefts, abnormalities of the nuclear membrane, and signs of functional failure, such as nuclear substance leak and the abnormal presence of cytoplasmic material in the nucleus (Frisch et al., 1975:545). The presence of dyserythropoiesis is not well explained. Suggested hypotheses are that it originates from the same etiological agent as produced the aplasia, as would be the case in benzole intoxication, that is relates to the preexisting clonal disease (nocturnal paroxystic hemoglobinuria, myelodysplasia/acute leukemia), and that it appears at the time of hemopoietic regeneration after treatment. The qualitative morphological abnormalities can also appear in the granulopoietic and megakaryocytic series. While the selective lesions of the erythroblast series have no special significance, those observed in the remaining hemopoietic series, especially in the megakaryocytes, may be predictive of the long-term appearance of a myelodysplastic syndrome/acute leukemia (De Planque et al., 1988:55).

Medullary biopsy is essential for the diagnosis of aplasia and contributes to the differential diagnosis (Burkhardt, 1966:326; Duhamel et al., 1978:17; Hernandez-Nieto and Rozman, 1980:4; Jamshidi and Swaim, 1971:335; January and Fowler, 1943:792; Kansu and Erslev, 1976:326; Marín, 1981:135; Marín and Rozman, 1983:291; Rozman et al., 1985:982; Te Velde and Haak, 1977:61), but is of no use for following the outcome of the disease. The specimen should be obtained from a bone area distant from that biopsied previously, and the size should be not less than 1 cm in length measured from the cortical area. In this way one eliminates the error of interpreting as pathological the subcortical fat area which exists in normal subjects, as well as evaluating lesion distribution heterogeneity by detecting subcortical hypercellular foci. Interpreting medullary cellularity from biopsy samples can vary depending on the patient's age and the interpretation method used, so that the measurement error amounts to 20% for specimens from normal individuals. The appropriate technique for preparing the sample is that described by Te Velde (Te Velde and Haak, 1977:61) using methacrylate, as it results in better preservation and less modification of cell structure than when paraffin is used. The characteristic image is that of hemopoietic tissue replaced by fat tissue in the presence of lymphoid, plasma, and macrophage cells in the absence of fibrosis, although some authors accept the presence of some reticulinic fibrosis. The lesion of the reticulinic structure is defined as an interstitial hemorrhage and interfibrillar edema; this latter lesion must be differentiated from medullary gelatinous transformation. Other characteristic features of aplasia are: (1) the presence of focal hyperplasia of erythroid and granulocytic cells at a similar maturation stage, with abundant mitoses and signs of dyserythropoiesis (Heimpel et al., 1975:235; Te Velde and Haak, 1977:61); and (2) increases of macrophage numbers and reticular iron. The frequency of the most common histopathological lesions observed in biopsied samples from a consecutive series of 113 patients from our unit (Rozman et al., 1985:982) is shown in Table 8.1. Three categories of hemopoietic cellularity decrease can be identified: stage I, a moderate decrease; stage II, clearly hypocellular bone marrow or irregularly distributed (like a chess board); stage III, empty bone marrow, in which only fat and stroma cells can be observed. The analysis of lymphoplasmocytic infiltration identified the following categories: stage 0, no infiltration; stage I, some isolated lymphoplasmocytic focus; stage II, marked infiltration together with nonaffected areas; and stage III, infiltration throughout the entire sample. Interstitial hemorrhage has been subdivided into the following categories: stage 0, absent or seen in less than 10% of the sample; stage I, observed in an area between 10 and 50% of the entire sample; and stage II, present in more that 50% of the sample. Interfibrillar edema, which is recognized as an eosinophilic, amorphous or finely granular substance, has been classified into the following categories: stage 0, absent; stage I, involving less than 50% of the interstitium; and stage II, involving more than 50% of the interstitium.

Table 8.1. Bone marrow histopathology of 113 patients. Hospital Clinic (1974–84). University of Barcelona, Spain

	Stage			
	0	I	II	III
Cellularity/fat tissue (%)	—	1	31	68
Lymphoplasmocytic infiltration (%)	13	35	37	15
Hemorrhage (%)	3	73	24	—
Edema (%)	7	60	33	—

Isotopic investigations of hemopoiesis

Patients with medullary aplasia are incapable of incorporating iron into their erythroblasts. This fact has been used to develop isotopic investigations to quantify the degree of erythropoietic failure. Using the isotope ^{59}Fe in the form of ferrous citrate has allowed the pattern of aplasia to be established, i.e., an increase in plasma iron levels, prolonged clearance of the isotope and reduced incorporation (Najean et al., 1965:639; Scott et al., 1959:119). Unfortunately, these tests are of little practical use, since they are very long and also require much time to be interpreted, but they may be used in the differential diagnosis of refractory anemias in which the plasma clearance of the isotope is normal. Simplifying the tests by using other isotopes, such as ^{52}Fe and ^{55}Fe, has not solved the problem either, given the difficulty in obtaining these isotopes and the degree of patient irradiation required (Anger and Van Dyke, 1964:1587; Chaudhuri et al., 1974:667). An alternative to the ferrokinetic studies is to use scintigraphy with indium-113 (^{113}In). This isotope is transported by plasma transferrin to the erythroid bone marrow. Its properties (half-life of 2.8 days, gamma emission of 0.17 and 0.25 MeV) allow it to be used in scintigraphy. This examination is useful for identifying the distribution of areas of residual hemopoiesis (Goodwin et al., 1971:75; Hosain et al., 1969; McNeil et al., 1974:647, 1976:599).

Proton magnetic resonance imaging and spectroscopy

Magnetic resonance imaging (MRI) can visualize bone marrow more clearly than other imaging techniques, since bone generates weak signals whereas fat in the marrow gives strong signals. Chemical shift imaging techniques can be used to explore the presence of protons in fat and water in the marrow. In bone marrow hypoplasia the hemopoietic cells are replaced by fat cells resulting in a shortening of the T1 phase of the MRI image (Kaplan et al., 1987:441; McKinstry et al., 1987:701; Olson et al., 1986:540). Localized hyperplastic areas within the abnormal marrow fat can be visualized (Yoshida et al., 1985:47). However, some children with aplastic anemia have a uniformly intense MRI signal from the femur, knee and hip similar to normal controls (Cohen et al., 1984:715; Kangarloo et al., 1986:205). Comparing the water-to-fat ratio quantitatively, it is feasible to discriminate between the different patterns. MRI is a noninvasive method of analyzing and quantifying the bone marrow content in aplastic anemia (Amano and Kumazaki, 1997:286), but further investigation is necessary to confirm the clinical relevance of this technique.

Follow-up and survival

The natural history of the disease is unpredictable but implies a high mortality, of greater than 70% 5 years after diagnosis. Fewer than 5% of patients go into a spontaneous remission once the etiological agent is eliminated (Bottiger and Westerholm, 1972:315; Cronkite, 1967:273; Lewis, 1965:1027; Li et al., 1972:153, Marín 1981:140; Najean et al, 1965:639; O'Gorman Hughes, 1973:361; Vincent and De Gruchy, 1967:977; Williams et al., 1973:195). Hemorrhage is the first cause of death, although it is usually accompanied by infection. The hemorrhage is caused by thrombocytopenia, while infection is the aggravating factor for hemorrhagic risk (Lewis, 1965:1027; Marín, 1981:140; Van der Weyden and Firkin, 1972:1; Williams et al., 1973:195). The most frequent infections are caused by bacteria, but the use of immunosuppressive treatments has changed the spectrum so that fungal infections are now frequently detected. The complications of long-term hemotherapeutic treatment, of mainly hemosiderosis and viral infections, and the development of a clonal disease such as a myelodysplastic syndrome/acute leukemia or nocturnal paroxysmal hemoglobinuria, cause long-term morbidity and mortality even in cured patients.

The actuarial survival curve is biphasic, suggesting two types of behavior. One group of patients, about 40%, die in the first 3 months after diagnosis. The remainder have a more or less chronic course which can last several years (Marín, 1981:140; Williams et al., 1973:195). This biphasic behavior is observed in all the general series, including our own (Figure 8.1) independent of the year of publication and the treatments received. Defining the parameters that differentiate between both groups is important for indicating the optimal treatment in each particular case, as is using a common language to communicate between the different health teams involved in managing these patients.

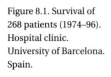

Figure 8.1. Survival of
268 patients (1974–96).
Hospital clinic.
University of Barcelona.
Spain.

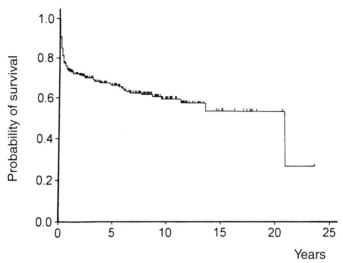

Prognosis identification

Disease severity, and consequently patient survival, are directly related to the degree of hemopoietic failure. It is impossible to quantify the degree of this failure directly, so its consequences and the reliability of some of the complementary investigations have been analyzed (Boggs and Boggs, 1976:71).

The prognostic value of symptoms

The clinical criteria of the acute, severe forms of aplasia are its spectacular symptoms, especially if they are mainly hemorrhagic, and the rapid onset, which prompt the patient to seek urgent medical attention (Camitta et al., 1979:504; Lewis, 1965:1027; Lynch et al., 1975:517; Marín, 1981:143; Najean and Bernard, 1965:1; Williams et al., 1973:195). Not all authors agree that females with aplasia have a better prognosis than males (Williams et al., 1973:195), or that children have a worse prognosis than adults (Lewis, 1965:1027; Li et al., 1972:153; Lorhman et al., 1976b:599; Marín, 1981:143; Najean and Bernard, 1965:1; Williams et al., 1973:195). Etiology does not seem to play any role (Camitta et al., 1979:504; Lewis, 1965:1027).

The prognostic value of peripheral blood cell counts

There is a direct relationship between the intensity of hemopoietic failure and the degree of peripheral blood cytopenia, but its evaluation is not easy. Transfusion is one of the first therapeutic measures to be performed before the diagnosis is made, and it distorts the hemoglobin levels and erythrocyte count. Furthermore, the degree of neutropenia and thrombocytopenia, which are less

Table 8.2. Clinical/biological data at diagnosis and prognostic impact for 268 patients. Hospital clinic (1974–96). University of Barcelona, Spain

Variable	Value	Prognosis (P)
Delay between time of first symptoms and diagnosis (days)	*61 (3–280)	<0.025
Anemic syndrome (%)	84	N.S.
Infection (%)	38	N.S.
Hemorrhage (%)	82	N.S.
Hemoglobin (g/l)	*73 (35–170)	N.S.
Total reticulocytes (100 ml)	*89 (0–1000)	<0.001
Corrected reticulocytes (%)	*0.19 (0–2.6)	<0.001
Mean corpuscular volume (fl)	*91 (74 118)	<0.005
Total leukocytes (10^9/l)	*2.4 (0.5–7.5)	<0.025
Granulocytes (10^9/l)	*0.75 (0–4.8)	<0.001
Monocytes (10^9/l)	*0.09 (0–1.0)	<0.001
Lymphocytes (10^9/l)	*1.5 (0.2–5.4)	N.S.
Platelets (10^9/l)	*16 (2–150)	<0.005
Erythrocyte sedimentation rate (mm/h)	*72 (5–175)	N.S.
Blood iron level (μg/ml)	*194 (50–370)	<0.05
Fetal hemoglobin (%)	*2 (0.5–8.5)	N.S.
Nonmyeloid cellularity (%)	*71 (15–98)	<0.005
^{59}Fe clearance (min)	#*172 (90–370)	<0.025
^{59}Fe incorporation (%)	#*48 (5–95)	<0.025

Notes:

* Median and range.

Data from 32 patients.

easily influenced, can change during an infection or because of an increased rate of destruction. When analyzed separately, the severity of neutropenia has been related to increased mortality (Killander et al., 1969:10; Lewis, 1965:1027; Marín, 1981:143; Mathé et al., 1970:131; Najean and Bernard, 1965:1; Williams et al., 1973:195). Some authors have pointed out that the total reticulocyte count is a more sensitive prognostic indicator than neutrophil and platelet counts (Lohrman et al., 1976a:647; Marín, 1981:145; Mathé et al., 1970:131; Williams et al., 1973:195). Using flow cytofluorimetry, Torok-Storb et al. (1985:1015) identified a population of small cells phenotypically associated with the erythroid lineage that was strongly associated with the response to immunomodulatory treatment. Combining the peripheral values of the three series has not been found to be very efficient, except when the degrees of reticulopenia, leukopenia

Table 8.3. Bone marrow histopathology of 113 patients. Prognosis. Hospital Clinic (1974–84), University of Barcelona, Spain

	Stage	O/E ratio	P
Cellularity/fat tissue	I+II versus III	0.54/1.35	<0.0025
Lymphoplasmocytic infiltration	0+I versus II+III	0.69/1.47	<0.0025
	0+I+II versus III	0.80/5.87	<0.0010
Hemorrhage			N.S.
Edema			N.S.

and thrombopenia are compared with survival at 4 months (Killander et al., 1969:10; Lynch et al., 1975:517). The increase in mean corpuscular volume is not correlated with the reticulocyte count and, in less severe forms, is associated with greater survival (Camitta et al., 1979:504; Marín, 1981:145). Mathé et al. (1970:131) described the worse prognosis of lymphocytosis. No data on monocyte, basophil and eosinophil counts are available.

In 1968, Bloom and Diamond (1968:304) described how a better prognosis is associated with an increase in fetal hemoglobin to levels above 400 mg/dl. This factor has been favorably considered by some pediatrics groups (Frish et al., 1975:545).

The prognostic value of the cytology and histopathology of medullary aplasia

Interest in myelograms and bone marrow biopsy is limited by the heterogeneous distribution of the aplastic lesion and the interpretation errors caused by the alterations that occur during sample obtention and processing. The only feature of the myelogram to be evaluated is nonmyeloid cellularity (Lynch et al., 1975:517; Marín, 1981:146; Najean and Pecking, 1979:564), the percentage of which correlates directly with disease severity. The degree of hemopoietic hypoplasia and the intensity of lymphoplasmocytic infiltration are usually accepted as prognostic factors (Frisch and Lewis, 1974:231; Lewis, 1965:1027; Li et al., 1972:153; Lynch et al., 1975:517, Marín and Rozman, 1983:291; Najean and Bernard, 1965:1; Te Velde and Haak, 1977:61; Williams et al., 1973:195), as also observed in our series (Rozman et al., 1985:982) (Table 8.3).

The prognostic value of isotope examinations

The utility of isotopes depends on problems associated with their application. In 1965 Najean described greater mortality 6 months after diagnosis when the incorporation of the iron isotope was equal or less than 11%, while life expectancy was above 1 year when clearance was greater than 43% (Najean and Bernard, 1965:1).

Table 8.4. Distribution percentiles of prognostic variables for 213 patients. Hospital clinic. University of Barcelona. Spain

Percentile	Reticulocytes (% corrected)	Granulocytes (10^9/l)	Platelets (10^9/l)	MVC (fl)
42.5	0.14	0.50	10	90
66	0.36	0.95	20	97
90	1.0	2.10	46	109

The utility of scintigraphy has also been described in a short series of 22 patients (McNeil et al., 1976:599).

Statistical prediction models

Since none of the prognostic elements analyzed is very reliable, some investigators have developed mathematical models based on association with criteria of high prognostic value, as shown by previous univariate analysis (Lynch et al., 1975:517; Najean and Pecking, 1979:564; Najean et al., 1979:343; Rozman et al., 1985:982; Wehinger and Lencer 1977:561). None of the prediction models has been accepted as a usual working tool, but they have allowed confirmation that they are no better than the experience of a competent physician.

International criteria

The most widely accepted criteria in publications and cooperative ventures are those established in 1975 (Camitta et al., 1975:355), based on the experience of Williams et al. (1973). These criteria combine data from peripheral blood and bone marrow and require the decrease of at least two of the peripheral cell values:

Neutrophils $\qquad$ $<0.5\times10^9$/l
Platelets $\qquad$ $<20\times10^9$/l
Anemia + reticulocytes corrected for packed cell volume $\qquad$ $<1\%$,

with the demonstration of hypocellularity in the myelogram calculated by the percentage of nonmyeloid cellularity (NMC) and the percentage of hemopoiesis reduction in the biopsied bone marrow sample:

Severe hypocellularity $\qquad$ $<25\%$ of NMC
Moderate hypocellularity (25–50%) $\qquad$ $>70\%$ of NMC.

   Two modifications of these criteria have been proposed. The first is the decrease in the percentage of reticulocytes (Rozman et al., 1987:955). In our experience 90% of 213 patients presented, at diagnosis, a corrected reticulocyte count below 1%, while only 42.5% exhibited a correlation between granulocyte and platelet counts and the criteria of severity (Table 8.4). The reticulocyte count should probably be lowered to around 0.15%. In this same study we were also able to confirm the prognostic implication of reductions in two or three peripheral-blood hematological values (Rozman et al., 1987:955).

The second modification (Gluckman et al., 1982:541) is to define the high-risk group as those having a neutropenia defined as counts lower than $0.2 \times 10^9/l$. This modification is being accepted, since the existence of this subgroup has been confirmed in the trials with new treatments.

Conclusion

Medullary aplasia does not have specific signs and symptoms and it is caused by hemopoietic failure. The intensity of clinical expression is directly related to the degree of pancytopenia. All patients present a low count of all three blood elements during the course of the disease. Anemia is accompanied by reticulopenia which may be absolute.

The most frequent cytopenia at diagnosis is thrombocytopenia. Although in less aggressive presentations neutrophil counts may be normal, neutropenia is generally the rule. Medullary biopsy is essential for the diagnosis. A myelogram is not a diagnostic test, but it is useful in the differential diagnosis. Aplastic anemia may be accompanied by dyserythropoiesis. While the selective lesions of the erythroblast series have no special significance, those observed in the remaining hemopoietic series, especially in the megakaryocytes, may be predictive of the long-term appearance of a myelodysplastic syndrome/acute leukemia. Isotopic investigations of hemopoiesis are of little practical use, since they are very long and also require much time to be interpreted, but they may be used in the differential diagnosis of refractory anemias. Magnetic resonance imaging (MRI) can visualize bone marrow more clearly than other imaging techniques, but further investigation is necessary to confirm the clinical relevance of this technique. The natural history of the disease is unpredictable but implies a high mortality, of greater than 70% 5 years after diagnosis. The actuarial survival curve is biphasic, suggesting two types of behavior. One group of patients, about 40%, die in the first 3 months after diagnosis. The remainder have a more or less chronic course which can last several years. Disease severity and consequently patient survival are directly related to the degree of hemopoietic failure. It is impossible to quantify the degree of this failure directly, but clinical, biological and other complementary investigations can be used, indirectly, in the prognostic analysis. The most widely accepted criteria in publications and cooperative ventures are those established in 1975 (Camitta et al., 1975:355).

References

Adam, W., Heimpel, H. and Kratt, E. (1973) Die Bestimmung der Thrombozytenlebenszeit mit 51Cr. II Untersuchungen über die Lebenszeit autologer Thrombozyten bei Patienten mit ausgeprägter Thrombozytopenie. *Blut*, **21**, 9.

Aksoy, M., Dinçol, K., Erdem, S., Akgün, T. and Dinçol, G. (1972) Details of blood changes in 32 patients with pancytopenia associated with long-term exposure to benzene. *British Industrial Medicine*, **29**, 56–63.

Alter, B. P., Rappeport, J. M., Huisman, T. H. J., Schroeder, W. A. and Nathan, D. G. (1976) Fetal erythropoiesis following bone marrow transplantation. *Blood*, **48**, 843–53.

Amano, Y. and Kumazaki, T. (1997) Proton MR imaging and spectroscopy evaluation of aplastic anemia: three bone patterns. *Journal of Computer Assisted Tomography*, **21**, 286–92.

Anger, H. O. and Van Dyke, D. C. (1964) Human bone marrow distribution shown in vivo by iron-52 and positron scintillation camera. *Science*, **144**, 1587–94.

Bacon, P. A., Sewell, R. and Crowther, D. (1975) Reactive lymphoid cells 'immunoblasts' in autoimmune and haematological disorders. *Clinical and Experimental Immunology*, **19**, 201–8.

Baldridge, C. W. (1935) Macrocytic anemia with aplastic features following the application of synthetic organic hair dye. *American Journal of Medical Science*, **189**, 759–64.

Bloom, G. E. and Diamond, L. X. (1968) Prognostic value of fetal hemoglobin levels in acquired aplastic anemia. *New England Journal of Medicine*, **278**, 304–7.

Boggs, D. R. and Boggs, S. S. (1976) The pathogenesis of aplastic anemia. A defective pluripotent hematopoietic stem cell with inappropiate balance of differentiation and selfreplication. *Blood*, **48**, 71–6.

Boivin, P. (1977) Red blood cell enzyme abnormalities in dyserythropoietic anaemias. In *Dyserythropoiesis*, ed. S. M. Lewis and R. L. Verwilghen, pp. 221. London: Academic Press.

Bottiger, L. E. and Westerholm, B. (1972) Aplastic anaemia I. Incidence and aetiology. *Acta Medica Scandinavica*, **192**, 315–18.

Burkhardt, R. (1966) Technische Verbesserungen und Auswendungsbereich der Histobiopsie von Knochenmark und Knochen. *Klinische Wochenschrift*, **44**, 326–34.

Camitta, B. M., Rappeport, J. M., Parkman, R. and Nathan, D. C. (1975) Selection of patients for bone marrow transplantation in severe aplastic anemia. *Blood*, **45**, 355–63.

Camitta, B. M., Thomas, E. D., Nathan, D. C., Gale, R. P., Kopeckyk. J., Rappeport, J. M., Santos, G., Gordon–Smith, E. C. and Storb, R. (1979) A prospective study of androgens and bone marrow transplantation for treatment of severe aplastic anemia. *Blood*, **53**, 504–14.

Chaudhuri, T. K., Ehrhardt, J. C. R., De Gowen, P. L. and Christie, J. H. (1974) ^{59}Fe whole body scanning. *Journal of Nuclear Medicine*, **15**, 667–73.

Clark, R. A., Johnson, F. L., Klebanoff, S. J. and Thomas, E. D. (1976) Defective neutrophil chemotaxis in bone marrow transplant patients. *Journal of Clinical Investigation*, **58**, 22–31.

Cohen, M. D., Klatte, E. C., Baehner, R., Smith, J. A., Martin–Simmerman, P., Carr, B. E., Provisor, A. J., Weetman, R. M., Coates, T. and Siddiqui, A. (1984) Magnetic resonance imaging of bone marrow in children. *Radiology*, **151**, 715–18.

Cronkite, E. P. (1967) Radiation-induced aplastic anaemia. *Seminars in Hematology*, **4**, 273–7.

De Planque, M. M., Kluin-Nelemans, H. C., Van Krieken, H. J. M., Kluin, P. M., Brand, A., Beverstock, G. C., Willemze, R. and Van Rood, J. J. (1988) Evolution of acquired severe aplastic anaemia to myelodysplasia and subsequent leukemia in adults. *British Journal of Haematology*, **70**, 55–62.

Dreyfus, S. (1959) A propos de 81 observations de pancytopénies idiopathiques chroniques sans splénomégalie. *Revue d'Hematologie*, **14**, 62–70.

Duhamel, G., Muratone, R., Bryon, P. A. and Horschowski, N. (1978) Les lésions histologiques de la moelle dans l'aplasie médullaire. *Nouvelle Revue Francaise d'Hématologie Blood Cells*, **20**, 16–31.

Frisch, B. and Lewis, S. M. (1974) The bone marrow in aplastic anaemia:diagnostic and prognostic features. *Journal of Clinical Pathology*, **27**, 231–41.

Frisch, B., Lewis, S. M. and Sherman, D. (1975) The ultrastructure of dyserythropoiesis in aplastic anaemia. *British Journal of Haematology*, **29**, 545–52.

Geary, C. G., Dawson, D. W., Sitlani, P. K., Allison, H. A. and Leyland, M. J. (1974) An association between aplastic anaemia and sideroblastic anaemia. *British Journal of Haematology*, **27**, 337–44.

Gluckman, E., Devergie, A., Poros, A. and Degoulet, P. (1982) Results of immunosuppression in 170 cases of severe aplastic anaemia. Report of the European Group of Bone Marrow Transplant (EGBMT). *British Journal of Haematology*, **51**, 541–50.

Goodwin, D. A., Goode, R., Brown, L. and Imbornone, C. J. (1971) ^{111}In-labelled transferrin for the detection of tumours. *Radiology*, **100**, 175–9.

Gruppo, R. A., Lampkin, B. C. and Granger, S. (1977) Bone marrow cellularity determination: comparison of the biopsy, aspirate and buffy coat. *Blood*, **49**, 29–31.

Hasselbach, R. C. and Thomas, J. W. (1960) Aplastic anaemia. *Canadian Medical Association Journal*, **82**, 1253–63.

Heimpel, H. and Kubanek, B. (1975) Pathophysiology of aplastic anemia. *British Journal of Haematology, Supplement*, **31**, 57–69.

Heimpel, H., Rehbock, C. and Von Eimeren, A. (1975) Verlauf und Prognose der Panmyelopathie und der isolierten aplastischen Anämie. *Blut*, **30**, 235–54.

Hellriegel, K. P., Züger, D. and Gross, R. (1977) Prognosis in acquired aplastic anemia; an approach in the selection of patients for allogenic bone marrow transplantation. *Blut*, **34**, 11–18.

Hernandez-Nieto, L. and Rozman, C. (1980) In *Biopsia medular en la clínica hematológica*, ed. L. Hernandez-Nieto and C. Rozman, p. 4. Barcelona: Salvat Editores.

Hosain, F., McIntyre, P. A., Pouluse, K., Stern, H. S. and Wagner, H. (1969) Binding of trace amounts of ionic indium-113 to plasma transferrin. *Clinica Chimica Acta*, **24**, 69–75.

Huhn, D., Fateh-Moghadam, A., Demmler, K., Kroseder, A. and Ehrhart, H. (1975) Hëmatologische und immunologische Befunde bei der Knochenmarkaplasie. *Klinische Wochenschrift*, **53**, 7–15.

Jamshidi, K. and Swaim, W. R. (1971) Bone marrow biopsy with unaltered architecture: a new biopsy device. *Journal of Laboratory and Clinical Medicine*, **77**, 335–42.

January, L. E. and Fowler, W. M. (1943) Aplastic anemia. *American Journal of Clinical Pathology*, **10**, 792–801.

Kangarloo, H., Dietrich, R. B., Taira, R. T., Gold, R. H., Lenarsky, C., Boechat, M. I., Feig, S. A. and Salusky, I. (1986) MR imaging of bone marrow in children. *Journal of Computer Assisted Tomography*, **10**, 205–9.

Kansu, E. and Erslev, A. J. (1976) Aplastic anaemia with 'hot pockets'. *Scandinavian Journal of Haematology*, **17**, 326–34.

Kaplan, P. A., Asleson, R. J., Klassen, L. W. and Duggan, M. J. (1987) Bone marrow patterns in aplastic anemia: observations with 1. 5-T MR imaging. *Radiology*, **164**, 441–4.

Killander, A., Lundmark, X. M. and Sjolins, S. (1969) Idiopathic aplastic anemia in children. Results of androgen treatment. *Acta Paediatrica Scandinavica*, **58**, 10–14.

Kleeberg, U., Heimpel, H., Kleihauer, E. and Olischlager, A. (1971) Relativer Glutathion und/oder Pyruvatekinasemangel in den Erythrozyten bei Panmyelopathien und akuten Leukämien. *Klinische Wochenschrift*, **49**, 557–8.

Lewis, S. M. (1965) Course and prognosis in aplastia anemia. *British Medical Journal*, **1**, 1027–34.

Lewis, S. M. (1969) Studies of the erythrocyte in aplastic anaemia and other dyserythropoietic states. *Nouvelle Revue Francaise d'Hématologie Blood Cells*, **9**, 49–64.

Lewis, S. M. and Verwilghem, R. L. (1973) Dyserythropoiesis and dyserythropoietic anemias. *Progress in Hematology*, **8**, 99–129.

Lewis, S. M. and Verwilghem, R. L. (1977) Dyserythropoiesis: definition, diagnosis and assessment. In *Dyserythropoiesis*, ed. S. M. Lewis and R. L. Verwilghem, p. 3. London: Academic Press.

Lewis, S. M., Dacie, J. V and Tills, D. (1961) Comparison of the sensitivity to agglutination and haemolysis by a high-titre cold antibody of the erythrocytes of normal subjects and of patients with a variety of blood diseases including P.N.H. *British Journal of Haematology*, **7**, 64–73.

Li, F. P., Alter, B. P. and Nathan, D. G. (1972) The mortality of acquired aplastic anemia in children. *Blood*, **40**, 153–62.

Lohrman, H., Niethaurmer, D., Kern, P. and Heimpel, H. (1976*a*) Identification of high-risk patients with aplastic anaemia in selection for allogenic bone marrow transplantation. *Lancet*, **II**, 647–50.

Lohrman, H., Kern, P., Niethaurmer, D. and Heimpel, H. (1976*b*) Identification of high-risk patients with aplastic anaemia. *British Journal of Haematology*, **34**, 599–612.

Lynch, R. E., Williams, D. M., Reading, J. C. and Cartwright, S. E. (1975) The prognosis in aplastic anemia. *Blood*, **45**, 517–28.

Marín, P. (1981) Aplasia medular: análisis de los factores pronósticos. PhD thesis. University of Barcelona.

Marín, P. and Rozman, C. (1983) Prognostic value of the bone marrow biopsy in aplastic anaemia. In *Abstracts Book of the Seventh Meeting of International Society for Haematology, European and African Division*, p. 291.

Mathé, G., Amiel, S. L., Schwarzenberg, L., Choay, J., Trolard, P., Schneider, M., Hayat, M., Schlumberger, J. R. and Jasmin, C. (1970) Bone marrow grafts in man after conditioning by antilymphocyte serum. *British Medical Journal*, **2**, 131–6.

McGibbon, B. H. and Mollin, D. L. (1965) Sideroblastic anaemia in man: observations on seventy cases. *British Journal of Haematology*, **11**, 59–68.

McKinstry, C. S., Steiner, R. E., Young, A. T., Jones, L., Swirsky, D. and Aber, V. (1987) Bone marrow in leukemia and aplastic anemia: MR imaging before, during and after treatment. *Radiology*, **162**, 701–7.

McNeil, B. J., Holman, B. L., Button, L. N. and Rosenthal, D. S. (1974) Use of indium chloride scintigraphy in patients with myelofibrosis. *Journal of Nuclear Medicine*, **15**, 647–51.

McNeil, B. J., Rappeport, J. M. and Nathan, D. C. (1976) Indium chloride scintigraphy: an index of severity in patients with aplastic anemia. *British Journal of Haematology*, **34**, 599–604.

Najean, Y. and Bernard, J. (1965) Prognosis and evolution of the idiopathic pancytopenias. *Seminars in Haematology*, **5**, 1–13.

Najean, Y. and Pecking, A. (1979) Prognostic factors in acquired aplastic anemia. A study of 352 cases. *American Journal of Medicine*, **67**, 564–71.

Najean, Y., Bernard, J., Wainberger, M., Dresch, C., Boiron, M. and Seligmann, M. (1965) Evolution et prognostic des pancytopenies idiopathiques. *Nouvelle Revue Francaise d'Hématologie Blood Cells*, **5**, 639–56.

Najean, Y., Ardaillon, N., Caen, J., Larrieu, M. J. and Bernard, J. (1966) Survival of radiochromium labelled platelets in thrombocytopenias. *Blood*, **4**, 1071–8.

Najean, Y., Ardaillon, N. and Faille, S. (1973) Etude retrospective de 135 cas de thrombopenie chronique avec durée de vie normale des plaquetes. *Nouvelle Revue Francaise d'Hématologie Blood Cells*, **13**, 529–37.

Najean, Y., Pecking, A. and Le Danvic, M. (1979) Androgen therapy of aplastic anaemia. A prospective study of 352 cases. *Scandinavian Journal of Haematology*, **22**, 343–51.

O'Gorman Hughes, D. W. (1973) Aplastic anaemia in childhood: a reappraisal. II. Idiopathic and acquired aplastic anemia. *Medical Journal of Australia*, **2**, 361–9.

Olson, D. O., Shields, A. F., Scheurich, C. J., Porter, B. A. and Moss, A. A. (1986) Magnetic resonance imaging of the bone marrow in patients with leukemia, aplastic anemia and lymphoma. *Investigative Radiology*, **21**, 540–6.

Rasche, H. (1975) Blutgerinnungsfaktor XIII und Fibrinstabilisie Rung (1975). *Klinische Wochenschrift*, **53**, 1137–45.

Rozman, C., Marín, P., Grañena, A., Nomdedeu, B., Montserrat, E., Feliu, E. and Vives Corrons, J. L. (1981) Prognosis in acquired aplastic anaemia. A multivariate analysis of 80 cases. *Scandinavian Journal of Haematology*, **26**, 321–9.

Rozman, C., Marín, P., Brugués, R. and Feliu, E. (1985) Valor pronóstico de la histopatología medular en la anemia aplástica. *Sangre*, **30**, 982–92.

Rozman, C., Marín, P., Nomdedeu, B. and Montserrat, E. (1987) Criteria for severe aplastic anemia. *Lancet*, **II**, 955–7.

Scott, J. L., Cartwright, G. E. and Wintrobe, M. M. (1959) Acquired aplastic anemia: an analysis of thirty-nine cases and review of the pertinent literature. *Medicine Baltimore*, **38**, 119–29.

Shahidi, N. T., Gerald, P. and Diamond, L. K. (1962) Alkali-resistant hemoglobin in aplastic anemia of both acquired and congenital types. *New England Journal of Medicine*, **266**, 117–23.

Territo, M. C., Gale, R. P. and Cline, M. J. (1977) Neutrophil function in bone marrow transplant recipients. *British Journal of Haematology*, **35**, 245–50.

Te Velde, J. and Haak, H. L. (1977) Aplastic anemia: histological investigation of methacrylate embedded bone marrow biopsy specimens; correllation with survival after conventional treatment in 15 adult patients. *British Journal of Haematology*, **35**, 61–9.

Torok-Storb, B., Doney, K., Sale, G., Thomas, E. D. and Storb, R. (1985) Subsets of patients with aplastic anemia identified by flow microfluorometry. *New England Journal of Medicine*, **312**, 1015–22.

Twomey, J. J., Douglas, L. C. and Sharkey, O. (1973) The monocytopenia of aplastic anemia. *Blood*, **41**, 187–95.

Van der Weyden, M. and Firkin, B. G. (1972) The management of aplastic anaemia in adults. *British Journal of Haematology*, **22**, 1–7.

Vincent, P. L. and De Gruchy, G. C. (1967) Complications and treatment of acquired aplastic anemia. *British Journal of Haematology*, **13**, 977–84.

Wehinger, H. and Lencer, E. (1977) Zur Prognose dar Panmyelopthiese; die Formel von Lynch. *Monatsschrift Kinderheilkunde*, **125**, 561–3.

Williams, D. M., Lynch, R. E. and Cartwright, G. E. (1973) Drug-induced aplastic anemia. *Seminars in Hematology*, **10**, 195–223.

Yoshida, H., Asai, S., Yashiro, N. and Iio, M. (1985) MRI of bone marrow. *Radiation Medicine*, **3**, 47–55.

Part III

Treatment of acquired aplastic anemia

9

Supportive treatment of patients with severe aplastic anemia

Per Ljungman

Huddinge University Hospital, Sweden

Introduction

The survival of patients with severe aplastic anemia (SAA) has improved greatly over the last few decades. Several factors have contributed to this improvement, including better immunosuppressive therapy, better results following allogeneic bone marrow transplantation (BMT), and improved supportive therapies. The major causes of mortality in patients with SAA are infections, bleedings, and graft-versus-host disease (GVHD) in patients who have undergone allogeneic BMT. This chapter covers transfusion therapy and the management of infection.

Prevention and treatment of infections

Risk of infections

The risk of infection in patients with SAA is determined by several factors. The most important factor is the number of leukocytes during the different phases of the disease. In a study including 150 patients, the absolute neutrophil count (ANC) and the absolute monocyte count at diagnosis were correlated to the development of febrile episodes (Weinberger et al., 1992). In another small series of patients the monocyte count and total leukocyte count were associated with the risk of infection (Keidan et al.,1986). T-cell defects must also be considered as a risk factor for infection in patients who receive immunosuppressive therapy with antilymphocyte/antithymocyte globulin (ALG/ATG) combined with cyclosporin. In one randomized study the risk of infectious complications was higher in patients receiving ATG combined with prednisone than in patients treated with cyclosporin alone. Recently it was suggested in a pilot study that the addition of granulocyte colony-stimulating factor (G-CSF) to ATG and cyclosporin can reduce the risk of severe infectious complications (Bacigalupo et al., 1995).

Patients who undergo allogeneic BMT experience varying risks of infection at different periods after transplantation. During the first phase – the aplastic period – the risk of infection depends mainly on the number of neutrophil granulocytes, but also on damage to body barriers through the conditioning regimen before the transplantation. However, other factors also participate including depression of macrophage, T-cell and natural killer (NK) cell functions. During the second phase – the acute GVHD phase – the depression of the T-cell function dominates. This stage varies in length from a few weeks for patients who have received a matched graft from an HLA-identical sibling donor, and who do not develop acute GVHD, to many months for patients receiving an unrelated graft and who have GVHD. The third stage is characterized by B-cell dysfunction frequently combined with T-cell dysfunction in patients with chronic GVHD. This phase may not develop at all in some patients but may, on the other hand, continue for decades in patients with severe chronic GVHD. Each of these periods has characteristic infections and the physician must recognize these differences and manage the patients accordingly.

Types of infections in SAA patients

Very few studies have looked exclusively at patients with SAA either after immunosuppression or allogeneic BMT. In one large series of aplastic anemia patients treated with immunosuppression, bacteria and fungi were the most common causes of microbiologically documented infection (Weinberger et al., 1992). The pattern of bacterial infections was similar to the pattern found in patients with chemotherapy-induced neutropenia, including the common occurrence of infections associated with central venous lines. Infections were also the most frequent causes of death (62% of the deaths) in this study. Fungal infections were the commonest causes of fatal infections, and the severity of neutropenia and monocytopenia were risk factors for the development of fungal infection. Infections caused by viruses and parasites were less common in this series. Several case reports also describe infections with different fungal species in patients with aplastic anemia, supporting the high risk of fungal infection in these patients (Aquino et al., 1995; Machet et al., 1995; Munoz et al., 1997; Nussbaum and Hall, 1994).

Prevention of infections

Infectious agents can be transmitted in the hospital environment. Many centers try to treat neutropenic patients, including those with aplastic anemia, in single rooms with varying additional routines for infection prevention early after BMT and during intensive immunosuppressive therapy for aplastic anemia. Highly controlled environments such as laminar air flow (LAF) rooms have been used for

BMT patients, and reduce acute GVHD and mortality (Navari et al., 1986; Storb et al., 1983). However, it has been difficult to prove that any of these methods is definitely superior to the others. It is likely that control of room air quality through filtration (HEPA) is important for reducing the transmission of pathogens such as aspergillus. Also contaminated water can be important in spreading infections with *Pseudomonas* spp., *Legionella* spp. and possibly fungi such as aspergillus. Furthermore, reducing the risk of pathogen transmission from staff and family members by restricting access to individuals with symptoms of infection, such as respiratory viruses, combined with careful hand-washing routines is also important. Another important part of management both during immunosuppressive therapy and after BMT is the care of the central venous lines, to reduce the risk of developing infections with Gram-positive cocci, in particular coagulase-negative staphylococci.

Antibacterial chemoprophylaxis

The most commonly used prophylactic antibacterial agents used for those with neutropenia belong to the quinolone group. Neutropenic patients treated with these agents have a lower risk of developing Gram-negative infections and have a fever for a shorter period; however, their survival is not improved (Cruciani et al., 1996). Today, many centers are reluctant to use antibacterial prophylaxis because of the risk of development of resistance.

There have been no studies of antifungal prophylaxis exclusively in SAA patients undergoing immunosuppressive therapy without BMT. Nonabsorbable antifungal agents such as nystatin and oral amphotericin B were used extensively in neutropenic and stem-cell transplant patients, but their efficacy is not proven. Prophylaxis with fluconazole (400 mg/day) has been tested in two randomized trials in allogeneic BMT patients; both trials revealed that this treatment reduces the risk of developing invasive fungal infections, mainly with candida (Goodman et al., 1992; Slavin et al., 1995). Lower doses of fluconazole are commonly used, but this has not been proven to be effective for BMT patients. Fluconazole is ineffective against aspergillus infections. In centers where aspergillus is a major problem different strategies have been tried, such as low-dose intravenous amphotericin B or a nasal spray containing amphotericin B. None of these was shown to be effective in a randomized controlled trial. Itraconazole has some efficacy against aspergillus, but until now poor and erratic absorption has limited its usefulness. New formulations are in clinical testing that may be more effective as prophylactic agents.

In allogeneic stem-cell transplant patients prophylactic measures against *Pneumocystis carinii* are indicated either by trimethoprim–sulfamethoxazole or by pentamidine.

Antiviral prophylaxis

Antiviral prophylaxis against *Herpes simplex* virus (HSV) infection is indicated in seropositive BMT patients (Ljungman et al., 1986*a*; Saral et al., 1981). There are no data about the need for prophylaxis against HSV in nonBMT SAA patients, although the risk of HSV infection is increased in patients receiving therapy that depresses T-cell function.

Cytomegalovirus (CMV) infection is an important cause of morbidity and mortality after allogeneic BMT. The patient's CMV serostatus is an important risk factor for developing CMV disease (Ljungman et al., 1990). Thus, prevention of CMV infection in seronegative SAA patients who may at sometime need an allogeneic BMT is indicated. Therefore, SAA patients should be given either screened blood products from seronegative blood donors or leukocyte-depleted blood products (Bowden et al., 1993). Antiviral chemoprophylaxis against CMV is more controversial. According to the results of a randomized trial, high-dose acyclovir improves survival (Prentice et al., 1994). Prophylactic ganciclovir reduces the risk of CMV disease but does not improve survival (Goodrich et al., 1993; Winston et al., 1993). Prophylactic immune globulin is expensive and, although it probably reduces CMV disease, seems to be less effective than other available procedures (Bass et al., 1993).

Diagnosis of infection

Investigation of fever

Fever without known cause (FUO) is a frequent problem in the management of neutropenic and BMT patients. A fever that persists after adequate broad-spectrum antibacterial therapy has been given for 3–5 days requires further diagnostic procedures to be performed, directed against fungal and viral infections. In many centers it is policy to start antifungal therapy with amphotericin B after 3–5 days of FUO (Pizzo et al., 1984). Diagnosing fungal infections is still very difficult, and no technique sensitive and specific enough to be reliable exists at the time of writing. New techniques are being developed and promising results were obtained in studies using polymerase chain reaction (PCR), but it is too early to assess whether they will be major improvements (Einsele et al., 1997). Thus, antifungal therapy is frequently started if there is a prolonged fever. Fever occurring later after BMT, when the patient has engrafted, can also cause diagnostic problems. Probably the most common cause in patients not on antiviral prophylaxis is CMV, but other herpes viruses and adenovirus can also cause fever at this stage. Diagnostic procedures for CMV have developed greatly recently, with the so-called antigenemia test and PCR for CMV DNA being used increasingly (Boeckh et al., 1992; Einsele et al., 1991*a,b*; van Son and The, 1989). The rapid culture techniques are reliable for diagnosing active CMV infection but are less sensitive. Serology for CMV has no place in diagnosing ongoing CMV infection after transplant and should only be used for immunity assessment before the transplant. Attributing a fever reliably to any of the other viral infections is much more difficult and these diagnoses should be interpreted as diagnoses of exclusion.

Investigation of patients with pulmonary infiltrates

Patients who present with pulmonary infiltrates are also difficult to diagnose. The radiographic pattern is rarely diagnostic for the differential diagnosis of infiltrates. A computerized tomography (CT) scan is more sensitive but still mostly unspecific. However, the appearance of the CT scan may suggest fungal pneumonia, in particular invasive aspergillosis (Saugier et al., 1993; McWhinney et al., 1993). Since so many different infectious agents may cause pneumonia in severely immunocompromised patients, such as those with SAA, it is important to make a correct diagnosis. Today the procedure used in most centers is the broncho-alveolar lavage, which is safe and reasonably easy for the patient. However, it is important to recognize its drawbacks. First it is not particularly good at establishing the diagnosis of aspergillus pneumonia and other fungal pneumonias. Second, it can yield false-positive results, in particular in CMV and other viral infections (Ruutu et al., 1990). Therefore, other procedures are frequently carried out as well as broncho-alveolar lavage, such as protected brushing and trans-bronchial-directed biopsies. Finally open lung biopsy can be considered in some cases. However, these more invasive procedures may be difficult to perform safely in SAA patients with persistent severe thrombocytopenia.

Treatment of infection

Treatment of bacterial infections

The treatment of bacterial infections is usually rather straightforward and any of several combinations of broad-spectrum antibacterial agents can be used. In many centers it is practice to add a glycopeptide antibiotic, such as vancomycin, to the initial combination if the patient remains febrile after 48–72 h. However, this practice should be avoided, since the Gram-positive bacteria for which a glycopeptide agent is the only alternative are rarely rapidly fatal and initiation of vancomycin can usually wait until a Gram-positive infection is documented and the sensitivity pattern of the bacteria is known (Schimpff et al., 1994). This restrictive policy is recommended by authorities in several countries because of the risk of developing vancomycin-resistant bacteria, in particular enterococci and staphylococci.

Treatment of fungal infections

Amphotericin B was for a long time the only broad-spectrum antifungal drug available and remains the cornerstone of therapy in many centers. The main problem with amphotericin B is nephrotoxicity but the newly developed lipid formulations of amphotericin B have been shown to be less nephrotoxic. Thus, the lipid formulations' main advantage is that larger amounts of amphotericin B can be administered. Several questions are still not resolved, however, including the optimal dosing of these formulations and whether the antifungal efficacy is different compared to that of standard amphotericin B. The mortality from mold infections such as aspergillus and fusarium is still high, despite the introduction of lipid formulations of amphotericin B, and new more effective drugs are needed. Recently case reports describing a successful outcome with the combination of amphotericin B with granulocyte transfusions were published, and this may be an alternative for patients who do not respond to antifungal therapy alone (Catalano et al., 1997; Clarke et al., 1995).

Fluconazole has been used mostly for prophylaxis in transplant patients but can also be used for treating *Candida* infections. However, *Candida* species other than *albicans*, in particular *C. krusei*, are frequently resistant to fluconazole and some species, for example *C. lusitaniae*, can also be resistant to amphotericin B (Wingard, 1995). Thus, determining antifungal resistance is becoming increasingly important. Fluconazole has no effect against aspergillus infections. Itraconazole has some efficacy against aspergillus but its use has been hampered by its poor and erratic absorption. Thus, itraconazole has not been useful as primary therapy against aspergillus infections but may be considered as secondary prophylaxis after induction therapy with amphotericin B. However, new formulations of itraconazole with better absorption are being tested. New antifungal agents are on the horizon including voraconazole, which has a broad spectrum of antifungal activity in vitro, and liposomal nystatin.

Treatment of viral infections

HSV infections after BMT can be difficult to diagnose and differentiate from mucositis caused by the conditioning regimen. As described above prophylaxis is recommended for patients at risk of HSV reactivation. If HSV disease occurs it can usually be treated with acyclovir or famciclovir. Acyclovir resistance is uncommon but should be considered if HSV disease is diagnosed despite adequate prophylaxis (Reusser et al., 1996). It should be remembered that if HSV is resistant to acyclovir there is also resistance to famciclovir and ganciclovir. Foscarnet has been shown to be effective against acyclovir-resistant HSV strains (Safrin et al., 1991).

For several years now, it has been recognized that preventing CMV disease in BMT patients is essential because the results of treating proven CMV disease, in particular pneumonia, are poor (Boeckh et al., 1996b; Ljungman et al., 1992). Antiviral prophylaxis is described above. The other widely used strategy is the so-called preemptive therapy. The first studies with this strategy were hampered by a lack of sensitivity of the diagnostic assays, allowing CMV disease to develop before the signal tests became positive (Goodrich et al., 1991; Schmidt et al., 1991). Later developments of sensitive diagnostic methods allowing antiviral therapy to be initiated before the development of CMV disease have increased the value of this strategy. Either antigenemia detecting the pp65 protein or PCR for CMV DNA can be used as the basis for preemptive therapy (Boeckh et al., 1996*a*, 1997; Einsele et al., 1995; Ljungman et al., 1996). One advantage of the preemptive therapy strategy compared to prophylaxis is that fewer patients require therapy, thereby reducing the cost and the risk of side-effects. Two antiviral drugs are available for preemptive therapy, ganciclovir and foscarnet. Each of the drugs has advantages and disadvantages, and at the time of writing a randomized comparative study is being done by the Infectious Diseases Working Party of the European Group for Blood and Marrow Transplantation (EBMT). CMV infections in nontransplanted SAA patients seem to be rare and routine preventive strategies are not warranted, with the exception of avoiding primary infection with the use of leukocyte-depleted blood products.

The therapy results for established CMV pneumonia are still unsatisfactory. The mortality in recently published reports was at least 50% (Boeckh et al., 1996*b*; Ljungman et al., 1992). Standard therapy of CMV pneumonia is ganciclovir combined with intravenous immune globulin, but it should be stated that no controlled study has assessed the impact of adding the intravenous immune globulin to antiviral therapy. On the other hand, there are no data to support the addition of immune globulin to antiviral chemotherapy for other forms of CMV disease such as gastrointestinal disease (Ljungman et al., 1998). Recently several centers have reported an increased frequency of late CMV disease occurring many months after the transplant (Boeckh et al., 1996*b*; Krause et al., 1997). Late CMV disease probably develops because of a continued deficiency of specific immune responses against CMV, and it is most common in unrelated and mismatched transplant recipients (Boeckh et al., 1996*b*; Krause et al., 1997). In a recently performed risk factor analysis we found that in patients monitored by PCR and treated preemptively with antiviral therapy the probability of developing CMV disease was 1% in patients who underwent BMT with an HLA-identical sibling donor, while it was 5.6% in patients with an unrelated donor or mismatched family donors (Ljungman et al; unpublished data). There is no difference in mortality whether CMV pneumonia occurs during the first 100 days or later after transplantation (Boeckh et al., 1996*b*). Recipients of unrelated grafts also seem to have an increased risk of developing previously rare forms of CMV disease such as retinitis and central nervous system (CNS) disease (Ljungman et al., unpublished observation).

Varicella-zoster virus (VZV) infections are common in BMT patients (Ljungman et al., 1986*b*; Locksley et al., 1985). The most frequent form of VZV infection is localized Herpes zoster but disseminated forms occur. Primary varicella infection can occur in severely immunocompromised patients including those with aplastic anemia. Previously intravenous acyclovir has been the recommended therapy for localized Herpes zoster infection, although many centers have used oral acyclovir (Ljungman et al., 1989). Recently two drugs with better pharmacological properties have been introduced, famciclovir and valaciclovir, and, although no controlled trial has been completed, the pharmacokinetic data predict that they would be effective. Intravenous acyclovir is strongly recommended for treating primary varicella or disseminated Herpes zoster in immunocompromised patients.

It has been well documented from several small descriptive studies that respiratory virus infections can be severe after BMT (Harrington et al., 1992; Ljungman, 1997; Wendt et al., 1992; Whimbey et al., 1996). The most serious of these infections is that caused by respiratory syncytial virus (RSV), which, in a series of reports, has been shown to have a mortality of 40–80% in patients with RSV pneumonia (Harrington et al., 1992; Ljungman, 1997; Whimbey et al., 1995, 1996). Also parainfluenza virus, in particular type-3 and influenza A and B infections, can cause fatal infections in stem-cell-transplant patients (Aschan et al., 1989; Lewis et al., 1996; Ljungman, 1997; Ljungman et al., 1993; Wendt et al., 1992; Whimbey et al., 1994). The mortality in parainfluenza virus infections has been reported to be approximately 30%, while in influenza A infections the experience varies, with mortality ranging from 14% to 50%. Many centers have tried ribavirin, either inhaled or parenteral, for treating patients with upper-respiratory symptoms caused by RSV or parainfluenza viruses, or as therapy for established pneumonia. However, no controlled clinical trials for these therapies has been completed. It is important to realize that infections with respiratory viruses can be easily transmitted between individuals and therefore the risk for nosocomial spread is substantial. There are no data about the risk of severe respiratory virus infections in aplastic anemia patients who undergo immunosuppressive therapy without BMT.

Pneumococcus is the most important pathogen in long-term survivors after allogeneic BMT, causing sinus and respiratory tract infections, meningitis and fulminant shock (Winston et al., 1979). Infections are more common in patients with severe chronic GVHD but can occur also in other patients. There are several studies of currently available polysaccharide-based vaccines, all showing poor antibody responses particularly when given within the first 7 months after BMT, or to patients with ongoing immunosuppressive therapy (Aucotourier et al., 1987; Hammarström et al., 1993; Winston et al., 1983). Thus, other preventive strategies, for example long-term prophylaxis with antibacterial agents such as penicillin, should be considered.

Transfusion support

Support with blood components is essential for patients with aplastic anemia, regardless of whether these patients undergo immunosuppressive therapy or

BMT. The possibilities for transfusion support include erythrocyte, platelet, and granulocyte transfusions.

Erythrocyte transfusions are life-saving for patients with SAA. Platelet transfusions are frequently given to patients with aplastic anemia after immunosuppressive therapy and BMT. The optimal use of platelets for SAA patients is not clearly defined, and centers have their own platelet level standards to indicate whether a transfusion is required. Platelet survival diminishes during ALG therapy (Gratama et al., 1984); therefore, intensified platelet support is used in many centers in association with ALG therapy. Granulocyte transfusions were frequently used in the early 1980s. Navari et al. (1986) showed that prophylactic granulocyte transfusions during BMT improved survival compared to patients receiving conventional treatment. However, the outcome was inferior to isolation in LAF rooms and the practice of prophylactic granulocyte transfusions is not used today. The efficacy of therapeutic granulocyte transfusions was hampered by the difficulty of harvesting enough granulocytes to influence the outcome of infections. However, granulocyte transfusions may make a comeback as a therapeutic option with the possibility of harvesting large numbers of granulocytes from G-CSF-stimulated volunteer donors. No controlled studies of their effectiveness have been published.

Even though blood transfusions save lives, there are significant problems associated with their use. These include induction of alloimmunization, transfusion-associated GVHD, transmission of infectious agents, and the development of complications caused by iron overload.

Transfusions and risk for graft rejection after BMT

A greater number of pretransplant blood transfusions is associated with an increased risk of marrow rejection in SAA patients undergoing HLA-identical BMT (Anasetti et al., 1986; Deeg et al., 1986). Blood transfusions from unrelated donors were found to be associated with the development of cytotoxic T-lymphocytes against nonHLA antigens expressed on donor cells (Kaminski et al., 1990). Also multitransfused SAA patients have increased numbers of autoreactive cytotoxic cells (Kaminski et al., 1992). In dogs, irradiation of blood products reduces the risk of becoming sensitized to minor histocompatibility antigens (Bean et al., 1994).

Alloimmunization after transfusion

One common problem in multitransfused patients, including patients with aplastic anemia, is that they develop alloimmunization to leukocytes present in the blood products, by generating either HLA or nonHLA antibodies. Alloimmunization can result in a decreased response to given platelet transfusions and the development of febrile transfusion reactions to erythrocyte transfusions. Alloimmunization can be detected by lymphocytotoxicity testing. The risk of platelet refractoriness is higher in women who have been pregnant and increases with the number of platelet transfusions (Brand et al., 1988; Klingemann et al., 1987). The risk of becoming immunized by filtered platelet transfusions was calculated in one study to be 2.7% in patients who had not been pregnant or received nonleukocyte-depleted transfusions, while 31% of patients with either of these risk factors developed HLA antibodies (Novotny et al., 1995). Leukocyte filtration performed before storage at the blood bank is more effective than bedside filtration and is therefore recommended.

Using leukocyte-depleted blood products possibly reduces the risk of developing alloimmunization, but the results of the relevant studies vary. A small pilot study of the use of leukocyte-depleted blood products in patients with SAA showed that their use reduced the risk of developing platelet refractoriness when compared with historical controls (Killick et al., 1997). Similar results were obtained in a study of children with leukemia and SAA (Saarinen et al., 1993). In a randomized study including women with leukemia who had previously been pregnant, leukocyte depletion did not decrease the risk of becoming refractory to platelets (Sintnicolaas et al., 1995).

Transmission of infectious agents

Many infectious agents can be transmitted through transfusions, including bacteria, parasites, and viruses. During the 1990's the number of tests performed on blood products has increased significantly, reducing the risk of transmitting human immunodeficiency virus (HIV), hepatitis B and C. Many countries routinely test blood donors for human T-cell lymphotropic virus 1 (HTLV-1). Despite these tests, new viruses transmittable by blood products will probably be identified in the next few years, including a virus causing nonA, nonB, nonC transfusion-associated hepatitis. Recently there has also been a debate regarding the risk of blood-borne transmission of the agent that causes the human form of bovine spongiform encephalopathy.

Cytomegalovirus (CMV) can be transmitted through blood products. The risk of transmission from a erythrocyte unit that has not been depleted of leukocytes has been calculated to be approximately 3%. It is probably the monocytes that transmit CMV (Einhorn and Öst, 1984; Söderberg et al., 1993). Since CMV is associated with significant morbidity and also mortality after BMT, it is clearly indicated to try and prevent patients who are seronegative for CMV from contracting the infection from transfusions. Two methods prove effective at reducing the risk of transfusion-associated CMV: using screened CMV-seronegative blood donors and using leukocyte-depleted blood products. In a randomized study, Bowden et al. (1993) showed that these two modalities are similarly effective at preventing

CMV infection in BMT patients. Worldwide, the majority of blood donors are seropositive for CMV; therefore, blood banks have difficulty in producing enough screened seronegative blood products. Thus, many hospitals use leukocyte-depleted blood products instead for patients with SAA, which has additional potential advantages as outlined below. No data support there being an additional benefit in using both screened and filtered blood products. Since CMV is transmitted by leukocytes, granulocyte transfusions from CMV-seropositive donors to CMV-seronegative patients should be avoided because of high risk of transmitting CMV (Hersman et al., 1982).

The potential additional advantages of using leukocyte-depleted blood products are that the risks of transmitting other viruses associated with leukocytes are reduced. One such leukocyte-associated virus is HTLV-1, which is the etiological agent for adult T-cell leukemia (ATL), and progressive HTLV-1-associated myelopathy. Leukocyte filtration can reduce the number of HTLV-1-infected cells (Al et al., 1993). Other viruses that are associated with leukocytes and therefore presumably can be transferred by blood transfusions include Epstein–Barr virus (EBV), human herpesvirus type 6 (HHV-6) and human herpesvirus type 8 (HHV-8 or Kaposi's sarcoma-associated herpesvirus). Although the clinical relevance of transmitting these agents is unknown, the possibility can be regarded as an additional indication for using leukocyte-depleted blood products.

Transfusion-associated GVHD

GVHD is a rare but extremely serious complication of blood transfusions. It can occur in immunocompetent patients but is more common in immunosuppressed patients who are unable to reject immune-competent T-cells from the blood products. Fatal transfusion-associated GVHD in a patient with aplastic anemia has been reported, and since current immunosuppressive therapy includes therapy to reduce T-cell function it is important to reduce the risk of transfusion-associated GVHD by irradiating all blood products. Furthermore, as described above, irradiation probably decreases the risk of becoming sensitized to minor histocompatibility antigens, giving additional support to the practice (Bean et al., 1994).

Iron overload

Patients receiving large numbers of erythrocyte transfusions are at risk of developing complications associated with iron overload. Therefore, their iron stores must be assessed and chelation therapy with desferrioxamine introduced before complications develop. Venesection may be considered for patients who have been successfully treated with BMT or have become transfusion free after immunosuppressive therapy.

Conclusion

During the last few decades the survival of patients with aplastic anemia has improved. One major contributing factor to this improvement is the development of supportive care. Advances have been made both in the prevention and treatment of infections and in the utilization of blood product support. Further advances can be expected in the future.

References

Al, E., Visser, S., Broersen, S., Stienstra, S. and Huisman, J. (1993) Reduction in HTLV-1 infected cells in blood by leukocyte filtration. *Annals of Hematology*, **67**, 295–300.

Anasetti, C., Doney, K., Storb, R. et al. (1986) Marrow transplantation for severe aplastic anemia. Long-term outcome in fifty 'untransfused' patients. *Annals of Internal Medicine*, **104**, 461–6.

Aquino, V., Norvell, J., Krisher, K. and Mustafa, M. (1995) Fatal disseminated infection due to *Exserohilum rostratum* in a patient with aplastic anemia. *Clinical Infectious Diseases*, **20**, 176–8.

Aschan, J., Ringdén, O., Ljungman, P., Andersson, J., Lewensohn-Fuchs. I. and Forsgren, M. (1989) Influenza B in transplant patients. *Scandinavian Journal of Infectious Diseases*, **21**(3), 349–50.

Aucotourier, P., Barra, A., Intrator, I. et al. (1987) Long lasting IgG subclass and antibacterial polysaccharide antibody deficiency after allogeneic bone marrow transplantation. *Blood*, **70**, 779–85.

Bacigalupo, A., Brochia, G., Corda, G. et al. (1995) Antilymphocyte globulin, cyclosporin and granulocyte colony-stimulating factor in patients with acquired severe aplastic anemia (SAA). A pilot study by the EBMT SAA working party. *Blood*, **85**, 1348–53.

Bass, E., Powe, N., Goodman, S. et al. (1993) Efficacy of immune globulin in preventing complications of bone marrow transplantation: a meta-analysis. *Bone Marrow Transplantation*, **12**, 179–83.

Bean, M., Gordon, T., Appelbaum, F. et al. (1994) Gamma irradiation of pretransplant blood transfusions from unrelated donors prevents sensitization to minor histcompatibility antigens on dog leukocyte antigen-defined canine marrow grafts. *Transplantation*, **57**, 423–6.

Boeckh, M., Bowden, R. A., Goodrich, J. M., Pettinger, M. and Meyers, J. D. (1992) Cytomegalovirus antigen detection in peripheral blood leukocytes after allogeneic marrow transplantation. *Blood*, **80**(5), 1358–64.

Boeckh, M., Gooley, T. A., Myerson, D., Cunningham, T., Schoch, G. and Bowden, R. A. (1996*a*) Cytomegalovirus pp65 antigenemia-guided early treatment with ganciclovir versus ganciclovir at engraftment after allogeneic marrow transplantation: a randomized double-blind study. *Blood*, **88**(10), 4063–71.

Boeckh, M., Riddell, S., Cunningham, T., Myerson, D., Flowers, M. and Bowden, R. (1996*b*) Increased risk of late CMV infection and disease in allogeneic marrow transplant recipients after ganciclovir prophylaxis is due to a lack of CMV-specific T-cell responses. *Blood*, **302a**.

Boeckh, M., Gallez-Hawkins, G., Myerson, D., Zaia, J. and Bowden, R. (1997) Plasma poly-merase chain reaction for cytomegalovirus DNA after allogeneic marrow transplantation: comparison with polymerase chain reaction using peripheral blood leukocytes, pp65 antigenemia, and viral culture. *Transplantation*, **64**, 108–13.

Bowden, R., Cays, M., Schoch, G. et al. (1995) Comparison of filtered blood. (FB) to serone-gative blood products (SB) for prevention of cytomegalovirus (CMV) infection after marrow transplant. *Blood*, **86**, 3598–603.

Brand, A., Claas, F., Voogt, P., Wasser, M. and Bernisse, J. (1988) Alloimmunization after leukocyte-depleted multiple random donor platelet transfusions. *Vox Sanguinis*, **54**, 160–6.

Catalano, J. R. F., Scarpato, N., Picardi, M., Rocco, S. and Rotoli, B. (1997) Combined treat-ment with amphotericin B and granulocyte transfusions from G-CSF stimulated donors in an aplastic patient with invasive aspergillosis undergoing bone marrow transplanta-tion. *Haematologica*, **82**, 71–2.

Clarke, K., Szer, J., Shelton, M., Coghlan, D. and Grigg, A. (1995) Multiple granulocyte trans-fusions facilitating successful unrelated bone marrow transplantation in a patient with very severe aplastic anemia complicated by suspected fungal infection. *Bone Marrow Transplantation*, **16**, 723–6.

Cruciani, M., Rampazzo, R., Malena, M. et al. (1996) Prophylaxis with fluoroquinolones for bacterial infections in neutropenic patients: a meta-analysis. *Clinical Infectious Diseases*, **23**, 795–805.

Deeg, H., Self, S., Storb, R. et al. (1986) Decreased incidence of marrow rejection in patients with severe aplastic anemia changing impact of risk factors. *Blood*, **68**, 1363–8.

Einhorn, L. and Öst, Å. (1984) Cytomegalovirus infection of human blood cells. *Journal of Infectious Diseases*, **149**, 207.

Einsele, H., Steidle, M., Valbracht, A., Saal, J., Ehninger, G. and Müller, C. (1991*a*) Early occurrence of HCMV infection after BMT as demonstrated by the PCR technique. *Blood*, **77**, 1104–10.

Einsele, H., Ehninger, G., Steidle, M. et al. (1991*b*) Polymerase chain reaction to evaluate antiviral therapy for cytomegalovirus disease. *Lancet*, **ii**, 1170–2.

Einsele, H., Ehninger, G., Hebart, H. et al. (1995) Polymerase chain reaction monitoring reduces the incidence of cytomegalovirus disease and the duration and side effects of antiviral therapy after bone marrow transplantation. *Blood*, **86**, 2815–20.

Einsele, H., Hebart, H., Roller, G. et al. (1997) Detection and identification of fungal patho-gens in blood by using molecular probes. *Journal of Clinical Microbiology*, **35**, 1353–60.

Goodman, J., Winston, D., Greenfield, R. et al. (1992) A controlled trial of fluconazole to prevent fungal infections in patients undergoing bone marrow transplantation. *New England Journal of Medicine*, **326**, 845–51.

Goodrich, J., Bowden, R., Fisher, L., Keller, C., Schoch, G. and Meyers, J. (1993) Ganciclovir prophylaxis to prevent cytomegalovirus disease after allogeneic marrow transplant. *Annals of Internal Medicine*, **118**, 173–8.

Goodrich, J. M., Mori, M., Gleaves, C. A. et al. (1991) Early treatment with ganciclovir to prevent cytomegalovirus disease after allogeneic bone marrow transplantation. *New England Journal of Medicine*, **325**, 1601–7.

Gratama, J., Brand, A., Jansen, J., Zwaan, F., Valentijn, R. and Bermisse, J. (1984) Factors influencing platelet survival during antilymphocyte globulin treatment. *British Journal of Haematology*, **57**, 5–15.

Hammarström, V., Pauksen, K., Azinge, J., Öberg, G. and Ljungman, P. (1993) The influence of graft versus host reaction on the response to pneumococcal vaccination in bone marrow transplant patients. *Journal of Supportive Care in Cancer*, **1**, 195–9.

Harrington, R., Hooton, T., Hackman, R. et al. (1992) An outbreak of respiratory syncytial virus in a bone marrow transplant center. *Journal of Infectious Diseases*, **165**, 987–93.

Hersman, J., Meyers, J., Thomas, E., Buckner, C. D. and Clift, R. (1982) The effect of granulocyte transfusions on the incidence of cytomegalovirus infection after allogeneic marrow transplantation. *Annals of Internal Medicine*, **96**, 149–52.

Kaminski, E., Hows, J., Goldman, J. and Batchelor, J. (1990) Pretransfused patients with severe aplastic anaemia exhibit high numbers of cytotoxic T lymphocyte precursors probably directed at non-HLA antigens. *British Journal of Haematology*, **76**, 401–5.

Kaminski, E., Hows, J., Goldman, J. and Batchelor, J. (1992) Lymphocytes from multi-transfused patients exhibit cytotoxicity against autologous cells. *British Journal of Haematology*, **81**, 23–6.

Keidan, A., Tsatalas, C., Cohen, J., Cousins, S. and Gordon–Smith, E. (1986) Infective complications of aplastic anemia. *British Journal of Haematology*, **63**, 503–8.

Killick, S., Win, N., Marsh, J. et al. (1997) Pilot study of HLA alloimmunization after transfusion with pre-storage leucodepleted blood products in aplastic anemia. *British Journal of Haematology*, **97**, 677–84.

Klingemann, H., Self, S., Banaji, M. et al. (1987) Refractoriness to random donor platelet transfusions in patients with aplastic anemia: a multivariate analysis of data from 264 cases. *British Journal of Haematology*, **66**, 115–21.

Krause, H., Hebart, H., Jahn, G., Muller, C. and Einsele, H. (1997) Screening for CMV-specific T-cell proliferation to identify patients at risk of developing late onset CMV disease. *Bone Marrow Transplantation*, **19**, 1111–16.

Lewis, V., Champlin, R., Englund, J. et al. (1996) Respiratory disease due to parainfluenza virus in adult bone marrow transplant recipients. *Clinical Infectious Diseases*, **23**, 1033–7.

Ljungman, P. (1997) Respiratory virus infections in bone marrow transplant recipients: the European perspective. *American Journal of Medicine*, **102** [Suppl. 3A].

Ljungman, P., Wilczek, H., Gahrton, G. et al. (1986a) Long-term acyclovir prophylaxis in bone marrow transplant recipients and lymphocyte proliferation responses to herpes virus antigens in vitro. *Bone Marrow Transplantation*, **1**(2), 185–92.

Ljungman, P., Lönnqvist, B., Gahrton, G., Ringdén, O., Sundqvist, V. A. and Wahren, B. (1986b) Clinical and subclinical reactivations of varicella-zoster virus in immunocompromised patients. *Journal of Infectious Diseases*, **153**(5), 840–7.

Ljungman, P., Lönnqvist, B., Ringdén, O., Skinhöj, P. and Gahrton, G. A. (1989) Randomized trial of oral versus intravenous acyclovir for treatment of herpes zoster in bone marrow transplant recipients. Nordic Bone Marrow Transplant Group. *Bone Marrow Transplantation*, **4**(6), 613–15.

Ljungman, P., Niederwieser, D., Pepe, M. S., Longton, G., Storb, R. and Meyers, J. D. (1990) Cytomegalovirus infection after marrow transplantation for aplastic anemia. *Bone Marrow Transplantation*, **6**(5), 295–300.

Ljungman, P., Engelhard, D., Link, H. et al. (1992) Treatment of interstitial pneumonitis due to cytomegalovirus with ganciclovir and intravenous immune globulin: experience of European Bone Marrow Transplant Group. *Clinical Infectious Diseases*, **14**(4), 831–5.

Ljungman, P., Andersson, J., Aschan, J. et al. (1993) Influenza A in immunocompromised patients. *Clinical Infectious Diseases*, **17**(2), 244–7.

Ljungman, P., Loré, K., Aschan, J. et al. (1996) Use of a semi-quantitative PCR for cytomegalovirus DNA as basis for preemptive therapy in allogeneic bone marrow transplant recipients. *Bone Marrow Transplantation*, **17**, 583–7.

Ljungman, P., Cordonnier, C., Einsele, H. et al. (1998) Use of intravenous immune globulin in addition to antiviral therapy in the treatment of CMV gastrointestinal disease in allogeneic bone marrow transplant recipients: a report from the European Group for Blood and Marrow Transplantation (EBMT). *Bone Marrow Transplantation*, **21**, 473–6.

Locksley, R., Flournoy, N., Sullivan, K. and Meyers, J. (1985) Infection with varicella-zoster virus after marrow transplantation. *Journal of Infectious Diseases*, **152**, 1172–8.

Machet, M., Diot, E., Stephanov, E. et al. (1995) Cutaneous candidiasis due to *Candida parapsilosis* occurring in the course of idiopathic aplastic anemia. *Annals de Pathologie*, **15**, 276–9.

McWhinney, P. H., Kibbler, C. C., Hamon, M. D. et al. (1993) Progress in the diagnosis and management of aspergillosis in bone marrow transplantation: 13 years' experience. *Clinical Infectious Diseases*, **17**(3), 397–404.

Munoz, F., Demmler, G., Travis, W., Ogden, A., Rossmann, S. and Rinaldi, M. (1997) *Trichoderma longibrachum* infection in a pediatric patient with aplastic anemia. *Journal of Clinical Microbiology*, **35**, 499–503.

Navari, R., Buckner, C., Clift, R. et al. (1986) Prophylaxis of infection in patients with aplastic anemia receiving marrow transplants. *American Journal of Medicine*, **76**, 564–72.

Novotny, V., van Doorn, R., Witvliet, M., Claas, F. and Brand, A. (1995) Occurrence of allogeneic HLA and non-HLA antibodies after transfusion of prestorage filtered platelets and red blood cells. *Blood*, **85**, 1736–41.

Nussbaum, F. and Hall, W. (1994) Rhinocerebral mucormycosis: changing patterns of disease. *Surgical Neurology*, **41**, 152–6.

Pizzo, P., Robichaud, K., Gill, F. and Witebsky, F. (1984) Empiric antibiotic and antifungal therapy for cancer patients with prolonged fever and granulocytopenia. *American Journal of Medicine*, **72**, 101–7.

Prentice, H. G., Gluckman, E., Powles, R. L. et al. (1994) Impact of long-term acyclovir on cytomegalovirus infection and survival after allogeneic bone marrow transplantation. European Acyclovir for CMV Prophylaxis Study Group. *Lancet*, **343**(8900), 749–53.

Reusser, P., Cordonnier, C., Einsele, H. et al. (1996) European survey of herpesvirus resistance to antiviral drugs in bone marrow transplant recipients. Infectious Diseases Working Party of the European Group for Blood and Marrow Transplantation (EBMT). *Bone Marrow Transplantation*, **17**(5), 813–17.

Ruutu, P., Ruutu, T., Volin, L., Tukiainen, P., Ukkonen, P. and Hovi, T. (1990) Cytomegalovirus is frequently isolated in bronchoalveolar lavage fluid of bone marrow transplant recipients without pneumonia. *Annals of Internal Medicine*, **112**(12), 913–16.

Saarinen, U., Koskimies, S. and Myllylä, G. (1993) Systemic use of leukocyte-free blood components to prevent alloimmunization and platelet refractoriness in multitransfused children with cancer. *Vox Sanguinis*, **65**, 286–92.

Safrin, S., Crumpacker, C., Chatis, P. et al. (1991) A controlled trial comparing foscarnet with vidarabine for acyclovir-resistant mucocutaneous herpes simplex in the acquired immunodeficiency syndrome. The AIDS Clinical Trials Group. *New England Journal of Medicine*, **325**(8), 551–5.

Saral, R., Burns, W., Laskin, O. and Santos, G. (1981) Acyclovir prophylaxis of herpes simplex virus infections. *New England Journal of Medicine*, **305**, 603–67.

Saugier, V. P., Devergie, A., Sulahian, A. et al. (1993) Epidemiology and diagnosis of invasive pulmonary aspergillosis in bone marrow transplant patients: results of a 5 year retrospective study. *Bone Marrow Transplantation*, **12**(2), 121–4.

Schimpff, S. C., Scott, D. A. and Wade, J. C. (1994) Infections in cancer patients: some controversial issues. *Support Care in Cancer*, **2**(2), 94–104.

Schmidt, G. M., Horak, D. A., Niland, J. C., Duncan, S. R., Forman, S. J. and Zaia, J. A. (1991) A randomized, controlled trial of prophylactic ganciclovir for cytomegalovirus pulmonary infection in recipients of allogeneic bone marrow transplants; the City of Hope–Stanford–Syntex CMV Study Group. *New England Journal of Medicine*, **324**, 1005–11.

Sintnicolaas, K., van Marwijk Kooij, M. and van Prooijen, H. et al. (1995) Leukocyte depletion of random single-donor platelet transfusions does not prevent secondary human leukocyte antigen-alloimmunization and refractoriness: a randomized prospective study. *Blood*, **85**, 824–8.

Slavin, M. A., Osborne, B., Adams, R. et al. (1995) Efficacy and safety of fluconazole prophylaxis for fungal infections after marrow transplantation – a prospective, randomized, double-blind study. *Journal of Infectious Diseases*, **171**(6), 1545–52.

Söderberg, C., Larsson, S., Bergstedt–Lindqvist, S. and Möller, E. (1993) Definition of a subset of human peripheral blood mononuclear cells that are permissive to human cytomegalovirus infection. *Journal of Virology*, **67**(6), 3166–75.

Storb, R., Prentice, R., Buckner, C. et al. (1983) Graft-versus-host disease and survival in patients with aplastic anemia treated by marrow grafts from HLA-identical siblings. Beneficial effect of a protective environment. *New England Journal of Medicine*, **308**, 302–7.

van Son, W. and The, T. H. (1989) Cytomegalovirus infection after organ transplantation: an update with special emphasis on renal transplantation. *Transplant International*, **2**(3), 147–64.

Weinberger, M., Elattar, I., Marshall, D. et al. (1992) Patterns of infection in patients with aplastic anemia and the emergence of *Aspergillus* as a major cause of death. *Medicine (Baltimore)*, **71**(1), 24–43.

Wendt, C., Weisdorf, D., Jordan, M. et al. (1992) Parainfluenza virus respiratory infection after bone marrow transplantation. *New England Journal of Medicine*, **326**, 921–6.

Whimbey, E., Elting, L., Couch, R. et al. (1994) Influenza A virus infections among hospitalized adult bone marrow transplant recipients. *Bone Marrow Transplantation*, **13**, 437–40.

Whimbey, E., Champlin, R., Englund, J. et al. (1995) Combination therapy with aerosolized ribavirin and intravenous immunoglobulin for respiratory syncytial virus disease in adult bone marrow transplant recipients. *Bone Marrow Transplantation*, **16**, 393–9.

Whimbey, E., Champlin, R. E., Couch, R. B. et al. (1996) Community respiratory virus infections among hospitalized adult bone marrow transplant recipients. *Clinical Infectious Diseases*, **22**(5), 778–82.

Wingard, J. (1995) Importance of *Candida* species other than *C. albicans* as pathogens in oncology patients. *Clinical Infectious Diseases*, **20**, 115–25.

Winston, D., Schiffman, L., Wang, D. et al. (1979) Pneumococcal infection after human bone marrow transplantation. *Annals of Internal Medicine*, **91**, 835–41.

Winston, D., Ho, W., Schiffman, G. et al. (1983) Pneumococcal vaccination of recipients of bone marrow transplants. *Archives of Internal Medicine*, **143**, 1735–7.

Winston, D., Ho, W., Bartoni, K. et al. (1993) Ganciclovir prophylaxis of cytomegalovirus infection and disease in allogeneic bone marrow transplant recipients. *Annals of Internal Medicine*, **118**, 179–84.

10

Immunosuppressive treatment of aplastic anemia

André Tichelli

University Hospitals, Basel

Hubert Schrezenmeier

Free University of Berlin

and

Andrea Bacigalupo

Ospedale San Martino, Genova

Introduction

Treatment of patients with aplastic anemia aims to improve peripheral blood counts so that the patients no longer require transfusions and are not at risk of opportunistic infections. In contrast to bone marrow transplantation, where the defective organ is replaced by healthy marrow, immunosuppressive treatment will not cure the disease but rather aims to eliminate the 'autoaggressive' cells responsible for the aplastic marrow resulting in pancytopenia. Today, immunosuppressive regimens for aplastic anemia include antilymphocyte globulin (ALG) and cyclosporin. In the present chapter the term ALG is used for all antilymphocyte serums, antilymphocyte and antithymocyte globulin (ATG). The use of ALG goes back to Mathé's early studies. He used ALG as a conditioning regimen before marrow infusion for four accidentally irradiated patients (Mathé et al., 1970). Although no engraftment was observed, two of the four patients survived, presenting with autologous regeneration of hemopoiesis. Similar observations were made by Speck and Kissling, in a study of rabbits with benzene-induced aplasia (Speck and Kissling, 1971). Control animals died, whereas animals treated with ALG and infusion of HLA-haploidentical marrow recovered autologous bone marrow function. These observations clearly indicate that ALG alone is not sufficient to allow engraftment of allogeneic marrow. Nevertheless, recovery of hemopoiesis seemed possible after treatment with ALG. The evidence that autologous reconstitution can occur under experimental and clinical circumstances uncovered new possibilities for treating patients with aplastic anemia.

Lessons from the clinical trials

Effectiveness of ALG

The clinical effectiveness of ALG was first apparent in individual patients who showed evidence of autologous reconstitution of hemopoiesis (Jeannet et al., 1976). Since the early results were promising, a small number of European centers started ALG treatment with or without marrow infusion. ALG's effectiveness was demonstrated by reproducing the early results: survival was improved compared with historical data for patients treated with support alone (Delgado-Lamas et al., 1989; Doney et al., 1981; Fairhead et al., 1983; Gluckman et al., 1978; Jansen et al., 1982; Marmont et al., 1983; Rothmann et al., 1982; Silingardi and Torelli, 1979; Speck et al., 1977, 1978). Since that time, few controlled, randomized trials and a number of large single-center and multicenter retrospective studies evaluating ALG in the treatment of aplastic anemia have been published in Europe and the USA (Table 10.1). The criticism that most of the responses after ALG treatment are spontaneous remissions can no longer be sustained.

The proof of ALG's effectiveness was definitively demonstrated by two prospective trials. In the UCLA study, 42 newly diagnosed patients with severe aplastic anemia were randomized to either receive ALG or be followed as controls (Champlin et al., 1983). Only patients who received ALG responded. The hemopoiesis of 11 of the 21 patients receiving ALG had, and remained, improved at 3 months compared to none of 21 control patients ($P<0.0005$). Twelve control patients subsequently received ALG, and six improved. Overall 53% of the patients treated with ALG responded eventually. Furthermore, the survival of responders was significantly better. Two-year survival for responders was 100%, as compared to 14% for nonresponders ($P=0.0001$).

The second randomized trial was conducted by the Aplastic Anemia Study Group, who compared the treatments with ALG, HLA-haploidentical marrow, and androgen with androgen alone (Camitta et al, 1983). Regimen including ALG resulted in a 2-year probability of survival of 76% compared to 31% in the control group ($P<0.002$). As in the previous trial, the response rate was higher in the ALG-treated group. Twenty of 29 patients treated with ALG responded completely or partially, compared to 7 of 37 in the control group ($P<0.01$). The blood counts of nonresponders gradually improved. Reticulocyte and neutrophil counts usually began to increase 4–10 weeks after ALG administration, while platelet count increases followed 1–2 months after this. It was common for the blood counts of responders not to recover completely, suggesting that hemopoietic stem cells or components of the marrow microenvironment are damaged permanently. Thus, it is definitively established that treating with ALG improves the hemopoietic response and survival.

Table 10.1. Large trials of treatment of aplastic anemia with antilymphocyte globulin (ALG)

Center	Study design	ALG regimen	Additional treatment	Total number/ response (%)	Survival	Message
UCLA (Champlin et al., 1983)	Prospective, randomized	20 mg/kg × 8 days	Steroids	41 (53%)	—	Improved response with ALG
Severe Aplastic Anemia Group (Camitta et al., 1983)	Multicenter, randomized	40 mg/kg × 4 days	Steroids, androgens	42 (69%)	76% at 2 years	Improved survival with ALG
EMBT (Gluckman et al., 1982)	Multicenter retrospective	Various	Various	170 (32%)	52% at 4 years	Influence of blood counts on survival
EBMT (Bacigalupo et al., 1988)	Multicenter retrospective	Various	Various	509 (—)	61% at 6 years	Comparison between BMT and immuno-suppression
Hammersmith (Marsh et al., 1987)	Single-center, retrospective	3.76 mg/kg × 5 days	Steroids, androgens	64 (33%)	53% at 6 years	Influence of disease severity
Basel (Speck et al., 1986)	Single-center	40 mg/kg × 5 days	Steroids, androgens, ±haplo-BM	72 (74%)	65% at 8 years	Relapse and late complications may occur
Seattle (Doney et al., 1997)	Single-center, retrospective	15 mg/kg × 10 days	Steroids, androgens, ±GM-CSF	227 (44%)	38% at 15 years	BMT for young SAA with matched related donor
Genoa (Marmont et al., 1983)	Single-center, retrospective	40 mg/kg × 5 days	Steroids, androgens, haplo-BM	42 (57%)	60% at 5 years	Sequential ALG for refractory or relapsed SAA
UCLA (Paquette et al., 1995)	Single-center, retrospective	20mg/kg × 8 days	Steroids	155	48% at 6 years	Superior long-term outcome with BMT rather than ALG
NHLBI (Young et al., 1988	Multicenter prospective	15mg/kg per day × 10 vs 28 days	Steroids	77 (48%)	58% at 1 year	ALG administration for 28 days does not improve response

Notes:

BMT = bone marrow transplantation; GM-CSF = granulocyte/macrophage colony-stimulating factor; SAA = severe aplastic anemia.

The impact of severity of disease

The following studies have tackled questions concerning immunosuppression in aplastic anemia. First, an attempt to find factors predicting hemopoietic reconstitution after immunosuppression was undertaken. The SAA Working Party of the EBMT evaluated variables correlating with survival in 170 patients treated with immunosuppression. Blood counts at the time of treatment as well as after immunosuppression correlated with survival (Gluckman et al., 1982, 1984). Indeed, patients with neutrophil counts below 0.2×10^9/l and reticulocyte counts below 20×10^9/l had a 1-year survival of 40%, compared to 70% in patients with higher counts ($P = 0.0001$). An improvement of blood counts 2 months after treatment correlated with an improved survival of 80%, compared to 30% in slow or nonresponders. Unexpectedly, patients treated within the first month of diagnosis had a decreased chance of survival. This last result could be the consequence of selection bias, explained by the rapid death of patients with very severe aplastic anemia who were treated early after diagnosis.

Other studies show the strong correlation between disease severity and survival after immunosuppression. Of 64 patients treated with ALG between 1980 and 1985 in the Hammersmith Hospitals, overall actuarial survival at 6 years was 53%, with 79% survival for nonsevere, and 36% for severe, aplastic anemia (Figure 10.1). The neutrophil and platelet counts before treatment were highly predictive, whereas gender, age, and etiology were not. In addition, the mean corpuscular volume (MCV) of red blood cells was shown to be a simple and early factor predicting the response to ALG treatment. Responders had higher MCV values at 1, 2, and 4 weeks after treatment (Marsh et al., 1987). However, there is a large overlap in MCV between responders and nonresponders, which raises questions about the usefulness of such a parameter in decision making. In the UCLA retrospective study of the long-term outcome of aplastic anemia following immunosuppression, the most important pretreatment predictor of survival was disease severity (Paquette et al., 1995). The survival of patients with moderate aplastic anemia was significantly better than that of patients with severe or very severe disease ($P = 0.04$). The 6-year actuarial survival rates of the three groups were 71%, 48% and 38%, respectively.

A second EBMT retrospective study evaluated survival as a function of disease severity, by correlating disease severity with age for patients treated with immunosuppression or bone marrow transplantation (Bacigalupo et al., 1988). This study was the first to demonstrate that immunosuppression is a true alternative treatment to bone marrow transplantation (Figure 10.2): overall 6-year survival among patients receiving both types of treatment is similar. Furthermore, Cox regression analysis demonstrates that low neutrophil counts and increasing age are both inversely correlated with survival. Immunosuppression is superior to transplantation for patients with neutrophil counts above 0.2×10^9/l and who are

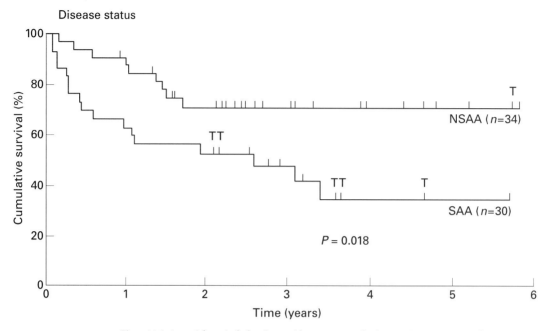

Figure 10.1. Actuarial survival of patients with nonsevere aplastic anemia (NSAA) is significantly higher than that of patients with severe aplastic anemia (SAA). Taken from Marsh et al., 1987; with permission.

older than 20 years of age (82% versus 62%; $P=0.002$). In contrast, outcome of bone marrow transplantation is better for patients with very low neutrophil counts ($<0.2 \times 10^9$/l) and who are younger than 20 (64% versus 38%; $P=0.01$). Comparable results are obtained by large single-center studies (Doney et al., 1990; Marmont et al., 1983; Speck et al., 1986).

Cyclosporin

What is currently the best immunosuppressive treatment for aplastic anemia? Although there is no longer any doubt about the efficacy of ALG, cyclosporin's discovery raised the possibility of an alternative immunosuppressive treatment that is cheaper and less toxic. Cyclosporin has been used successfully as an immunomodulatory drug to treat patients with various autoimmune diseases, such as rheumatoid arthritis, noninfectious uveitis or Sjögren's syndrome. In the early 1980s anecdotal reports claimed that cyclosporin effectively treats patients with severe aplastic anemia who did not respond to ALG (Bridges et al., 1987; Finlay et al., 1984; Seip and Vidnes, 1985; Stryckmans et al., 1984). However, larger studies

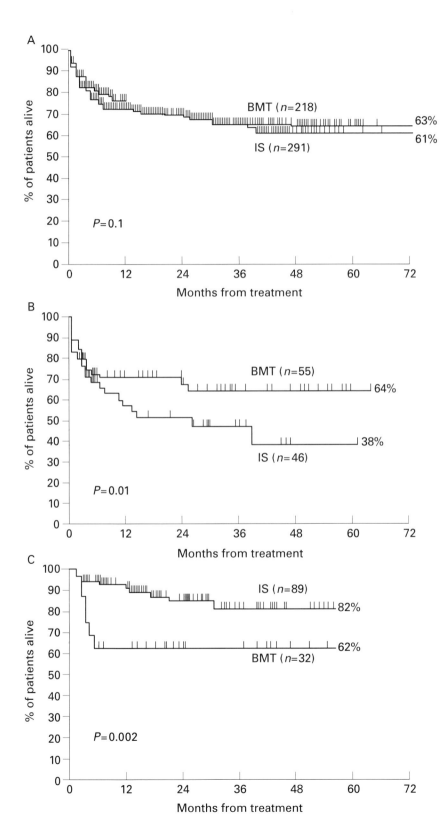

Figure 10.2A–C. Actuarial survival of patients with aplastic anemia treated with bone marrow transplantation (BMT) or immunosuppression (IS). When all patients are included (Figure 2A) no difference is observed; in patients under 20 years of age with fewer than $0.2 \times 10^9/l$ granulocytes (Figure 2B) BMT is clearly better than IS; in patients over 20 years of age and with more than $0.2 \times 10^9/l$ granulocytes (Figure 2C) IS is superior to BMT. Taken from Bacigalupo et al., 1988, with permission.

which followed these reports were not conclusive. Cyclosporin produced no response in a South African study of 12 consecutive adults with severe aplastic anemia prospectively randomized to receive cyclosporin alone or in combination with ALG and then followed for 36 months. Two of these patients responded during the second phase of the study, following addition of corticosteroids and androgens 3 months after starting the treatment with cyclosporin (Jacobs et al., 1985).

In contrast, in a study of 23 children with aplastic anemia, 12 responded to cyclosporin and androgens. The hematological response was better in newly diagnosed patients. Seven of ten patients not previously treated with ALG responded, as compared to only five of 13 pretreated patients. The blood counts of one of the patients clearly depended on cyclosporin (Shahidi et al., 1990). Similar results were obtained in the National Institutes of Health study, in which 22 patients were treated with ALG and cyclosporin, with or without corticosteroids. Eight patients responded, and all but one no longer required transfusions. The addition of prednisone resulted in prompter and fuller hematological improvement (Leonard et al., 1989). However, no patient with neutrophil counts below $0.2 \times 10^9/l$ responded to cyclosporin. Two of nine patients with Diamond–Blackfan, and two of four patients with pure red cell aplasia responded with hematological improvement (Leonard et al., 1989). An Austrian study showed similar results in 15 patients with transfusion-dependent severe aplastic anemia treated with combined immunosuppression consisting of ALG and high-dose methylprednisolone. Eleven of 15 patients have since become transfusion-independent, one of whom was followed for too short a period for evaluation and three patients died of bleeding or infection (Hinterberger-Fischer et al., 1989).

A French Co-operative Study, which compared ALG with cyclosporin as a first-line therapy for severe aplastic anemia, proved cyclosporin's efficacy definitively (Table 10.2). Patients were randomized to receive ALG and prednisone or cyclosporin alone. At 3 months, patients who had either not responded, or had done so only minimally, received the alternative therapy to assess the value of sequential immunosuppression in the treatment of severe aplastic anemia. One hundred and nineteen patients were randomized: 25 were excluded, of whom 3 were misdiagnosed and 22 did not follow the cross-over protocol. Ninety-four patients were analyzed: 46 patients received cyclosporin, and 48 ALG. The actuarial survival was 66.7%, with a median follow-up time of 19 months. There was no significant difference in survival between the groups. At 12 months, the actuarial survival was 70% in the cyclosporin-treated group, and 64% in the ALG-treated group, giving complete and partial responses of 31.6% and 30%, respectively. The main prognostic factor was the absolute neutrophil counts at entry. Patients with neutrophil counts less than $0.2 \times 10^9/l$ had a significantly poorer survival compared to patients whose neutrophil counts were higher than $0.2 \times 10^9/l$ ($P=0.0001$). The main complication was infection, which occurred more frequently and was also more likely

Table 10.2. Large trials of treatment of aplastic anemia with antilymphocyte globulin (ALG) in combination with cyclosporin and/or granulocyte colony-stimulating factor (G-CSF)

Center	Study design	ALG regimen	Cyclosporin (CSA)	Total number/response (%)	Survival	Message
German Aplastic Anemia Study Group (Frickhofen et al., 1991)	Multicenter, randomized ALG vs ALG + CSA	0.75 mg/day ×8 days	12 mg/kg per day	84 (70%)	64% at 41 months	Improved response with combination ALG+ CSA
Cooperative Group on the Treatment of AA (Gluckman et al., 1992a–c)	Multicenter randomized ALG vs CSA	12 mg/kg per day ×5	6 mg/kg per day	119 (30%)	70% (CSA) at 1 year	No difference between ALG or cyclosporin
South Africa (Jacobs et al., 1985)	Single-center randomized ALG vs ALG + CSA	15 mg/kg per day ×5	12.5 mg/kg ×7 days 6.25 mg/kg per day[†]	12 (0%)	—	No response of CSA with or without ALG
NIH Study (Leonard et al., 1989)	Single-center	No ALG	12 mg/kg per day* 15 mg/kg per day**	22 (36%)	—	CSA may be effective in patients refractory to ALG
Austrian Study (Hinterberger-Fischer et al., 1989)	Single-center	No ALG	$	14 (73%)	—	CSA may be effective in patients refractory to ALG
University of Wisconsin–Madison (Shahidi et al., 1990)	Single-center	13/23 with ALG	7 mg/kg per day	23 (52%)	58% at 5 years	Study on children
EBMT on nonsevere AA (Marsh et al., 1997)	Multicenter randomized	10 mg/kg per day ×5	5 mg/kg per day	42 (48%) CSA 47 (63%) ALG + CSA	—	Improved response in nonsevere AA with ALG+ CSA
EBMT (Bacigalupo et al., 1995)	Pilot, multicenter prospective with G-CSF	15 mg/kg per day ×5	5 mg/kg per day + 5 µg/kg per day ×90[‡]	40 (82%)	92% at 2 years	Addition of G-CSF is well tolerated

Notes:

*Adults; **children; [†]dose of cyclosporin after 7 days of treatment; [‡]G-CSF; $dose to maintain trough serum levels of 200–300 ng/ml.

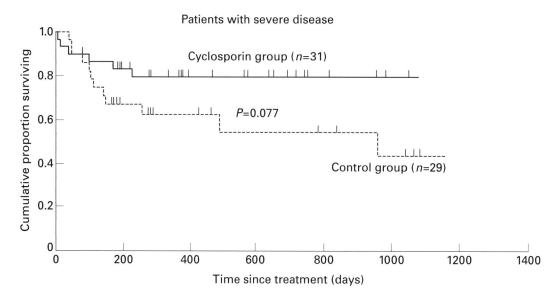

Figure 10.3. Actuarial survival of patients with severe disease treated with antilymphocyte globulin (ALG) plus cyclosporin is significantly higher than that of those treated with ALG alone (control group). Taken from Frickhofen et al., 1991, with permission.

to be lethal during ALG therapy. In this French Co-operative study, initial treatment of aplastic anemia with either cyclosporin or ALG followed by cross-over therapy for nonresponders produced comparable responses and survival rates (Esperou et al., 1989; Gluckman et al., 1992*b,c*).

Intensification of immunosuppression

Would intensifying the immunosuppression improve results? This question was first addressed by the German Aplastic Anemia Study Group. Since patients not eligible for bone marrow transplantation respond best to ALG or cyclosporin, it seemed reasonable to investigate the combination of both immunosuppressants. In a randomized multicenter trial, ALG and methylprednisolone, with or without cyclosporin, were compared (Frickhofen et al., 1991). Eighty-four patients were included in the study: 43 were treated with cyclosporin and 41 were controls. Partial or complete remission was greater at 6 months after treatment with ALG and cyclosporin, as compared to ALG alone (70% versus 46%; $P < 0.03$), mainly because patients with severe disease responded better (Figure 10.3). However, the groups did not differ in kinetics of response or the quality of remission. The actuarial survival of all patients at 41 months was 64% in the cyclosporin group and 58% in the control arm ($P = 0.16$). The inability to translate the increased response rate into prolonged survival is not really surprising. Indeed nonresponding or relapsing patients received an alternative treatment.

Since the German Aplastic Anemia Study Group study, others have demonstrated that although cyclosporin increases the response rate to ALG in the first 3–6 months, it does not improve survival compared to ALG alone (Fuhrer et al., 1994; Marsh and Gordon-Smith, 1995). In a National Institutes of Health study, 55 patients were included in a trial of 4 days of ALG together with 6 months of cyclosporin. Sixty-seven percent of patients had responded at 3 months, and 78% at 1 year. Actuarial survival was 86% at 1 year and 72% at 2 years (Rosenfeld et al., 1995). However, patients relapsed more frequently in all trials of intensive immunosuppression. The details are discussed in the section entitled, 'Relapses and nonresponses'. Despite the high relapse rate observed, these data support the use of an immunosuppressive regimen that involves both ALG and cyclosporin as first-line therapy for severe aplastic anemia.

In an ongoing prospective trial from the EBMT, patients with nonsevere aplastic anemia and neutrophil counts $\geqslant 0.5 \times 10^9/l$ were randomized to compare cyclosporin alone, administered in out-patients, with combined cyclosporin and ALG therapy (Marsh et al., 1997). The end point of the study was the response at 6 months. One hundred and seventeen patients were randomized, of whom 89 (42 in the cyclosporin group, 47 in the combination group) were followed up for more than 6 months. At 6 months, 20 (48%) patients in the cyclosporin group and 30 (64%) in the combination arm were transfusion-independent. More patients in the cyclosporin group needed further treatment with ALG (37%) compared with those in the ALG and cyclosporin group (11%). There was no difference in survival between the two arms. As for patients with a severe form of aplastic anemia, the combination of ALG and cyclosporin produced a better response than cyclosporin alone in patients with nonsevere disease. However, since nonresponding patients can be salvaged by a second course of immunosuppression, it has yet to be proven which of the two treatments is the most cost effective and produces the best outcome. Indeed, cyclosporin can be given in out-patient clinics, whereas ALG cannot. Furthermore, unlike those with severe aplastic anemia, patients with a neutrophil count above $0.5 \times 10^9/l$ have a much lower risk of developing an overwhelming infection. It is conceivable that, with rigorous monitoring, these particular patients may start with cyclosporin alone, with any who do not respond progressing to cyclosporin plus ALG therapy.

Adjuncts to immunosuppression

Other ways to intensify treatment have been investigated over the last 20 years. Some have now been clearly proven not to improve results and are no longer used; others are still being investigated. To complete the overview of immunosuppressive treatment in aplastic anemia, the results of these studies are presented briefly. In the late 1970s, based on experimental and clinical results, the simultaneous infusion of HLA-haploidentical marrow was thought to be necessary for autologous hemopoietic regeneration (Jeannet et al., 1976). The role of marrow infusion was obvious in rabbits with experimental benzene-induced aplasia, where ALG alone was ineffective (Finlay et al., 1984). It was thought initially that the aplastic anemia remitted more completely if ALG treatment was supplemented with marrow infusion. Indeed, some patients responded to ALG and haploidentical marrow infusion after a first course of ALG alone had failed (Speck et al., 1977, 1986). However, studying a larger number of patients demonstrated definitively that bone marrow infusion has no beneficial effect (Doney et al., 1981, 1984; Gluckman et al., 1982; Speck et al., 1986). Meanwhile, it has become clear that repeatedly immunosuppressing patients refractory to the first course of ALG may improve their recovery. The efficacy of repetitive immunosuppression will be discussed in detail in the section entitled 'Relapses and nonresponses'.

Corticosteroids were used long before ALG to treat aplastic anemia. Today, most ALG protocols include medium-dose corticosteroids (1mg/kg per day) in order to reduce the side-effects and serum sickness of ALG treatment (Bacigalupo et al., 1986). No controlled studies have been carried out to investigate whether adding corticosteroids improves the recovery. However, Young and Speck (1984) showed, in a retrospective analysis, that ALG and corticosteroids are not superior to ALG alone. Bacigalupo et al. (1979, 1980) showed that high-dose methylprednisolone induces hematological remission in aplastic anemia. Since then, a number of centers have given patients high doses of methylprednisolone to intensify immunosuppression, but with inconsistent results (Doney et al., 1987; Hinterberger-Fischer et al., 1986; Kojima et al., 1992; Novitzky et al., 1991, 1992; Speck et al., 1986). Later, in a controlled randomized study, high-dose methylprednisolone was compared to the normal dose of corticosteroids in patients treated with ALG and androgens. Thirty-three percent of the patients receiving the normal dose and 48% of the patients given high-dose methylprednisolone responded to ALG treatment ($P = 0.33$). Actuarial survival at 4 years was 43% and 47%, respectively ($P = 0.99$). There were no differences in acute toxicity, cause of death or late hematological complications (Doney et al., 1997). However, in the long term, corticosteroids produced more aseptic necrosis of the femur (Doney et al., 1997). These results confirm that using high doses of corticosteroids is no longer justified and that the normal dose should be given just for a short period to reduce the toxicity of ALG infusion and serum sickness.

Shahidi and Diamond (1959, 1961) were the first to show that combined therapy with testosterone and corticosteroids induces remission of acquired and congenital aplastic anemia. In nine of 17 children with acquired disease, a sustained remission was obtained with androgens. The remaining patients died from bleeding or infection. The blood counts remained steady, even though the androgen therapy was stopped when remission stabilized. Similar treatment was given to seven patients with congenital aplastic anemia, in six of whom the hemoglobin concentration and neutrophil counts rose satisfactorily. The efficacy of androgen treatment in marrow failure was confirmed by further small, retrospective studies (Alexanian et al., 1972; Desposito et al., 1964; Sanchez-Mesal et al., 1963). Consequently, most ALG protocols initially include androgens. In a single-center nonrandomized trial (Speck et al., 1986), some of the patients were declared to be clearly dependent of androgens for the maintenance of their blood counts. However, in the first prospective study from UCLA (Champlin et al., 1985), adding androgens did not improve the patients' response to ALG. Fifty-three patients with moderate to severe aplastic anemia were prospectively randomized to receive ALG, with or without oral androgens. Eleven of 26 patients (42%) receiving ALG plus androgen responded, three patients with a complete, and eight with a partial response. Twelve of 27 patients (44%) receiving ALG plus placebo responded, five patients with a complete, and seven with a partial response ($P>0.05$). Survival was comparable in the two groups: actuarial survival at 2 years was 55% in patients receiving ALG plus androgen, compared with 50% in the ALG plus placebo group (Champlin et al., 1985). In contrast, a second study from Frankfurt (Kaltwasser et al., 1988) showed that patients given ALG combined with androgens responded better, and more of them survived, compared with those not given the androgens. Thirty patients were prospectively randomized to be treated with 100 mg/kg ALG with or without the oral androgen methenolone (3 mg/kg). Eleven of the 15 patients receiving ALG (73%) and androgens responded, as did 4 of the 15 patients (27%) receiving ALG only. The difference in response rate was statistically significant ($P=0.01$). The survival probability, i.e., probability of being alive in 5 years, for patients receiving ALG plus androgen was 87%, compared to 43% for those receiving ALG only. However, the difference in survival rates between both groups did not reach statistical significance ($P=0.15$) (Kaltwasser et al., 1988).

A retrospective analysis by the EBMT group also showed the advantage of androgens given in association with ALG and corticosteroids (Bacigalupo et al., 1986). This retrospective analysis was followed by a randomized trial including 134 patients with acquired aplastic anemia (Bacigalupo et al., 1993a). Patients were given ALG (15 mg/kg per day) for 5 days and methylprednisolone for 1 month, and randomized either to receive ($n=69$) or not receive ($n=65$) oxymetholone (2 mg/kg per day) administered daily for 4 months. Early mortality in the two arms was comparable, 12/69 (17%) and 11/65 (17%), respectively, and correlated with the severity of the disease. The response rate at 3 months was significantly higher in patients receiving androgens (56% versus 40%; $P=0.04$); it was 78% versus 27% ($P=0.03$) in females with neutrophil counts less than 0.5×10^9/l. In a multivariate Cox analysis of patients with neutrophil counts $\leq0.5\times10^9$/l, the probability of responding without androgens was reduced compared to the androgen arm ($P=0.05$). However, survival was comparable in the two groups (71% versus 65%). Females with neutrophil counts $\leq0.5\times10^9$/l and receiving androgens had a slightly but not significantly improved survival (74% versus 50%,

$P=0.1$) compared to those not receiving androgens. These results demonstrate that supplementing ALG therapy with androgens as a first-line treatment of aplastic anemia may benefit a subgroup of patients, improving the response rate at 4 months but not survival. However, the effect of androgens as an adjunct to ALG in combination with cyclosporin has not yet been tested.

Splenectomy

What is the role of splenectomy as an adjuvant measure in the immunosuppressive treatment of aplastic anemia? Removal of the spleen is indicated if splenic sequestration outweighs the bone marrow's capacity to replace destroyed hemopoietic cells. The benefit of splenectomy is well established in several hematological diseases such as hereditary spherocytosis (Tchernia et al., 1994), idiopathic thrombocytopenic purpura (Dan et al., 1992) and autoimmune hemolytic anemia (Charleux et al., 1989). In aplastic anemia its role remains controversial. Before more specific treatment was available, splenectomy performed as a last resort did benefit a minority of patients (Grumet and Yankee, 1970; Heaton et al., 1957; Koch and Beaumont, 1967). Today, splenectomy has been replaced as a single therapeutic measure by more specific treatment.

Speck et al. (1996) evaluated, in a single center, the positive and adverse effects of splenectomy, studying 80 splenectomized, and 52 nonsplenectomized patients with severe aplastic anemia as a control group. All 132 patients were first treated with ALG, methylprednisolone, and androgens. The indications for splenectomy were prolonged transfusion requirements, a transient or incomplete response to ALG, or thrombocytopenia refractory to platelet transfusions. All patients survived splenectomy. Ten patients (12.5%) suffered from nonfatal surgical complications. Splenectomy induced a significant increase in the peripheral blood neutrophil, reticulocyte and platelet counts within 2 weeks, and all values continued to increase over the following weeks. Twenty-eight of 132 patients (21%) developed a late clonal disorder such as myelodysplastic syndrome or paroxysmal nocturnal hemoglobinuria, or both. The incidence was identical in both groups. Actuarial survival at 18 years after ALG was 51% for splenectomized patients and 61% for the control group ($P=$ n.s.). These data show that splenectomy is safe for patients with aplastic anemia. It increases peripheral blood counts immediately and, thereafter, hemopoiesis improves continuously. Therefore, splenectomy should be reconsidered for selective nontransplanted patients who have prolonged transfusion requirements despite otherwise optimal treatment.

Timing and quality of response

What type of response can be expected after immunosuppressive treatment? In those who respond, hemopoiesis improves gradually, and blood counts may never normalize for some. In contrast, hemopoiesis usually recovers quickly and completely following successful bone marrow transplantation. Patients who have been immunosuppressed have lower than normal platelet and neutrophil counts, their red blood cells are persistently macrocytic, they have raised levels of fetal hemoglobin and their bone marrow continues to show signs of disease, such as dysplasia of hemopoiesis, lymphocytosis and increased numbers of mast cells (Frickhofen et al., 1991; Marsh et al., 1987; Tichelli et al., 1992). Accordingly, most patients have residual abnormalities of hemopoiesis in vitro, with reduced capacities to grow hemopoietic progenitors (Nissen et al., 1980; Rudivic et al., 1985), and initiate long-term cultures (Alexanian et al., 1972; Marsh et al., 1990).

The time taken to respond to immunosuppression varies widely from 1 to 12 months. Neutrophil counts generally increase by 2 months after treatment, but patients continue to improve up to 1 year after treatment. Of those who do respond, 45% have done so by 3 months, and 70% by 6 months. Nissen et al. (1993) evaluated, in a single-center study, the speed of hematological recovery of 103 patients with severe aplastic anemia treated with ALG. During and shortly after treatment neutrophil counts rose transiently, probably because of the concomitant use of high-dose corticosteroids, and then fell back to pretreatment values. Thereafter, neutrophil counts increased gradually over nearly 50 weeks, and reticulocyte counts over 8 weeks. After 1 year, values varied broadly between individual patients. Platelet counts were the slowest to recover, but an overall increase was observed over nearly 2 years. Hemopoietic recovery was significantly delayed in girls younger than ten. This late recovery and the lack of clear criteria to define a response render a comparison between individual studies very difficult. Some patients' blood counts will never make more than a minimal improvement, increasing just enough to prevent bleeding or infections, freeing the patient from transfusions. In other patients, blood counts will recover to near normal values after immunosuppression. In a study, both cases may be assessed as a hematological recovery.

Mechanism of action of ALG and cyclosporin

Antilymphocyte globulin is a polyclonal IgG derived from the serum of animals immunized with human lymphocytes, produced by horse or rabbit immunization. Despite the general assumption that ALG acts essentially as an immunosuppressant, the mechanism underlying its therapeutic effect in aplastic anemia is not yet fully elucidated. In contrast, cyclosporin's mechanism of action is now well understood. The mechanisms of action of ALG and cyclosporin will now be discussed.

ALG acts mainly as an immunosuppressant, by inducing the destruction of cytotoxic lymphocytes that inhibit hemopoietic stem cells (Taniguchi et al., 1990). ALG contains antibodies that recognize multiple T-lymphocyte membrane antigens on human peripheral blood cells. These include antibodies against CD2, CD3, CD4, CD5, CD6, CD8, CD11, CD11a, CD18, CD25, CD28, CD45, and HLA-DR (Bonnefoy-Berard et al., 1991, 1992; Raefsky et al., 1986; Smith et al., 1985). Titration studies show the highest titer of antibodies towards CD6, CD16, CD18, CD38, CD40, and CD58, most of which are not T-cell specific. Interestingly, the antibodies to T-cell antigens CD3, CD4, CD8, CD11a, CD40 CD45, and CD54 are those that persist the longest in the plasma of transplanted rhesus monkeys (Rebellato et al., 1994). These results suggest that the persistence of ALG antibodies in vivo may be related to the prolonged anergy of circulating T-cells after ALG treatment. Recently, Teramura et al. (1997) presented in vitro evidence that ALG inhibits the CD8-positive cells that immunosuppress hemopoietic progenitor cells.

Functionally, the polyclonal ALG contains activating (antiCD3, antiCD2) and blocking (antiCD4, antiCD18, antiCD11a, and antiHLA-DR) antibodies. The blocking ability of ALG is attributed to the direct binding of monoclonal antibodies to T-cell and natural killer cell antigens, as well as to the interleukin-2 (IL-2) receptor (Raefsky et al., 1986). Treating cells with ALG blocks the binding of monoclonal antibodies directed against either lymphocyte differentiation or histocompatibility antigens (Greco et al., 1983). Whatever the source of lymphocytes used, ALG reacts with both T- and B-cell lines, and contain antibodies specific for T- and B-cells. Administering ALG reduces the number of circulating lymphocytes rapidly. Six patients with aplastic anemia received five doses of ALG every second day. Following the first dose, the absolute number of helper T-lymphocytes reduced significantly and rapidly. ALG treatment did not significantly change the absolute numbers of mononuclear cells, suppressor T-lymphocytes and cells bearing HLA-DR antigen (Lopez-Karpovitch et al., 1989).

Today, various ALG preparations are available commercially. However, the antibody specificity varies widely within batches and preparations (Smith et al., 1985). ALG products from five different sources were compared using flow cytometry to define their specific antibody content: three horse (Upjohn ATGAM; Minnesota MALG; Merieux ATG), and two rabbit (Merieux ATG; Fresenius ATG) preparations. Fresenius uses a Jurkat cultured cell line as its immunogen, whereas all other manufacturers employ at least some human lymphocytes. The three horse products have similar activity to most antigens tested. Fresenius rabbit ATG has the lowest activity against most antigens (especially CD4), whereas the activity of the Merieux rabbit product is similar to that of the horse ALG (Bourdage and Hamlin, 1995).

There is now clear evidence that ALG also acts as an immunostimulator in patients with aplastic anemia. Indeed, besides its known immunosuppressive mechanism, ALG has a mitogenetic effect on lymphocytes, and can induce cell proliferation and enhance colony-stimulating activity in vitro (Gascon et al., 1985; Kawano et al., 1988). The production of GM-CSF by T-cells increases after ALG treatment as compared to the conventional mitogen phytohemagglutinin, and this promotes colony-forming unit (CFU-GM) growth. In contrast, tumor necrosis factor-α and interferon-γ levels are higher in phytohemagglutinin-primed T-cell supernatants, producing significant inhibition of CFU-GM. The ALG-driven T-cell release of hemopoietic growth factors is dose dependent (Tong et al., 1989, 1991). If this effect is beneficial in patients with marrow failure, then higher doses of ALG or repeated courses may be more effective in patients with aplastic anemia. However, as for the cytotoxic effect of various ALG products, there are marked differences in stimulatory activity between preparations (Kawano et al., 1989, 1990).

A possible immunoregulatory role for ALG was initially suggested following the observation of in vitro lymphokine production, especially IL-2, in patients with aplastic anemia. IL-2 is a soluble glycoprotein factor produced by T-cells that is required for the in vitro proliferation and differentiation of T-lymphocytes, natural killer cells and antibody production by B-cells. ALG naturally elevated in vitro IL-2 production by cells from 12 of 17 patients with aplastic anemia as well as IL-2 receptor expression on peripheral lymphocytes in 11 of 15 cases. Cells from patients with aplastic anemia responded more to ALG compared with cells from those without disease (Gascon et al., 1985). Other studies proved that T-cells stimulated by ALG in vitro re. ease IL-1, IL-2, IL-6 and interferon-γ, which then participate in both the immune response and hemopoiesis (Barbano et al., 1988; Rameshwar and Gascon, 1992). These properties of ALG may be relevant to the treatment of aplastic anemia and support the hypothesis of its having an immune modulatory mechanism of action.

ALG preparations are potent T-cell activators but, unlike other T-cell mitogens, including OKT3, they do not induce polyclonal B-cell activation with subsequent differentiation into immunoglobulin-secreting cells. The absence of a B-cell response can be attributed to a direct potent antiproliferative effect on B-cells (Bonnefoy-Berard et al., 1992). This in vitro effect may be relevant to some properties of ALG observed in vivo. The low incidence of lymphoproliferative disorders reported in heart allograft recipients who received ALG as compared with the group treated with OKT3 may be related to the antiproliferative activity of ALG on B-cells (Swimmen et al., 1990).

The fact that patients treated with ALG show lasting improvement suggests that ALG directly stimulates the proliferation of an early hemopoietic cell capable of self-renewal. ALG has been shown to have a direct stimulatory effect on progenitor cells via antiCD45RO activity present in the ALG preparation (Huang et al., 1987). An indirect effect of ALG on progenitor cells via release of cytokines from lymphocytes and stroma cells is also possible.

Despite its name, ALG is not specific for a particular cell type (Greco et al., 1983), but binds to virtually all circulating lymphocytes, granulocytes, and platelets, as well as to bone marrow cells. ALG also binds to visceral tissues, including thymus and testis cell membranes, and the nuclear and cytoplasmic components of tonsil, kidney, liver, breast, lung, and intestine. Some of the acute toxicity that happens during immunosuppressive treatment may be explained by the reactivity of ALG with nonlymphocyte cells. However, improvement in the standardization of commercially available ALG preparations should increase the specificity against lymphocytes.

Monoclonal antibodies have not been applied successfully to treat patients with aplastic anemia. Doney et al. (1985) showed that 1 of 12 patients who received monoclonal antibodies recovered partially, compared to 4 of 13 patients treated with ALG. Similar results have been obtained with various antiT-cell antibody preparations, which can induce significant lymphopenia (Champlin et al., 1984; Jansen et al., 1984). ALG's broad antibody specificity and its additional multiple biological properties are probably necessary for the successful treatment of aplastic anemia. For these reasons, specific antiT-cell antibody preparations have not found use in clinical practice.

Cyclosporin is an effective immunosuppressive drug. Current data suggest that cyclosporin is not cytotoxic but selectively inhibits IL-2 production by T-cells. This prevents the secondary production of other T-cell cytokines, including macrophage migration inhibition factor (MIF), macrophage procoagulant activity, interferon-γ and granulocyte-macrophage colony stimulating factor (GM-CSF). Biologically, cyclosporin inhibits inducible gene transcription in T-cells. By blocking the transcription of the IL-2 gene, cyclosporin impairs the IL-2-driven proliferation of activated helper T and cytotoxic T-lymphocytes (Erlanger, 1993; Schreiber and Crabtree, 1992; Wong et al., 1993). Cyclosporin is not myelosuppressive at immunosuppressive doses and, since it is not lymphocytotoxic, its immunosuppressive effects reverse when therapy ends.

Treatment schedules

Today, the combination of ALG and cyclosporin is considered to be the regimen of choice for treating patients with aplastic anemia who are not eligible for marrow transplantation. ALG is obtained from the serum of animals immunized with human lymphocytes. A number of different preparations are available, derived from either horse or rabbit, and they differ in the source of human lymphocytes used for immunization, being human thymocytes, thoracic duct lymphocytes, and B- or T-lymphoblastoid or lymphoma cell lines. Most centers use horse-derived ALG to treat aplastic anemia patients (Table 10.3). However, when a second course is necessary, some centers prefer to change the type of ALG and employ rabbit-derived serum (Bacigalupo et al., 1995; Marsh et al., 1987). European preparations such as Merieux ATG (Lyon, France) and Swiss Serum and Vaccine Institute ALG (Bern, Switzerland) appear to have equivalent efficacy to ATGAM (Upjohn ATG, USA) which is mainly used in the USA.

Table 10.3. ALG preparations used to treat aplastic anemia

Preparations	Species	Immunogen	Clinical experience in aplastic anemia
Upjohn ATGAM	Horse	Thymus	Most American centers (Paquette et al., 1995; Young et al., 1988)
Merieux ATG	Horse	Thymus	Most European centers (Bacigalupo et al., 1995; Marsh et al., 1987; Frickhofen et al., 1991; Gluckman et al., 1992a–c)
Merieux ATG	Rabbit	Thymus	Second ATG course in Italy, UK (Bacigalupo et al., 1995; Marsh et al., 1987)
Swiss Serum and Vaccine Institute ALG	Horse	Thoracic duct lymphocytes	UK; Basel, randomized trial of the AA Study Group (Speck et al., 1986; Fairhead et al., 1983; Camitta et al., 1983)
Minnesota MALG	Horse	Cultured lymphoblasts and thymus	Minnesota USA (Miller et al., 1983)
Fresenius ATG	Rabbit	Jurkat cell line	No experience in aplastic anemia
Ahlbulin ALG, Green Cross Co., Osaka, Japan			Japan (Kojima et al., 1992)

The crude serum is treated to obtain the immunoglobulin fraction. Specific absorption with various human tissues to remove unwanted specificities against antigens other than peripheral lymphocytes are performed. Preparations of ALG manufactured today are more specific and therefore produce fewer unexpected reactions against tissues other than lymphocytes. Nevertheless, there is still little standardization of the different commercial preparations.

The doses and duration of treatment used in the different trials vary considerably and have not been systematically compared. In a multicenter randomized trial there was no difference between a 10-day and 28-day regimen of ALG (Young et al., 1988), despite a trend towards a more rapid, frequent and complete remission with the longer treatment. Other schedules have not been compared. There are few clinical data that allow extrapolation of the optimal dosage and treatment duration. The great variability in response among clinical trials is caused by differences in patient selection, criteria for hematological improvement and the efficacy of the supportive care, rather than variations in the type, dose and duration of ALG treatment. Since no single-dose regimen has a proven superiority, it seems convenient to apply one of the high-dose, short duration schedules originally applied in Europe.

ALG causes severe sclerosis of peripheral veins; therefore, it should be diluted in 0.9% normal saline and has to be applied through a central venous catheter

(Marsh and Gordon-Smith, 1988). It makes no difference to acute toxicity whether the daily dose of serum is infused over a short period of time (1 hour) or over 12–18 hours (Ermakov et al., 1998). Intradermal injection of animal protein before the first injection in order to predict anaphylaxis is no longer used because of its low sensitivity and specificity.

Today, the prospective trials of the EBMT use horse ALG at a dose of 10mg/kg per day for 5 days. However, the optimal schedule has not been definitively resolved. For instance, intensification of immunosuppression by combining ALG and cyclosporin has been shown to produce higher response rates (Frickhofen et al., 1991). Therefore, there is good reason to believe that repeated sequential courses of ALG can improve outcome, even in responding patients. However, this topic has not yet been evaluated.

Cyclosporin is administered orally, in one single dose or divided into two equal daily portions. The optimal dose for the treatment of aplastic anemia has not been evaluated prospectively. In most trials, the dose of cyclosporin ranges between 6 and 12mg/kg per day (Frickhofen et al., 1991; Gluckman et al., 1992*b,c*; Jacobs et al., 1985; Leonard et al., 1989). However, it has not been demonstrated that higher doses are more efficient. In order to prevent renal toxicity, especially for long-term treatment, schedules with higher doses require frequent monitoring of blood cyclosporin and creatinine levels. Although the optimal duration of cyclosporin treatment is unknown, it is usually administered for at least 6–12 months. Few patients show dependence on the drug and blood counts drop as soon as the medication stops. Continuous administration of cyclosporin over years may be justified for cyclosporin-dependent patients, as well as for relapsing patients who respond to repeated courses of immunosuppression.

Adverse events of ALG

ALG's acute side-effects and toxicity include immediate allergic reaction, serum sickness, a transient negative effect on blood counts and toxicity caused by concomitant treatments. The immediate effects occur when ALG is infused, and include fever, rigors, rash, bronchospasm, and hypotension. These appear most commonly during the first 2 days of treatment and usually respond promptly to corticosteroids and antihistamines (Doney et al., 1987). The nonoccurrence of anaphylaxis after the test doses does not rule out the risk of an allergic reaction occurring during ALG infusion.

Febrile reactions which nearly invariably occur during the first administration of ALG may be impossible to distinguish clinically from a fever caused by sepsis. If there is doubt, patients should be treated for infection without delay. In a retrospective review, blood cultures from 39 consecutive patients with aplastic anemia who developed fever during ALG infusion were compared with those of 38 patients with acute leukemia. Four aplastic anemia patients had positive blood cultures as compared to 57/66 episodes among leukemia patients ($P = 0.0001$) (Dearden et al., 1998). These results suggest that fevers developing during ALG treatment are often not caused by infections. Therefore, it may be reasonable to consider discontinuing intravenous antibiotics after 48 hours if fever does not persist, no other clinical evidence of infections is observed, and blood cultures are negative.

Nonallergic toxicity can manifest as defibrination or cardiac arrhythmia, such as bradyarrhythmia and ventricular fibrillation. It is probably caused by unwanted specificity against antigens other than peripheral blood lymphocytes, and therefore depends on the type of ALG preparation applied. Life-threatening acute reactions rarely mean that ALG treatment must be withheld, but the treatment may be fatal even in the prepared medical setting (Bielory et al., 1988*b*). The incidence of acute reactions is not higher after repeated courses of ALG than after a single course (Tichelli et al., 1998). ALG derived from a particular species can be used for more than one course of treatment for aplastic anemia patients, and the risk always remains the same as that of the initial treatment. Despite this, it is often suggested that ALG derived from a different source should be used for the second course of treatment (Bacigalupo et al., 1995; Marsh et al., 1987). Acute reactions of the immediate hypersensitivity type are tolerable after re-exposure and are reversible.

Serum sickness may occur 5–14 days after beginning ALG treatment and lasts for 8–12 days (Bielory et al., 1988*a*). It is caused by circulating immune complexes formed between circulating animal protein and antispecies antibody produced by the patient's immune system. Serum sickness is characterized by fever, rash, arthralgia, myalgia, lymphadenopathy, serositis (pericarditis, pleurisy), and proteinuria. Atypical lymphocytes and plasma cells may be found in peripheral blood. The rash may be an urticarial or a maculopapular eruption on the trunk, as well as on the palmar and plantar surface of the hands and feet, respectively. The incidence of serum sickness is between 50% and 90%, with no clear correlation with the duration of ALG regimen (Bielory et al., 1986; Doney et al., 1987; Tichelli et al., 1998).

Acute-phase reactant values such as the erythrocyte sedimentation rate, and C-reactive protein and beta-2 microglobulin levels increase during the course of serum sickness. There is also an increase in serum levels of IgG, IgM, IgA, and IgE, and circulating immune complexes, as measured by the C1q-binding assay, and a decrease in complement levels (C3, C4, and CH50). Studying biopsied samples of lesioned skin reveals the presence of immune deposits (IgM, IgE, IgA and C3) in dermal vasculature (Bielory et al., 1988*a*). A direct correlation between increases in immune complex levels, decreases in serum complement levels, and the development of the clinical signs and symptoms of serum sickness could be demonstrated. However, the development of serum sickness is not prerequisite for a hemopoietic response with ALG (Bielory et al., 1986).

Increasing the number of treatment courses with ALG does not increase the incidence of serum sickness. However, manifestations appear significantly earlier after repeated exposure (median day 6) than after the initial exposure (median day 13; $P = 0.008$) (Tichelli et al., 1998). To prevent serum sickness, corticosteroids are usually included in the ALG regimen. If serum sickness appears despite this prophylaxis, symptoms usually respond within a few days to an increased dose of corticosteroids applied intravenously. However, the effectiveness of such a treatment is difficult to judge, as the illness is self-limited.

Antilymphocyte globulin causes an immediate leucopenia due to an abrupt decrease in the numbers of lymphocytes and neutrophils. Following the first dose of ALG the absolute and relative numbers of helper T-lymphocytes significantly and transiently reduce. In contrast the number of suppressor T-lymphocytes remains unchanged throughout the treatment (Lopez-Karpovitch et al., 1989). This effect on blood counts is probably the result of the animal immunoglobulins binding directly to circulating cells. Even though fever is a common acute reaction to ALG, a neutropenic patient may become pyrexic because of a bacterial or fungal infection. Therefore, immediate broad spectrum antibiotic therapy is recommended, in case of infection. For a long time, thrombocytopenia occurring during ALG treatment caused major concern. Despite daily prophylactic platelet transfusions, thrombocyte counts could not be maintained at an acceptable level, so that life-threatening bleeds were not rare. With improved manufacturing processes, commercially available ALG products do not usually contain specific antiplatelet antibodies. Ideally the platelet counts should be maintained during the whole course of ALG treatment above $20 \times 10^9/l$.

Antilymphocyte globulin is usually applied in combination with other drugs. It may be associated with androgens, normal or high-dose corticosteroids, cyclosporin or growth factors. Haploidentical bone marrow is no longer infused. Any of these drugs can be toxic on their own, or reinforce the side-effects of ALG. It is often difficult to make the distinction between symptoms caused by the disease itself and those secondary to ALG and concomitant drugs.

Side-effects of androgens include impotence in men, virilism, hirsutism and amenorrhea in women, and acne in both sexes. Most of these side-effects are largely dose dependent and reversible as soon as the drug is discontinued. In a series of 61 men treated with norethandrolone for more than 1 year, six developed gynecomastia, two of them requiring surgical correction. Malignant transformation has not been observed (Tichelli et al., 1988a). Hepatic tests are frequently abnormal during androgen treatment, but malignant transformations only occur rarely. In a series of 111 patients treated with androgens, four developed a hepatic tumor (Speck et al., 1990). Histology showed a liver carcinoma in one (Serke et al., 1986), and a hepatic adenoma in the others.

Toxicity associated with high-dose corticosteroids includes mild gastritis, hypertension, hyperglycemia, and aseptic necrosis (Doney et al., 1987). Avascular necrosis of bone has been studied retrospectively in patients with aplastic anemia treated with ALG followed by high-dose methylprednisolone. The cumulative incidence of necrosis is 21% and develops at a median of 14 months after the beginning of corticosteroid treatment. The hip is most commonly involved. In contrast, there are no cases of avascular necrosis of bone in a historical group of 61 patients with aplastic anemia treated with an identical regimen of ALG but used at a low dose in a short course (Marsh et al., 1993).

The combination of ALG and cyclosporin leads to significantly more liver toxicity, but reduces febrile reactions and the symptoms of serum sickness. Late effects of cyclosporin in aplastic anemia patients are gingival hyperplasia, hypertrichosis, tremor and nephrotoxicity (Frickhofen et al., 1991). Gingival hyperplasia worsens with inadequate dental hygiene, leading to gingival infections, and can be prevented by regular and careful dental care (Seymour and Jacobs, 1992). Other types of cyclosporin-related toxicity reported are hypertension, myalgia, fatigue, infection, seizures, and paresthesias (Leonard et al., 1989).

Growth factors applied in combination with ALG are usually well tolerated (Bacigalupo et al., 1995). Fatigue, fever, headache or myalgia are common and dose dependent, but rarely require the treatment to be stopped (Champlin et al., 1989; Ganser et al., 1990, 1992; Nissen et al., 1988). However, long-term complications may cause concern. Indeed, the occurrence of late clonal disease after immunosuppressive treatment for aplastic anemia is now well established (De Planque et al., 1988; Tichelli et al., 1988*b*). In several cases of patients treated with G-CSF in Japan, aplastic anemia evolved into myelodysplastic syndrome or clonal cytogenetic monosomy 7 (Imashuku et al., 1995; Ohsaka et al., 1995; Tsuzuki et al., 1997; Yamazaki et al., 1997). These results suggest that there is a possible link between the administration of G-CSF and transformation of aplastic anemia into myelodysplastic syndrome.

Immunosuppression in elderly patients

In allogeneic stem-cell transplantation, age is a major risk factor for transplant-related mortality. As a consequence, an upper age limit for transplantation for patients with aplastic anemia is set in many centers between the ages of 40 and 50. Immunosuppressive treatment with ALG and/or cyclosporin is therefore commonly used as a first-line strategy for older patients. However, data are scarce and so far no study has specifically addressed the outcome for elderly patients with aplastic anemia. At the EBMT Meeting of 1997, The Severe Aplastic Anemia Working Party presented a mutlicenter study, based on the retrospective data of patients recorded until January 1995 (Tichelli et al., 1997). The data of this study have now been updated for December 1997 (Tichelli at al, 1999). There were 810 patients with nonconstitutional aplastic anemia treated with immuno-

Figure 10.4. Patients with aplastic anemia treated with immunosuppression and included in the EBMT SAA registry between 1974 and 1995. The patients are represented according to age at first immunosuppression and calendar period (patients treated before 1980, between 1980 and 1989, and between 1990 and 1995). The white column represents patients aged 20–49 years, the gray column patients 50–59 years and the black column patients 60 years and older.

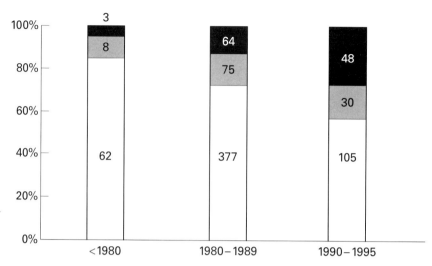

suppression in 56 centers. All 772 patients older than 19 years were included in the study. There were 438 males and 372 females, between 20 and 83 years old (median age 36 years). In order to evaluate the dependence of outcome on age, with special emphasis on advanced age, patients were stratified into three groups: two groups of patients older than 50 years (127 patients between 50 and 59 years; 115 patients ⩾60 years) and a reference group (568 patients between 20 and 49 years). The severity of disease, the number of courses of immunosuppression and splenectomy status were the same for all three groups. Neither were there any differences in gender, etiology, type of immunosuppression, and duration of treatment.

Between 1974 and 1997, the number of patients 50 years or older treated with immunosuppression increased. Before 1980, 8% of the patients were ⩾50 years, this value was 27% between 1980 and 1989, and 43% after 1990 (Figure 10.4). As of June 1997, 258 of 810 patients had died. A higher incidence of death was found in patients 50 years or older (28% for 20–49 years; 39% for 50–59 years; 43% for ⩾60 years; $P=0.04$). The probability of being alive at 5 years was 72% (20–49 years), 57% (50–59 years), and 50% (⩾60 years; $P<0.001$) (Figure 10.4). Overall the main cause of death was directly related to aplastic anemia, i.e., bleeding, infection. The excess number of deaths of patients 50 years or older was mainly caused by bleeding and infection (23% for 20–49 years; 32% for 50–59 years; 31% for ⩾60 years; $P=0.02$). Response to immunosuppressive therapy in all patients at 12 months was 62%; no difference was seen among the age groups. At 15 years, 70 of 810 patients developed a late clonal complication (25 myelodysplastic syndrome, 28 paroxysmal nocturnal hemoglobinuria, 14 solid tumors, 3 myelodysplastic syndrome together with paroxysmal nocturnal hemoglobinuria or solid tumor). Overall no difference was observed between the three age groups. Interestingly, no paroxysmal nocturnal hemoglobinuria was reported in patients older than 60.

Multivariate Cox regression analysis revealed that age (RR 1.8; CI 95% 1.3–2.5) and severity of disease (RR 3.4; CI 95% 2.5–4.7) increased the relative risk, but that gender, the type and number of courses of immunosuppression and splenectomy did not. When Cox regression analysis was performed separately on data from the three age groups, the severity of disease increased the relative risk for those in the 20–49 years and 50–59 years patient groups, but not in the $\geqslant$60 years patient group.

The Tichelli et al. (1999) study is the only one to have looked at the outcome for elderly patients whose aplastic anemia is treated with immunosuppression. It reveals that it is feasible and effective to immunosuppress those aged 50 years or more. More than 50% of patients older than 50 years were alive at 6 years after treatment. Their response rate and the time taken to respond are not different from those of younger patients. There is no reason to withhold treatment from older patients or to set an upper age limit for treating patients with aplastic anemia. The decision of whether to immunosuppress elderly patients should depend rather more on the individual's general medical condition.

Relapses and nonresponses

Sixty to eighty percent of patients with newly diagnosed acquired aplastic anemia respond to immunosuppressive treatment. However, in contrast to bone marrow transplantation, response to immunosuppression is often slow and incomplete. Patients retain their hematological abnormalities. Blood counts are lower than normal, red blood cells show macrocytosis and bone marrow morphology continues to show stigmata of the disease (De Planque et al., 1989b; Marsh et al., 1987; Nissen et al., 1982, 1993; Speck et al., 1986). The capacities for in vitro proliferation and initiation of long-term bone marrow cultures are grossly decreased (Marsh et al., 1990). These observations support the fact that patients are not cured from their disease after treatment with immunosuppression. It is therefore not surprising that relapse of aplastic anemia and late hematological complications may occur.

Relapses after an initial response to immunosuppression have been described to occur soon after the efficacy of ALG therapy has been established (Fairhead et al., 1983; Hinterberger-Fischer et al., 1986; Miller et al., 1983; Speck et al., 1981). When re-treating relapsed patients with additional courses of immunosuppression, a second remission can be induced in more than half of the patients (Frickhofen et al., 1986; Speck et al., 1986). In a series of 139 patients with aplastic anemia, 16 patients presented with recurrent aplasia after an initial response to immunosuppression. All five patients re-treated with ALG had a second remission. In contrast, five of six patients who were re-treated with corticosteroids or androgens did not respond at all, and one responded only partially (Doney et al.,

1990). More details can be obtained from the prospective randomized study of the German Aplastic Anemia Study Group, which compares treatment with ALG and methylprednisolone with or without cyclosporin (Frickhofen et al., 1991). Ten of the 52 patients who responded initially then relapsed 4–37 months after the first immunosuppression. Three relapsing patients were randomly allocated to the cyclosporin-treated group, and seven to the control arm. Two of three patients from the cyclosporin-treated group relapsed late and only after discontinuation of the drug. After re-treatment, the remission of both depended on cyclosporin. Overall seven of the ten relapsed patients responded to a second course of immunosuppressive therapy. Other single-center trials confirm the high incidence of relapse, with an actuarial risk of 36% at 2 years, but most relapsed patients respond to additional immunosuppression (Marsh and Gordon-Smith, 1995; Rosenfeld et al., 1995).

A multicenter study conducted by the EBMT SAA Working Party retrospectively evaluated the relapse of aplastic anemia after immunosuppression (Schrezenmeier et al., 1993). Of the 358 responding patients, 74 patients relapsed at a mean of 25 months after initial immunosuppression. The actuarial risk of relapse in these patients is 35.2% at 10 years. The risk of relapse was higher in patients responding within 120 days from immunosuppression (48%) compared to patients responding between 120 and 360 days (40%) and only 20% for slow responders (>360 days). The time between diagnosis and treatment was greater for patients who relapsed compared with those who did not. Age, gender and severity of the disease cannot predict relapse. Thirty-nine of the 74 (53%) relapsing patients responded to a second course of immunosuppression. The actuarial survival of relapsing patients responding to a second treatment is similar to that of patients who respond but do not relapse.

Despite the improved response rate with intensive immunosuppression, 20–30% of the patients still fail to respond to the initial course of treatment. Today, there is no consensus on how to treat patients who do not respond to ALG. Since treatment protocols including ALG yield the best results irrespective of additional immunosuppressive drugs, a second trial with ALG appears a logical approach (Frickhofen et al., 1991; Young and Barrett, 1995). However, doubts about repeating a previously unsuccessful treatment, fear of anaphylactic reactions and serum sickness after repeated exposure to ALG as well as concerns about overimmunosuppression prevent repeated use of ALG, and so far few data are available (Doney et al., 1990; Marsh and Gordon-Smith, 1988; Marsh et al., 1994; Means, Jr. et al., 1988; Rosenfeld et al., 1995; Socié et al., 1993).

Many centers apply a second course of ALG to patients who failed to respond to initial treatment. Almost half of the patients can respond to a second course of ALG (Doney et al., 1990; Facon et al., 1991; Marmont et al., 1983; Marsh and Gordon-Smith, 1995; Paquette et al., 1995; Pulver and Flaum, 1987). Preliminary data of a retrospective study of the EBMT SAA Working Party demonstrate that patients who do not respond to an initial course of immunosuppression have a good chance of responding to a second course (Schrezenmeier et al., 1998). In a cohort of 806 patients, 47% responded to the first course of treatment, and 43% to a second course given when the first failed. Furthermore, there was no difference in survival between the patients who did respond to immunosuppression, regardless of how many treatments they had received. The actuarial survival of 377 patients who responded to one course was 80.4%, as compared to 68.5% out of 72 patients who required a second course.

The immediate risk of repeated ALG must be considered. Re-treating patients with aplastic anemia with antihuman ALG derived from the same species as used in the first course does not increase the risk associated with the treatment. Acute reactions of the immediate hypersensitivity type are tolerable after re-exposure and reversible in all cases. The incidence and severity of serum sickness are similar in naive and previously exposed patients. Manifestations of serum sickness appear significantly earlier after repeated exposure (median of day 6) than after the initial exposure (Tichelli et al., 1998). This earlier occurrence of serum sickness after repeated exposures is compatible with a second set response.

Finally, sequential immunosuppression may lead to an increased risk of infections or the late onset of cancer. So far, there is no evidence of increased morbidity or mortality caused by infections after repeated immunosuppression of those with aplastic anemia (H. Schrezenmeier, personal observation) (Tichelli et al., 1998). However, because of the retrospective nature of most studies, there is selection bias involved in deciding who should be immunosuppressed again. It is likely that good-risk patients were selected for repeated treatment whereas bad-risk patients were not. In a small multicenter prospective trial involving 22 patients, the outcome of one course of ALG was compared with that of two courses. Both treatment modalities were well tolerated and both had similar response rates (Matloub et al., 1997). However, the small number of patients does not allow treatment efficacy to be evaluated. Patients with aplastic anemia treated with immunosuppression are at risk of developing myelodysplastic syndrome and leukemia (De Planque et al., 1989a; Marsh and Geary, 1991; Tichelli et al., 1988b). In a large cohort of patients this risk is highly increased relative to that in a general population. Among factors studied, treatment with multiple courses of immunosuppressive therapy were found to correlate with an increased risk of hematological cancer. In contrast, the risk of developing solid tumors was not increased by repeated immunosuppression (Socié et al., 1993).

These data demonstrate that relapse is a relevant problem associated with immunosuppressive treatment of aplastic anemia. However, relapsed patients respond to additional courses of immunosuppression and relapse is not associated with significantly poorer survival. Single case reports suggest that, for relapsing patients, continuing immunosuppression over the long-term may prevent further relapses. Likewise, the refractory state after a first course of immunosuppression can be successfully re-treated with a similar protocol. There is a good chance of responding to a second course of immunosuppression, even for those who do not respond to the first course.

Does bone marrow transplantation have a place in the treatment of patients resistant to immunosuppression? In this respect, one crucial question is whether postponing bone marrow transplantation until after one course of immunosuppression exposes the patient to an increased risk. In a multicenter retrospective EBMT study, the survival of previously untreated patients was higher than that of pretreated patients. Nevertheless, the 6-year survival of patients pretreated with immunosuppression was still 49%, compared to 64% for previously untreated patients (Bacigalupo et al., 1990). Other trials have reported individual patients undergoing bone marrow transplantation after failing to respond to ALG. In the UCLA study five patients subsequently received a bone marrow transplantation and two of them survived (Paquette et al., 1995).

A different therapeutic approach was recently evaluated. In a retrospective study, the aim was to compare bone marrow transplantation with immunosuppression, followed by a 'rescue' transplant if immunosuppression was ineffective (Lawlor et al., 1997). Seven of nine transplanted patients, and 16/18 patients treated with immunosuppression ceased being dependent on transfusions, including three of four patients who received a rescue transplantation. Actuarial survival was 75% in the bone marrow transplantation group and 92% in the immunosuppression group ($P=0.15$). Certainly both treatment modalities led to equivalent rates of transfusion independence and survival probabilities, but in a limited number of patients.

A comparable strategy was used in a prospective trial where adult patients were initially treated with immunosuppression, regardless of the availability of a bone marrow donor. Only those who did not respond were considered for bone marrow transplantation (Crump et al., 1992). Thirty-one consecutive patients who fulfilled the age criteria for allogeneic bone marrow transplantation were treated with ALG and high-dose corticosteroids. The overall response rate to immunosuppression was 58% (18/31). Nine of 14 patients with donors received secondary bone marrow transplantation, seven patients because they did not respond to ALG and two because of serious infections. Seven grafts were obtained from related and two from unrelated donors. This strategy resulted in an 80% 5-year actuarial survival rate for 31 patients. Two patients died of infection, two died from complications of bone marrow transplantation, and one remained dependent on transfusions.

Both studies demonstrate that transplantation is feasible after pretreatment with immunosuppression. However, there are still strong arguments against a sequential approach designing immunosuppression as the first-line treatment and bone marrow transplantation as the salvage option. First, bone marrow transplantation, but not immunosuppression, can prevent early deaths caused by severe pancytopenia. In a series of 56 ALG-treated patients who fulfilled the age criteria but were treated with immunosuppression, 14 patients (25%) died

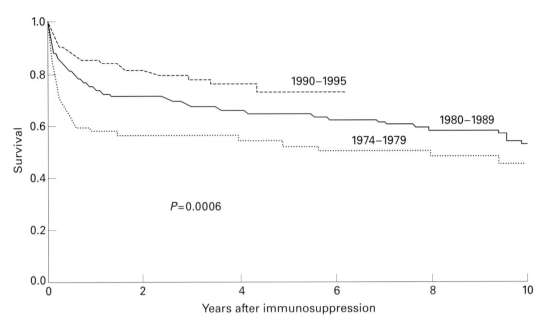

Figure 10.5. Actuarial survival according to calendar year of first treatment for patients with aplastic anemia treated with immunosuppression: $52 \pm 6\%$ for treatment between 1974 and 1979, $65 \pm 2\%$ for treatment between 1980 and 1989, and $77 \pm 3\%$ for treatment between 1990 and 1995 ($P=0.0006$). Data from the EBMT SAA registry.

within 100 days of beginning immunosuppression (Paquette et al., 1995). Second, postponing transplantation leads to a longer exposure to blood products and therefore to higher transplant-related mortality in cases of a secondary transplantation. Third, the long-term outcome of a sequential strategy has to be compared to that of first-line transplantation. This is particularly important for young patients, whose longer life expectancy will increase their risk of a late clonal complication in immunosuppressed patients.

A realistic option for young patients refractory to immunosuppression and who lack an HLA-matched sibling donor is an allogeneic bone marrow transplant from an alternative donor (Hows et al., 1992, 1998; Margolis et al., 1996). This topic is discussed in detail in Chapter 13. Nevertheless, the choice of second-line treatment will be directly influenced by the time needed to assess the response to the first course of immunosuppression and find an unrelated matched volunteer, as well as by the risk associated with the delay before re-treating the aplastic anemia patient.

New approaches to immunosuppressive treatment

The outcome for aplastic anemia patients treated with immunosuppression improved greatly between the 1970s and 1990s (Figure 10.5). Five-year survival probabilities are $52 \pm 6\%$ for patients treated between 1974 and 1979, $65 \pm 2\%$ for patients treated between 1980 and 1989, and $77 \pm 3\%$ for patients treated between 1990 and 1995 ($P = 0.0006$) (unpublished data of the EBMT). Despite this improvement, unresolved questions remain. Therefore, new approaches are being investigated. The contribution of these therapies as an alternative to immunosuppression for patients who lack an HLA-matched donor has to be viewed critically. The preliminary results of treating with high-dose cyclophosphamide and the combination of immunosuppression and G-CSF are discussed in this chapter.

Cyclophosphamide is a potent immunosuppressive agent that is used in most current conditioning regimens of bone marrow transplantation required for aplastic anemia (Gluckman et al., 1992a; Hows et al., 1989; Storb et al., 1997). After successful marrow transplantation patients usually recover normal hemopoiesis, and hemopoietic engraftment in these patients is of the donor type. Despite the improved outcome of transplantation, graft rejection remains a real problem for patients with aplastic anemia (Deeg et al., 1986). Nevertheless, even after graft rejection patients do not invariably die from the consequences of pancytopenia. There are patients with aplastic anemia in whom autologous marrow recovery has occurred after cyclophosphamide conditioning and marrow infusion (Sensenbrenner et al., 1977; Speck et al., 1976; Territo, 1977). Furthermore, recovery from aplastic anemia after treatment with cyclophosphamide alone has been reported (Baran et al., 1976). Since no single center has treated enough cases to perform a clinical trial, a survey conducted by the member of the American Society of Hematology analyzed cumulative data on the effectiveness of cyclophosphamide in patients with severe aplastic anemia (Griner, 1980). Seventy-three patients from 50 centers have been reported, but only three remissions have been observed. Doses of cyclophosphamide of the reported cases ranged from 100mg daily for up to 4 months to 30mg/kg daily for 4 days. Twenty-five percent of patients received cyclophosphamide in doses approaching those used for conditioning prior to marrow transplantation. The three patients with aplastic anemia described in this survey achieved a hematological remission with moderate to high doses of cyclophosphamide (40–120mg/kg) without bone marrow transplantation.

More recently the results relating to ten patients with severe aplastic anemia who did not have an HLA-identical sibling were published (Brodsky et al., 1996). The patients were treated with high-dose cyclophosphamide, receiving 45mg/kg per day over four consecutive days, with or without cyclosporin. A complete remission was achieved in seven patients. Six patients were alive and in continuous remission 7.3–17.8 years after treatment, and one died from acquired immunodeficiency syndrome (AIDS) 44 months after treatment with cyclophosphamide. The high-dose cyclophosphamide was well tolerated. In responders, a neutrophil count of 0.5×10^9/l was achieved at a median of 95 days (range 34–201 days), and the last platelet concentrate was transfused 85 days after treatment (median; range 35–151 days). None of the responders relapsed or developed a clonal disorder.

In contrast to what is observed after conventional immunosuppression with ALG and cyclosporin, all patients restored a complete hemopoiesis with normal peripheral blood counts, and only one patient had an elevated mean corpuscular volume (MCV). If residual abnormalities of hemopoiesis observed after ALG treatment reflect the persisting defect of stem cells, than these data may support the hypothesis that more intensive immunosuppression could eradicate the disease. Unlike those who respond to ALG and cyclosporin therapies, responders to high-dose cyclophosphamide would not be at risk of relapsing or of late clonal complication such as myelodysplastic syndrome or paroxysmal nocturnal hemoglobinuria. These data are encouraging, but preliminary. A trial with a larger number of patients needs to be performed. Furthermore, the high-dose cyclophosphamide may have drawbacks. The fear of treating a disease where the stem cells are already defective with a drug that could provoke a definitive aplasia is justified. Indeed, some patients have worsened pancytopenia for a prolonged period of time after exposure to cyclophosphamide (personal communications).

The use of growth factors will be reviewed separately. Here, only the study of the EBMT SAA Working Party evaluating the combination of immunosuppression and ALG, cyclosporin and G-CSF will be discussed. In a pilot trial involving 40 patients, the feasibility of combining G-CSF, at a dose of 5 μg/kg per day for 90 days, together with ALG and cyclosporin was tested. Patients with untreated severe aplastic anemia and with neutrophil counts of $\leq 0.5 \times 10^9$/l were eligible. Overall the treatment was well tolerated. Thirty-three patients (82%) had trilineage hemopoietic reconstitution and became independent of transfusions at a median interval of 115 days, four patients (10%) showed no recovery and three patients (8%) died early because of infection (Bacigalupo et al., 1995).

A next issue to consider, as for refractory autoimmune diseases, is the potential benefit of autologous stem-cell transplantation. However, the mobilization and collection of hemopoietic progenitor cells with preserved proliferation capacity in those with aplastic anemia might be difficult. Preliminary data show that patients with acquired severe aplastic anemia treated with ALG, methylprednisolone, cyclosporin and G-CSF can mobilize peripheral-blood hemopoietic progenitor cells. Cells with the phenotype and in vitro function of early hemopoietic progenitor cells are found, though in small numbers, in the peripheral blood of patients with severe aplastic anemia after treatment with immunosuppressants and prolonged G-CSF administration (Bacigalupo et al., 1993b, 1997). Whether mobilized progenitors are suitable for autologous reconstitution in these patients remains an open question.

Conclusion

Immunosuppressive treatment improves peripheral blood counts in patients with aplastic anemia. After successful treatment patients no longer require transfusions and become free from infections, but they are not cured from their disease. Nevertheless, immunosuppression is the treatment of choice for patients not eligible for bone marrow transplantation. Currently, the best results are obtained with a combination of ALG and cyclosporin. This combination leads to a survival probability at 2 years of 72%. Adding androgens and corticosteroids in normal or high doses to this combination has not further improved the results. There is a strong correlation between disease severity and survival after immunosuppression. Indeed, low neutrophil counts before treatment are related to a significantly lower survival. How patients with aplastic anemia respond to immunosuppressive treatment is independent of their age; however, age does influence survival, with older patients having an increased mortality. Nevertheless, there is no reason to withhold treatment from older patients solely because of their age. The decision to treat older patients should depend on their medical condition rather than a fixed age limit. In patients responding to immunosuppressive treatment, hemopoiesis improves gradually, and the time taken to respond varies widely from 1 to 12 months. However, blood counts may never normalize for some. Treatment with ALG and cyclosporin leads to immediate allergic reactions, serum sickness, a transient drop of blood counts and toxicity caused by concomitant treatments. The death rate is highest during the first year after treatment, and during this period the main causes of death are related to bleeding and severe infections. About 20–30% of patients fail to respond to an initial course of immunosuppression and a further 30% relapse after an initial response to immunosuppression. About half of these patients can respond to a second course of ALG. Re-treating aplastic anemia patients with ALG does not increase the risk associated with the treatment.

Acknowledgements

Our special thanks go to Aleksandra Wodnar Filipowicz for her critical comments on the manuscript and to Alois Gratwohl for his helpful discussions.

References

Alexanian, R., Nadell, J. and Alfrey, C. (1972) Oxymetholone treatment for anemia of bone marrow failure. *Blood*, **40**, 353–65.

Bacigalupo, A., Giordano, D., Vimercati, R. and Marmont, A. M. (1979) Bolus methylprednisolone in severe aplastic anemia. *New England Journal of Medicine*, **300**, 501–2.

Bacigalupo, A., Van Lint, M. T., Cerri, R., Giordano, D., Santini, G., Carrella, M., Damasio, E. E., Rossi, E., Risso, M., Vimercati, R., Podesta, M., Durando, A., Reali, G., Avanzi, G., Barbanti, M. and Marmont, A. M. (1980) Treatment of severe aplastic anemia with bolus of 6-methylprednisolone and antilymphocyte globulin. *Blut*, **41**, 168–71.

Bacigalupo, A., Van Lint, M. T., Congiu, M., Pittaluga, P. A., Occhini, D. and Marmont, A. M. (1986) Treatment of SAA in Europe 1970–1985: a report of the SAA Working Party. *Bone Marrow Transplantation*, **1**, 611–15.

Bacigalupo, A., Hows, J., Gluckman, E., Nissen, C., Marsh, J. C. W., Van Lint, M. T., Congiu, M., De Planque, M. M., Ernst, P., McCann, S., Ragavashar, A., Frickhofen, N., Würsch, A., Marmont, A. M. and Gordon–Smith, E. C. (1988) Bone marrow transplantation (BMT) versus immunosuppression for the treatment of severe aplastic anaemia: a report of the EBMT SAA Working Party. *British Journal of Haematology*, **70**, 177–82.

Bacigalupo, A., Hows, J., Würsch, A., Nissen, C., Gluckman, E., Devergie, A., Marsh, J. C., Van Lint, M. T., Congiu, M., Granena, A., De Planque, M. M., Ernst, P., McCann, S., Ragavashar, A., Frickhofen, N., Gordon–Smith, E. and Marmont, A. M. (1990) Treatment of severe aplastic anemia with bone marrow transplantation or immunosuppression: a report for the EBMT SAA Working Party. In *Aplastic anemia and other bone marrow failure syndromes*, N. T. Shahidi ed., p.115. Berlin: Springer-Verlag.

Bacigalupo, A., Chaple, A., Hows, J., Van Lint, M. T., McCann, S., Milligan, D., Chessells, J., Goldstone, A. H., Ottolander, J., Van't Veer, E. T., Comotti, B., Coser, P., Broccia, G., Bosi, A., Locascuilli, A., Catalano, L., Battista, R., Arcese, W., Carotenuto, M., Marmont, A. M. and Gordon–Smith, E. C. (1993*a*) Treatment of aplastic anaemia (AA) with antilymphocyte globulin (ALG) and methylprednisolone (MPred) with or without androgens: a randomized trial from the EBMT SAA working party. *British Journal of Haematology*, **83**, 145–51.

Bacigalupo, A., Piaggio, G., Podesta, M., Van Lint, M. T., Valbonesi, M., Lercari, G., Mori, P. G., Pasino, M., Franchini, E. and Rivabella, L. (1993*b*) Collection of peripheral blood hematopoietic progenitors (PBHP) from patients with severe aplastic anemia (SAA) after prolonged administration of granulocyte colony-stimulating factor. *Blood*, **82**, 1410–14.

Bacigalupo, A., Broccia, G., Corda, G., Arcese, W., Carotenuto, M., Gallamini, A., Locatelli, F., Mori, P. G., Saracco, P. and Todeschini, G. (1995) Antilymphocyte globulin, cyclosporin, and granulocyte colony-stimulating factor in patients with acquired severe aplastic anemia (SAA): a pilot study of the EBMT SAA Working Party. *Blood*, **85**, 1348–53.

Bacigalupo, A., Piaggio, G., Podesta, M., Tong, J., Pitto, A., Figari, O., Benvenuto, F., Vassallo, F., Tedone, E., Grassia, L., Van Lint, M. T., Gualandi, F. and Hoffman, R. (1997) Early hemopoietic progenitors in the peripheral blood of patients with severe aplastic anemia (SAA) after treatment with antilymphocyte globulin (ALG), cyclosporin-A and G-CSF. *Haematologica*, **82**, 133–7.

Baran, D. T., Griner, P. F. and Klemperer, M. R. (1976) Recovery from aplastic anemia after treatment with cyclophosphamide. *New England Journal of Medicine*, **295**, 1522.

Barbano, G. C., Schenone, A., Roncella, S., Ghio, R., Corcione, A., Mori, P. G., Ferrarini, M. and Pistoia, V. (1988) Anti-lymphocyte globulin stimulates normal human T cells to proliferate and to release lymphokines in vitro. A study at the clonal level. *Blood*, **72**, 956–63.

Bielory, L., Gascon, P., Lawley, T. J., Nienhuis, A., Frank, M. M. and Young, N. S. (1986) Serum sickness and haematopoietic recovery with antithymocyte globulin in bone marrow failure patients. *British Journal of Haematology*, **63**, 729–36.

Bielory, L., Gascon, P., Lawley, T. J., Young, N. S. and Frank, M. M. (1988*a*) Human serum sickness: a prospective analysis of 35 patients treated with equine anti-thymocyte globulin for bone marrow failure. *Medicine (Baltimore)*, **67**, 40–57.

Bielory, L., Wright, R., Nienhuis, A., Young, N. S. and Kalliner, M. A. (1988*b*) Antithymocyte globulin hypersensitivity in bone marrow failure patients. *Journal of the American Medical Association*, **260**, 3164–7.

Bonnefoy–Berard, N., Vincent, C. and Revillard, J. P. (1991) Antibodies against functional leukocyte surface molecules in polyclonal antilymphocyte and antithymocyte globulins. *Transplantation*, **51**, 669–73.

Bonnefoy–Berard, N., Flacher, M. and Revillard, J. P. (1992) Antiproliferative effect of antilymphocyte globulins on B cells and B-cell lines. *Blood*, **79**, 2164–70.

Bourdage, J. S. and Hamlin, D. M. (1995) Comparative polyclonal antithymocyte globulin and antilymphocyte/antilymphoblast globulin anti-CD antigen analysis by flow cytometry. *Transplantation*, **59**, 1194–200.

Bridges, R., Pineo, G. and Blahey, W. (1987) Cyclosporin A for the treatment of aplastic anemia refractory to antithymocyte globulin. *American Journal of Hematology*, **26**, 83–7.

Brodsky, R. A., Sensenbrenner, L. L. and Jones, R. J. (1996) Complete remission in severe aplastic anemia after high-dose cyclophosphamide without bone marrow transplantation. *Blood*, **87**, 491–4.

Camitta, B., O'Reilly, J. O., Sensenbrenner, L. L., Rappeport, J. M., Champlin, R. E., Doney, K., August, C., Hoffmann, R., Kirkpatrick, D., Stuard, R., Santos, G., Parkman, R., Gale, R. P. and Nathan, D. G. (1983) Antithoracic duct lymphocyte globulin therapy of severe aplastic anemia. *Blood*, **62**, 883–8.

Champlin, R., Ho, W. G., Feig, S. A., Lenarsky, C., Winston, D. J. and Gale, R. P. (1984) Lack of efficacy for intravenous monoclonal anti-T-cell antibody (T101) for aplastic anemia: a randomized controlled trial. *Blood*, **64**, 102A.

Champlin, R. E., Ho, W. G. and Gale, R. P. (1983) Antilymphocyte globulin treatment in patients with aplastic anemia. A prospective randomized trial. *New England Journal of Medicine*, **308**, 113–18.

Champlin, R. E., Ho, W. G., Feig, S. A., Winston, D. J., Lenarsky, C. and Gale, R. P. (1985) Do androgens enhance the response to antithymocyte globulin in patients with aplastic anemia? A prospective randomized trial. *Blood*, **66**, 184–8.

Champlin, R. E., Nimer, S. D., Ireland, P., Oette, D. H. and Golde, D. W. (1989) Treatment of refractory aplastic anemia with recombinant human granulocyte-macrophage-colony-stimulating factor. *Blood*, **73**, 694–9.

Charleux, H., Julien, M., Bonsquent, R., Ribardière, J. L., Marmuse, J. P. and Hakim, J. (1989) Splenectomy in hematologic diseases: indications, technics and early results. *Chirurgie*, **115**, 494–9.

Crump, M., Larratt, L. M., Maki, E., Curtis, J. E., Minden, M. D., Meharchand, J. M., Lipton, J. H. and Messner, H. A. (1992) Treatment of adults with severe aplastic anemia: primary therapy with antithymocyte globulin (ATG) and rescue of ATG failures with bone marrow transplantation. *American Journal of Medicine*, **92**, 596–602.

Dan, K., Gomi, S., Kuramoto, A., Maekawa, T. and Nomura, T. (1992) A multicenter prospective study on the treatment of chronic idiopathic thromocytopenic purpura. *International Journal of Hematology*, **55**, 287–92.

De Planque, M. M., Kluin–Nelemans, H. C., Van Krieken, H. J. M., Kluin, P. M., Brand, A., Beverstock, G. C., Willemze, R. and Van Rood, J. J. (1988) Evolution of acquired severe aplastic anaemia to myelodysplastic and subsequent leukaemia in adults. *British Journal of Haematology*, **70**, 55.

De Planque, M. M., Bacigalupo, A., Würsch, A., Hows, J., Devergie, A., Frickhofen, N., Brand, A. and Nissen, C. (1989*a*) Long-term follow-up of severe aplastic anaemia patients treated with antilymphocyte globulin. *British Journal of Haematology*, **73**, 121–6.

De Planque, M. M., Brand, A., Kluin–Nelemans, H. C., Eernisse, J. G., van der Burgh, F., Natarajan, A. T., Beverstock, G. C., Zwaan, F. E., Willemze, R. and van Rood, J. J. (1989*b*) Haematopoietic and immunologic abnormalities in severe aplastic anaemia patients treated with anti-thymocyte globulin. *British Journal of Haematology*, **71**, 421–30.

Dearden, C., Foukaneli, T., Lee, P., Gordon–Smith, E. and Marsh, J. C. (1998) The incidence and significance of fever during treatment with antilymphocyte globulin for aplastic anaemia. *Bone Marrow Transplantation*, **21** [Suppl. 1], S49–S49.

Deeg, H. J., Self, S., Storb, R., Doney, K., Appelbaum, F., Witherspoon, R. P., Sullivan, K. M., Sheehan, K., Sanders, J., Mickelson, E. and Thomas, E. D. (1986) Decreased incidence of marrow graft rejection in patients with severe aplastic anemia: changing impact factors. *Blood*, **68**, 1363–8.

Delgado–Lamas, J. L., Lopez–Karpovitch, X., Marin–Lopez, A., Romero–Garcia, F., Ruiz–Arguelles, G. J., Ruiz–Gonzalez, D. S., Taboada, C., Vazquez–Villegas, V. and Elena, Z. M. (1989) Low doses of high-potency antithymocyte globulin (ATG) in severe aplastic anemia: experience with the Mexican ATG. *Acta Haematologica*, **81**, 70–4.

Desposito, F., Akatsuka, J., Thatcher, L. G. and Smith, N. J. (1964) Bone marrow failure in pediatric patients. *Journal of Pediatrics*, **64**, 683–96.

Doney, K., Weiden, P., Buckner, C. D., Storb, R. and Thomas, E. D. (1981) Treatment of severe aplastic anemia using antilymphocyte globulin with or without an infusion of HLA haploidentical marrow. *Experimental Hematology*, **9**, 829–33.

Doney, K., Dahlberg, S. J., Monroe, D., Storb, R., Buckner, C. D. and Thomas, E. D. (1984) Therapy of severe aplastic anemia with anti-human thymocyte globulin and androgens: the effect of HLA-haploidentical marrow infusion. *Blood*, **63**, 342–8.

Doney, K., Martin, P., Storb, R., Whitehead, J., Smith, A. G., Hansen, J., Appelbaum, F., Buckner, C. D. and Thomas, E. D. (1985) A randomized trial of antihuman thymocyte globulin versus murine monoclonal antihuman T-cell antibodies as immunosuppressive therapy for aplastic anemia. *Experimental Hematology*, **13**, 520–4.

Doney, K., Storb, R., Buckner, C. D., McGuffin, R., Witherspoon, R. P., Deeg, H. J., Appelbaum, F., Sullivan, K. M. and Thomas, E. D. (1987) Treatment of aplastic anemia with antithymocyte globulin, high-dose corticosteroids, and androgens. *Experimental Hematology*, **15**, 239–42.

Doney, K., Kopecky, K., Storb, R., Buckner, C. D., Singer, J., Anasetti, C., Appelbaum, F., Beatty, P., Bensinger, W., Berenson, R., Clift, R., Deeg, H. J., Hansen, J., Hill, R., Loughran, T., Martin, P., Petersen, F. B., Sale, G., Sanders, J., Sullivan, K. M., Stewart, P., Weiden, P., Witherspoon, R. P. and Thomas, E. D. (1990) Long-term comparison of immunosuppressive therapy with antithymocyte globulin to bone marrow transplantation in aplastic anemia. In *Aplastic anemia and other bone marrow failure syndromes*, ed. N. T. Shahidi, p. 104. Berlin: Springer-Verlag.

Doney, K., Pepe, M., Storb, R., Bryant, E., Anasetti, C., Appelbaum, F. R., Buckner, C. D., Sanders, J., Singer, J., Sullivan, K. M., Weiden, P. and Hansen, J. (1992) Immunosuppressive treatment of aplastic anemia: results of a prospective randomized trial of antilymphocyte globulin (ATG), methylprednisolone, and oxymetholone to ATG, very high-dose methylprednisolone, and oxymetholone. *Blood*, **79**, 2566–71.

Doney, K., Leisenring, W., Storb, R. and Appelbaum, F. R. (1997) Primary treatment of acquired aplastic anemia: outcomes with bone marrow transplantation and immunosuppressive therapy. *Annals of Internal Medicine*, **126**, 107–15.

Erlanger, B. F. (1993) Do we know the site of action of cyclosporin? *Immunology Today*, **13**, 487–90.

Ermakov, B., Peters, C., Alexeitschik, A., Matthes–Martin, S., Ladenstein, R., Mann, G., Holter, W. and Gadner, H. (1998) Acute side effects of ATG with different infusion regimens. *Bone Marrow Transplantation*, **21** [Suppl. 1], S48.

Esperou, H., Devergie, A., Lehn, P., Lallemand, A. and Gluckman, E. (1989) A randomized study comparing cyclosporin A and antithymocyte globulin for treatment of severe aplastic anemia. *Nouvelle Revue Française d'Hématologie*, **31**, 65–8.

Facon, T., Walter, M. P., Fenaux, P., Morel, P., Dupriez, B., Gardin, C., Jouet, J. P. and Bauters, F. (1991) Treatment of severe aplastic anemia with antilymphocyte globulin and androgens: a report on 33 patients. *Annals of Hematology*, **63**, 89–93.

Fairhead, S. M., Chipping, P. M. and Gordon–Smith, E. (1983) Treatment of aplastic anaemia with antilymphocyte globulin (ALG). *British Journal of Haematology*, **55**, 7–16.

Finlay, J. L., Toretsky, J., Hoffman, R., Bruno, E. and Shahidi, N. T. (1984) Cyclosporin in refractory severe aplastic anemia. *Blood*, **64**, 104a.

Frickhofen, N., Heit, W., Raghavachar, A., Porzsolt, F. and Heimpel, H. (1986) Treatment of aplastic anemia with cyclosporin A, methylprednisolone, and antilymphocyte globulin. *Klinische Wochenschrift*, **64**, 1165–70.

Frickhofen, N., Kaltwasser, J. P., Schrezenmeier, H., Ragavashar, A., Vogt, H. G., Herrmann, F., Freund, M., Meusers, P., Salama, A. and Heimpel, H. (1991) Treatment of aplastic anemia with antilymphocyte globulin and methylprednisolone with or without cyclosporin. *New England Journal of Medicine*, **324**, 1297–304.

Fuhrer, M., Bender–Gotze, C., Ebell, W., Friedrich, W. and Kohne, E. (1994) Treatment of aplastic anemia – aims and development of the SAA 94 pilot protocol. *Klinische Padiatrie*, **206**, 289–95.

Ganser, A., Lindemann, A., Seipelt, G., Ottmann, O. G., Herrmann, F., Eder, M., Frisch, J., Schulz, G., Mertelsmann, R. and Hoelzer, D. (1990) Effects of recombinant human interleukin-3 in patients with normal hematopoiesis and in patients with bone marrow failure. *Blood*, **76**, 666–76.

Ganser, A., Lindemann, A., Ottmann, O. G., Seipelt, G., Hess, U., Geissler, G., Kanz, L., Frish, J., Schulz, G., Herrmann, F., Mertelsmann, R. and Hoelzer, D. (1992) Sequential in vivo treatment with two recombinant human hemopoietic growth factors (interleukin 3 and granulocyte macrophage colony stimulating factor) as a new therapeutic modality to stimulate hematopoiesis: results of a phase I study. *Blood*, **79**, 2583.

Gascon, P., Zoumbos, N. C., Scala, G., Djeu, J. Y., Moore, J. G. and Young, N. S. (1985) Lymphokine abnormalities in aplastic anemia: implications for the mechanism of action of antithymocyte globulin. *Blood*, **65**, 407–13.

Gluckman, E., Devergie, A., Faille, A., Barrett, A. J., Bonneau, M., Boiron, M. and Bernard, J. (1978) Treatment of severe aplastic anemia with antilymphocyte globulin and androgens. *Experimental Hematology*, **6**, 679–87.

Gluckman, E., Devergie, A., Poros, A. and Degoulet, P. (1982) Results of immunosuppression in 170 cases of severe aplastic anaemia. Report of the European Group of Blood and Bone Marrow Transplant. *British Journal of Haematology*, **51**, 541–50.

Gluckman, E., Marmont, A. M., Speck, B. and Gordon–Smith, E. (1984) Immunosuppressive treatment of aplastic anemia as an alternative treatment for bone marrow transplantation. *Seminars in Hematology*, **21**, 11–19.

Gluckman, E., Horowitz, M. M., Champlin, R. E., Hows, J., Bacigalupo, A., Biggs, J. C., Camitta, B., Gale, R. P., Gordon–Smith, E., Marmont, A. M., Masaoka, T., Ramsay, N. K., Rimm, A. A., Rozman, C., Sobocinski, K. A., Speck, B. and Bortin, M. M. (1992*a*) Bone marrow transplantation for severe aplastic anemia: influence of conditioning and graft-versus-host disease prophylaxis regimens on outcome. *Blood*, **79**, 269–75.

Gluckman, E., Esperou–Bourdeau, H., Baruchel, A., Boogaerts, M., Briere, J., Donadio, D., Leverger, G., Leporrier, M., Reiffers, J. and Janvier, M. (1992*b*) A multicenter randomized study comparing cyclosporin-A alone and antithymocyte globulin with prednisone for treatment of severe aplastic anemia. The cooperative group on the treatment of aplastic anemia. *Journal of Autoimmunity*, **5** [Suppl. A], 271–5.

Gluckman, E., Esperou–Bourdeau, H., Baruchel, A., Boogaerts, M., Briere, J., Donadio, D., Leverger, G., Leporrier, M., Reiffers, J. and Janvier, M. (1992*c*) Multicenter randomized study comparing cyclosporin-A alone and antithymocyte globulin with prednisone for treatment of severe aplastic anemia. *Blood*, **79**, 2540–6.

Greco, B., Bielory, L., Stephany, D., Hsu, S. M., Gascon, P., Nienhuis, A. and Young, N. (1983) Antithymocyte globulin reacts with many normal human cell types. *Blood*, **62**, 1047–54.

Griner, P. F. (1980) A survey of the effectiveness of cyclophosphamide in patients with severe aplastic anemia. *American Journal of Hematology*, **8**, 55–60.

Grumet, F. C. and Yankee, R. A. (1970) Long-term platelet support of patients with aplastic anemia: effect of splenectomy and steroid therapy. *Annals of Internal Medicine*, **73**, 1–7.

Heaton, L., Crosby, W. and Cohen, A. (1957) Splenectomy in the treatment of hypoplasia of the bone marrow, with a report of 12 cases. *Annals of Surgery*, **146**, 637–60.

Hinterberger–Fischer, M., Hinterberger, W., Hockern, P., Schmidmeier, W., Gadner, H., Geissler, K., Kos, M., Schwarzinger, I., Neumann, E. and Niessner, H. (1986) Treatment of severe aplastic anemia with combined immunosuppression (antithymocyte globulin and high-dose methylprednisolone). *Acta Haematologica*, **76**, 196–201.

Hinterberger–Fischer, M., Höcker, P., Lechner, K., Seewann, H. and Hinterberger, W. (1989) Oral cyclosporin-A is effective treatment for untreated and also previously immunosuppressed patients with severe marrow failure. *European Journal of Hematology*, **43**, 136–42.

Hows, J., Marsh, J. C., Yin, J. L., Durrant, S., Swirski, D., Worsley, A., Fairhead, S. M., Chipping, P. M., Palmer, S. and Gordon–Smith, E. (1989) Bone marrow transplantation for severe aplastic anaemia using cyclosporin: long term follow-up. *Bone Marrow Transplantation*, **4**, 11–16.

Hows, J., Szydlo, R., Anasetti, C., Camitta, B., Gajewski, J. and Gluckman, E. (1992) Unrelated donor marrow transplants for severe acquired aplastic anemia. *Bone Marrow Transplantation*, **10** (Suppl. 1), 102–6.

Hows, J., Camitta, B., Stone, J., Deeg, H. J. and Horowitz, M. M. (1998) Alternative donor BMT for acquired aplastic anaemia 1986–1993. *Bone Marrow Transplantation*, **21** [Suppl. 1], S47.

Huang, A. T., Mold, N. G. and Zhang, S. F. (1987) Antithymocyte globulin stimulates human hematopoietic progenitor cells. *Proceedings of the National Academy of Sciences of the USA*, **84**, 5942–6.

Imashuku, S., Hibi, S., Kataoka–Morimoto, Y., Yoshihara, T., Ikushima, S., Morioka, Y. and Todo, S. (1995) Myelodysplasia and acute myeloid leukaemia in cases of aplastic anaemia and congenital neutropenia following G-CSF administration. *British Journal of Haematology*, **89**, 188–90.

Jacobs, P., Wood, L. and Martell, R. W. (1985) Cyclosporin A in the treatment of severe acute aplastic anaemia. *British Journal of Haematology*, **61**, 267–72.

Jansen, J., Zwaan, F. and Haak, H. L. (1982) Antilymphocyte globulin treatment for aplastic anemia. *Scandinavian Journal of Hematology*, **28**, 341–51.

Jansen, J., Gratama, J. W., Zwaan, F. and Simonis, R. F. A. (1984) Therapy with monoclonal antibody OKT3 in severe aplastic anemia. *Experimental Hematology*, **12** [Suppl. 15], 46–7.

Jeannet, M., Speck, B., Rubinstein, A., Pelet, B., Wyss, M. and Kummer, H. (1976) Autologous marrow reconstitutions in severe aplastic anaemia after ALG pretreatment and HLA-A semi-incompatible bone marrow cell transfusion. *Acta Haematologica*, **55**, 129–39.

Kaltwasser, J. P., Dix, U., Schalk, K. P. and Vogt, H. (1988) Effect of androgens on the response to antithymocyte globulin in patients with aplastic anaemia. *European Journal of Haematology*, **40**, 111–18.

Kawano, Y., Nissen, C., Gratwohl, A. and Speck, B. (1988) Immunostimulatory effects of different antilymphocyte globulin preparations: a possible clue to their clinical effect. *British Journal of Haematology*, **68**, 115–19.

Kawano, Y., Takaue, Y., Watanabe, T., Ninomiya, T., Kuroda, Y., Nissen, C., Gratwohl, A. and Speck, B. (1989) Comparative study on in vitro lymphocytotoxicity and mitogenicity of different antilymphocyte globulin (ALG) preparations [in Japanese with English summary]. *Rinsho Ketsueki*, **30**, 327–31.

Kawano, Y., Nissen, C., Gratwohl, A., Wursch, A. and Speck, B. (1990) Cytotoxic and stimulatory effects of antilymphocyte globulin (ALG) on hematopoiesis. *Blut*, **60**, 297–300.

Koch, J. L. and Beaumont, T. (1967) Aplastic anemia and splenectomy. *Archives of Internal Medicine*, **119**, 305.

Kojima, S., Miyajima, Y., Fukuda, M., Matsuyama, T., Maeda, H., Yamamoto, K., Tsuzuki, S., Akatsuka, M., Sugihara, T. and Minami, S. (1992) Treatment of aplastic anemia with anti-lymphocyte globulin, high-dose methylprednisolone and androgen [in Japanese with English summary]. *Rinsho Ketsueki*, **33**, 11–16.

Lawlor, E. R., Anderson, R. A., Davis, J. H., Fryer, C. J., Pritchard, S. L., Rogers, P. C., Wu, J. K. and Schultz, K. R. (1997) Immunosuppressive therapy: a potential alternative to bone marrow transplantation as initial therapy for acquired severe aplastic anemia in childhood? *Journal of Pediatric Hematology/Oncology*, **19**, 115–23.

Leonard, E. M., Raefsky, E., Griffith, P., Kimball, J., Nienhuis, A. and Young, N. S. (1989) Cyclosporin therapy of aplastic anaemia, congenital and acquired red cell aplasia. *British Journal of Haematology*, **72**, 278–84.

Lopez–Karpovitch, X., Zarzosa, M. E., Cardenas, M. R. and Piedras, J. (1989) Changes in peripheral blood mononuclear cell subpopulations during antithymocyte globulin therapy for severe aplastic anemia. *Acta Haematologica*, **81**, 176–80.

Margolis, D., Camitta, B., Pietryga, D., Keever–Taylor, C., Baxter–Lowe, L. A., Pierce, K., Kupst, M. J., French, J. III, Truitt, R., Lawton, C., Murray, K., Garbrecht, F., Flomenberg, N. and Casper, J. (1996) Unrelated donor bone marrow transplantation to treat severe aplastic anaemia in children and young adults. *British Journal of Haematology*, **94**, 65–72.

Marmont, A. M., Bacigalupo, A. and Van Lint, M. T. (1983) Treatment for severe aplastic anemia with sequential immunosuppression. *Experimental Hematology*, **11**, 856–65.

Marsh, J. C. and Geary, C. G. (1991) Is aplastic anaemia a pre-leukaemic disorder? [editorial]. *British Journal of Haematology*, **77**, 447–52.

Marsh, J. C. and Gordon–Smith, E. (1988) The role of antilymphocyte globulin in the treatment of chronic acquired bone marrow failure. *Blood Review*, **2**, 141–8.

Marsh, J. C. and Gordon–Smith, E. C. (1995) Treatment of aplastic anaemia with antilymphocyte globulin and cyclosporin. *International Journal of Hematology*, **62**, 133–44.

Marsh, J. C., Chang, J., Testa, N. G., Hows, J. and Dexter, T. M. (1990) The hematopoietic defect in aplastic anemia assessed by long-term marrow culture. *Blood*, **76**, 1–10.

Marsh, J. C., Zomas, A., Hows, J. M., Chapple, M. and Gordon–Smith, E. C. (1993) Avascular necrosis after treatment of aplastic anaemia with antilymphocyte globulin and high-dose methylprednisolone. *British Journal of Haematology*, **84**, 731–5.

Marsh, J. C., Socié, G., Schrezenmeier, H., Tichelli, A., Gluckman, E., Ljungman, P., McCann, S. R., Raghavachar, A., Marin, P. and Hows, J. M. (1994) Haemopoietic growth factors in aplastic anaemia: a cautionary note. European Bone Marrow Transplant Working Party for Severe Aplastic Anaemia. *Lancet*, **344**, 172–3.

Marsh, J. C., Schrezenmeier, H., Marin, P., Ilhan, O., Ljungman, P., McCann, S., Socié, G., Tichelli, A., Hows, J., Ragavashar, A., Bacigalupo, A., Haas, O. and for the EBMT SAA Working Party (1997) Interim analysis of a prospective randomised study comparing cyclosporin with the combination of antithymocyte globulin and cyclosporin for the treatment of non-severe aplastic anaemia. *Bone Marrow Transplantation*, **19**, S89–S89.

Marsh, J. C. W., Hows, J., Bryett, K. A., Al–Hashimi, S., Fairhead, S. M. and Gordon–Smith, E. C. (1987) Survival after antilymphocyte globulin therapy for aplastic anemia depends on disease severity. *Blood*, **70**, 1046–52.

Mathé, G, Amiel, J. L., Schwarzenberg, L., Choay, J., Trolard, P., Schneider, M., Hayat, M., Schlumberger, J. R. and Jasmin, C. L. (1970) Bone marrow graft in man after conditioning with antilymphocyte serum. *British Medical Journal*, **2**, 131–6.

Matloub, Y. H., Smith, C., Bostrom, B., Koerper, M. A., O'Leary, M., Khuder, S., Smithson, W. A., Nickerson, H. J., Silberman, T., Hilden, J., Moertel, C. L., Month, S., Monteleone, P. and Ramsay, N. K. (1997) One course versus two courses of antithymocyte globulin for the treatment of severe aplastic anemia in children. *Journal of Pediatric Hematology/Oncology*, **19**, 110–14.

Means, R. T. Jr., Krantz, S. B., Dessypris, E. N., Lukens, J. N., Niblack, G. D., Greer, J. P., Flexner, J. M. and Stein, R. S. (1988) Re-treatment of aplastic anemia with antithymocyte globulin or antilymphocyte serum. *American Journal of Medicine*, **84**, 678–82.

Miller, W. J., Branda, R. F., Flynn, P. J., Howe, R. B., Ramsay, N. K. C., Condie, R. M. and Jacob, H. S. (1983) Antilymphocyte globulin treatment of severe aplastic anaemia. *British Journal of Haematology*, **55**, 17–25.

Nissen, C., Cornu, P., Gratwohl, A. and Speck, B. (1980) Peripheral blood cells from patients with aplastic anaemia in partial remission suppress growth of their own bone marrow precursors in culture. *British Journal of Haematology*, **45**, 233–43.

Nissen, C., Moser, Y., Bürgin, M., Oberholzer, M., Bannert, P., Corneo, M. and Speck, B. (1982) Aplastic anemia: low production of hemopoietic growth factors predicts failure or retarded recovery after immunosuppressive treatment. *Experimental Hematology*, **10** [Suppl. 12], 143–9.

Nissen, C., Tichelli, A., Gratwohl, A., Speck, B., Milne, A., Gordon–Smith, E. and Schaedelin, J. (1988) Failure of recombinant human granulocyte-macrophage colony-stimulating factor in aplastic anemia patients with very severe aplastic neutropenia. *Blood*, **72**, 2045–7.

Nissen, C., Gratwohl, A., Tichelli, A., Stebler, C., Wursch, A., Moser, Y., dalle Carbonare, V., Signer, E., Buser, M. and Ritz, R. (1993) Gender and response to antilymphocyte globulin (ALG) for severe aplastic anaemia. *British Journal of Haematology*, **83**, 319–25.

Novitzky, N., Wood, L. and Jacobs, P. (1991) Treatment of aplastic anaemia with antilymphocyte globulin and high-dose methylprednisolone. *American Journal of Hematology*, **36**, 227–34.

Novitzky, N., Mobara, G. and Jacobs, P. (1992) Antilymphocyte globulin and high-dose methylprednisolone improve survival in patients with aplastic anaemia without additional financial costs. *South African Medical Journal*, **81**, 254–7.

Ohsaka, A., Sugahara, Y., Imai, Y. and Kikuchi, M. (1995) Evolution of severe aplastic anemia to myelodysplasia with monosomy 7 following granulocyte colony-stimulating factor, erythropoietin and high-dose methylprednisolone combination therapy. *Internal Medicine*, **34**, 892–5.

Paquette, R. L., Tebyani, N., Frane, M., Ireland, P., Ho, W. G., Champlin, R. E. and Nimer, S. D. (1995) Long-term outcome of aplastic anemia in adults treated with antithymocyte globulin: comparison with bone marrow transplantation. *Blood*, **85**, 283–90.

Pulver, K. P. and Flaum, M. A. (1987) Refractory aplastic anemia: concomitant therapy with antithymocyte globulin and high-dose corticosteroids. *American Journal of Hematology*, **25**, 95–100.

Raefsky, E. L., Gascon, P., Gratwohl, A., Speck, B. and Young, N. S. (1986) Biological and immunological characterization of ATG and ALG. *Blood*, **68**, 712–19.

Rameshwar, P. and Gascon, P. (1992) Release of interleukin-1 and interleukin-6 from human monocytes by antithymocyte globulin: requirement for de novo synthesis. *Blood*, **80**, 2531–8.

Rebellato, L. M., Gross, U., Verbanac, K. M. and Thomas, J. M. (1994) A comprehensive definition of the major antibody specificities in polyclonal rabbit antithymocyte globulin. *Transplantation*, **57**, 685–94.

Rosenfeld, S. J., Kimball, J., Vining, D. and Young, N. S. (1995) Intensive immunosuppression with antithymocyte globulin and cyclosporin as treatment for severe acquired aplastic anemia. *Blood*, **85**, 3058–65.

Rothmann, S. A., Streeter, R. R., Bukowski, R. M. and Hewlett, J. S. (1982) Treatment of severe aplastic anemia with antithymocyte globulin. *Experimental Hematology*, **10**, 809–16.

Rudivic, R., Jovcic, G., Bilijanovic–Paunovic, L., Stojanovic, N., Mijoric, A. and Partivic Kentera, V. (1985) Myelopoiesis and erythropoiesis of bone marrow cells cultured in vitro in patients recovered from aplastic anaemia. *British Journal of Haematology*, **70**, 55–62.

Sanchez–Mesal, L., Torre–Lopez, J. and Derbez, R. (1963) Effect of oxymetholone in refractory anemia. *Archives of Internal Medicine*, **113**, 721–9.

Schreiber, S. L. and Crabtree, G. R. (1992) The mechanism of action of cyclosporin A and FK506. *Immunology Today*, **13**, 136–42.

Schrezenmeier, H., Hinterberger–Fischer, M., Hows, J., Ljungman, P., Locascuilli, A., Marin, P., Marsh, J. C., McCann, S., den Ottolander, G. J., Ragavashar, A., Socié, G., Tichelli, A., Van't Veer–Korthof, E., Bacigalupo, A. and for the EBMT SAA Working Party (1998) Second immunosuppressive treatment of patients with aplastic anemia not responding to the first course of immunosuppression: a report from the Working Party on Severe Aplastic Anemia of the EBMT. *Bone Marrow Transplantation*, **15**, S10.

Schrezenmeier, H., Marin, P., Raghavachar, A., McCann, S., Hows, J., Gluckman, E., Nissen, C., van't Veer–Korthof, E. T., Ljungman, P., Hinterberger, W., Van Lint, M. T., Frickhofen, N., Bacigalupo, A. and for the EBMT SAA Working Party (1993) Relapse of aplastic anaemia after immunosuppressive treatment: a report from the European Bone Marrow Transplantation Group SAA Working Party. *British Journal of Haematology*, **85**, 371–7.

Seip, M. and Vidnes, J. (1985) Cyclosporin in a case of refractory aplastic anemia. *Scandinavian Journal of Hematology*, **34**, 228–30.

Sensenbrenner, L. L., Steele, A. A. and Santos, G. (1977) Recovery of hematologic competence without engraftment following attempted bone marrow transplantation for aplastic anemia. *Experimental Hematology*, **5**, 51.

Serke, B., Dienemann, D., Speck, B., Zimmermann, T., Bear, U. and Huhn, D. (1986) Hepatocellular carcinoma and focal nodular hyperplasia associated with norethandrolone-therapy. *Blut*, **52**, 111–16.

Seymour, R. A. and Jacobs, D. J. (1992) Cyclosporin and the gingival tissues. *Journal of Clinical Periodontology*, **19**, 1–11.

Shahidi, N. T. and Diamond, L. K. (1959) Testosterone-induced remission in aplastic anemia. *Journal of Diseases in Childhood*, **98**, 293–303.

Shahidi, N. T. and Diamond, L. K. (1961) Testosterone-induced remission in aplastic anemia of both acquired and congenital types. *New England Journal of Medicine*, **264**, 953–67.

Shahidi, N. T., Wang, W., Shurin, S., Finlay, J. L., Sondel, P. and Dinndorf, P. (1990) Treatment of acquired aplastic anemia with cylcosporine and androgens. In *Aplastic anemia and other bone marrow failure syndromes*, ed. N. T. Shahidi, p. 155. New York: Springer-Verlag.

Silingardi, V. and Torelli, U. (1979) Recovery from aplastic anemia after treatment with antilymphocyte globulin. *Archives of Internal Medicine*, **130**, 582–3.

Smith, A. G., O'Reilly, J. O., Hansen, J. and Martin, P. (1985) Specific antibody-blocking activities in antilymphocyte globulin as correlates of efficacy for the treatment of aplastic anemia. *Blood*, **66**, 721–3.

Socié, G., Henry–Amar, M., Bacigalupo, A., Hows, J., Tichelli, A., Ljungman, P., McCann, S. R., Frickhofen, N., Van't Veer–Korthof, E. and Gluckman, E. (1993) Malignant tumors occurring after treatment of aplastic anemia. European Bone Marrow Transplantation-Severe Aplastic Anaemia Working Party. *New England Journal of Medicine*, **329**, 1152–7.

Speck, B. and Kissling, M. (1971) Successful bone marrow grafts in experimental aplastic anaemia using antilymphocyte serum for conditioning. *European Journal of Clinical Biological Research*, **10**, 1047–51.

Speck, B., Cornu, P., Jeannet, M., Nissen, C., Burri, H. P., Groff, P., Nagel, G. A. and Buckner, C. D. (1976) Autologous marrow recovery following allogeneic marrow transplantation in a patient with severe aplastic anemia. *Experimental Hematology*, **4**, 131–7.

Speck, B., Gluckman, E., Haak, H. L. and Van Rood, J. J. (1977) Treatment of aplastic anaemia by antilymphocyte globulin with or without allogeneic bone-marrow infusions. *Lancet*, **2**, 1145–8.

Speck, B., Gluckman, E., Haak, H. L. and Van Rood. J. (1978) Treatment of aplastic anaemia by antilymphocyte globulin with or without marrow infusion. *Clinical Haematology*, **7**, 611–21.

Speck, B., Gratwohl, A., Nissen, C., Leibundgut, U., Ruggero, O., Osterwalder, B., Burri, H. P., Cornu, P. and Jeannet, M. (1981) Treatment of severe aplastic anaemia with antilymphocyte globulin or bone marrow transplantation. *British Medical Journal*, **282**, 860–3.

Speck, B., Gratwohl, A., Nissen, C., Osterwalder, B., Würsch, A., Tichelli, A., Lori, A., Reusser, P., Jeannet, M. and Signer, E. (1986) Treatment of severe aplastic anemia. *Experimental Hematology*, **14**, 126–32.

Speck, B., Tichelli, A., Gratwohl, A. and Nissen, C. (1990) Treatment of severe aplastic anemia: a 12-year follow-up of patients after bone marrow transplantation or after therapy with antilymphocyte globulin. In *Aplastic anemia and other bone marrow failure syndromes*, ed. N. T. Shahidi, p. 96. New York: Springer–Verlag.

Speck, B., Tichelli, A., Widmer, E., Harder, F., Kissling, M., Würsch, A., Gysi, C. S., Signer, E., Bargetzi, M., Orth, B., Gratwohl, A. and Nissen, C. (1996) Splenectomy as an adjuvant measure in the treatment of severe aplastic anaemia. *British Journal of Haematology*, **92**, 818–24.

Storb, R., Leisenring, W., Anasetti, C., Appelbaum, F. R., Buckner, C. D., Bensinger, W. I., Chauncey, T., Clift, R. A., Deeg, H. J., Doney, K. C., Flowers, M. E. D., Hansen, J. A., Martin, P. J., Sanders, K. M. and Witherspoon, R. P. (1997) Long-term follow-up of allogeneic marrow transplants in patients with aplastic anemia conditioned by cyclophosphamide combined with antithymocyte globulin. *Blood*, **89**, 3890–1.

Stryckmans, P. A., Dumont, J., Velu, T. and Debusscher, L. (1984) Cyclosporin in refractory severe aplastic anemia. *New England Journal of Medicine*, **310**, 655–6.

Swimmen, L. J., Costanzo–Nordin, M., Fisher, S. G., O'Sullivan, E. J., Johnson, M. R., Heroux, A., Dizikes, G. J., Pifarre, R. and Fisher, R. I. (1990) Increased incidence of lymphoproliferative disorder after immunosuppression with the monoclonal antibody OKT3 in cardiac-transplant recipients. *New England Journal of Medicine*, **323**, 1723–6.

Taniguchi, Y., Frickhofen, N., Raghavachar, A., Digel, W. and Heimpel, H. (1990) Antilymphocyte immunoglobulins stimulate peripheral blood lymphocytes to proliferate and release lymphokines. *European Journal of Haematology*, **44**, 244–51.

Tchernia, G., Gauthier, F., Mielot, F., Dommergues, J. P., Yvart, J. and Chasis, J. (1994) Initial assessment of the beneficial effect of partial splenectomy in hereditary spherocytosis. *Blood*, **81**, 2014–20.

Teramura, M., Kobayashi, S., Iwabe, K., Yoshinaga, K. and Mizoguchi, H. (1997) Mechanism of action of antithymocyte globulin in the treatment of aplastic anaemia: in vitro evidence for the presence of immunosuppressive mechanism. *British Journal of Haematology*, **96**, 80–4.

Territo, M. C. (1977) Autologous bone marrow repopulation following high dose cyclophosphamide and allogeneic marrow transplantation in aplastic anemia. *British Journal of Haematology*, **36**, 305.

Tichelli, A., Gratwohl, A., Nissen, C., Würsch, A., Signer, E. and Speck, B. (1988*a*) Spätkomplikationen bei Patienten mit aplastischer Anämie. *Schweizerische Medizinische Wochenschrift*, **118**, 1528–32.

Tichelli, A., Gratwohl, A., Würsch, A., Nissen, C. and Speck, B. (1988*b*) Late haematological complications in severe aplastic anaemia. *British Journal of Haematology*, **69**, 413–18.

Tichelli, A., Gratwohl, A., Nissen, C., Signer, E., Stebler Gysi, C. and Speck, B. (1992) Morphology in patients with severe aplastic anemia treated with antilymphocyte globulin. *Blood*, **80**, 337–45.

Tichelli, A., Socié, G., Marsh, J. C., McCann, S., Hows, J., Schrezenmeier, H., Ragavashar, A., Ljungman, P., Marin, P., Gratwohl, A. and Bacigalupo, A. (1997) Immunosuppression and old age in patients with aplastic anaemia. *Bone Marrow Transplantation*, **19** [Suppl. 1], S90.

Tichelli, A., Passweg, J. R., Nissen, C., Bargetzi, M., Hoffmann, T., Wodnar–Filipowicz, A., Signer, E., Speck, B. and Gratwohl, A. (1998) Repeated treatment with horse antilymphocyte globulin for severe aplastic anaemia. *British Journal of Haematology*, **100**, 393–400.

Tichelli, A., Socié, G., Henry-Amar, M., Marsh, J. C., Passweg, J., Schrezenmeier, H., McCann, S., Hows, J., Ljungman, P., Marin, P., Raghavachar, A., Locasciulli A., Gratwohl, A. and Bacigalupo, A. (1999) Effectiveness of immunosuppressive therapy in older patients with aplastic anemia. *Annals of Internal Medicine*, **130**, 193–201.

Tong, J., Bacigalupo, A., Piaggio, G., Figari, O. and Marmont, A. (1989) Effect of antilymphocyte globulin (ALG) on bone marrow T/non-T cells from aplastic anaemia patients and normal controls. *British Journal of Haematology*, **73**, 546–50.

Tong, J., Bacigalupo, A., Piaggio, G., Figari, O., Sogno, G. and Marmont, A. (1991) In vitro response of T cells from aplastic anemia patients to antilymphocyte globulin and phytohemagglutinin: colony-stimulating activity and lymphokine production. *Experimental Hematology*, **19**, 312–16.

Tsuzuki, M., Okamoto, M., Yamaguchi, T., Ino, T., Ezaki, K. and Hirano, M. (1997) Myelodysplastic syndrome with monosomy 7 following combination therapy with granulocyte colony-stimulating factor, cyclosporin A and danazole in an adult patient with severe aplastic anemia [in Japanese with English summary]. *Rinsho Ketsueki*, **38**, 745–51.

Wong, R. L., Winlows, C. M. and Cooper, K. D. (1993) The mechanisms of action of cyclosporin A in the treatment of psoriasis. *Immunology Today*, **14**, 69–74.

Yamazaki, E., Kanamori, H., Taguchi, J., Harano, H., Mohri, H. and Okubo, T. (1997) The evidence of clonal evolution with monosomy 7 in aplastic anemia following granulocyte colony-stimulating factor using the polymerase chain reaction. *Blood Cells, Molecules, and Diseases*, **23**, 213–18.

Young, N. and Speck, B. (1984) Antithymocyte and antilymphocyte globulins: clinical trials and mechanism of action. *Progress in Clinical Biological Research*, **148**, 221–6.

Young, N. S. and Barrett, A. J. (1995) The treatment of severe acquired aplastic anemia. *Blood*, **85**, 3367–77.

Young, N. S., Griffith, P., Brittain, E., Elfenbein, G., Gardner, F., Huang, A., Harmon, D., Hewlett, J., Fay, J., Mangan, K., Morrison, F., Sensenbrenner, L. L., Shadduck, R., Wang, W., Zaroulis, C. and Zuckerman, K. (1988) A multicenter trial of antilymphocyte globulin in aplastic anemia and related diseases. *Blood*, **72**, 1861–9.

11

Role of cytokines in the treatment of aplastic anemia

Hubert Schrezenmeier

Free University of Berlin

The rationale and potential aims of growth factor treatment in aplastic anemia

The standard treatment of aplastic anemia is allogeneic stem-cell transplantation or immunosuppressive treatment. These approaches are discussed in more detail in Chapters 10, 12 and 13 of this volume. This chapter concentrates on the use of hemopoietic growth factors in aplastic anemia. Essentially there are four possible indications for the use of growth factors in aplastic anemia:

- Growth factors could be used *therapeutically* with the aim of inducing remission of the disease.
- Growth factors could be used as *adjuvant treatment* for patients receiving concomitant immunosuppressive treatment with the aim of improving the rate and quality of remissions after immunosuppression.
- Growth factors could be used as *supportive care* in order to reduce the risk of infection and bleeding associated with cytopenia.
- Growth factors could be used to *collect peripheral blood* stem cells for allogeneic (and possibly even autologous) stem-cell transplantation.

Hemopoietic growth factors have been used in all four settings. Growth factors exert several possible effects that provide the rationale for their use in the treatment of aplastic anemia:

1. a. Growth factors stimulate the proliferation and differentiation of the residual primitive hemopoietic progenitor cells in aplastic anemia (Bacigalupo et al., 1991, 1993*a*; Bagnara et al., 1992; Gibson et al., 1994; Scopes et al., 1995, 1996; Wodnar Filipowicz et al., 1992, 1997).

   b. Apoptotic activity in aplastic anemia bone marrow progenitor cells is accelerated (Maciejewski et al., 1995*a,b*; Philpott et al., 1995). Growth factors can exert antiapoptotic activity (Adachi et al., 1993; Philpott et al., 1997) and may therefore suppress the increased apoptotic activity in the bone marrow of those with aplastic anemia.

      By stimulating or improving the surival of early progenitor cells growth

factors may induce trilineage recovery. Stimulating the residual progenitor cell population or antiapoptotic effects might require supraphysio-
logical concentrations of hemopoietic growth factors.

2. Growth factors could stimulate committed progenitor cells, leading to a
    (cytokine-dependent) single-lineage response (see Tables 11.1–11.5). Increases
    in the numbers of neutrophils and platelets might reduce the incidence of
    infectious complications and hemorrhage, respectively. This could increase the
    number of patients surviving long enough to achieve a trilineage response to
    immunosuppressive treatment. Growth factors might also accelerate hemo-
    poietic recovery in patients responding to immunosuppressive treatment.

3. a. Immunosuppressive treatment with antithymocyte globulin (ATG) or anti-
        lymphocyte globulin (ALG) can induce the release of endogenous growth
        factors (Barbano et al., 1988; Kawano et al., 1988; Kojima et al., 1992a;
        Nimer et al., 1991; Taniguchi et al., 1990; Tong et al., 1991). Recombinant
        growth factors given at the same time as immunosuppressive treatment
        might synergize with the endogenous factors released by ATG/ALG.
    b. It has been hypothesized that the hemopoietic response of patients with
        aplastic anemia depends on the mobilization of progenitor cells, and the
        reseeding of these cells to the bone marrow (Bacigalupo et al., 1993b,
        1995). Torok–Storb et al. (1984) noted that ATG can induce progenitor
        cells to mobilize in some patients. The combination of ATG and growth
        factors might be more potent in its mobilizing capacity. For this reason
        combinations of immunosuppressive treatment and growth factors
        should be further investigated.
            By the effects on endogenous cytokines and the stem-cell mobilizing
        effect, growth factors might increase the response rate to conventional
        immunosuppressive treatment of aplastic anemia.

4. Circulating hemopoietic progenitor cells can be recovered after ATG treat-
    ment followed by granulocyte colony-stimulating factor (G-CSF) treatment
    in a proportion of patients with aplastic anemia (Bacigalupo et al., 1993b).
    The use of peripheral-blood progenitor cells for autotransplant in severe
    aplastic anemia might be considered (Koza et al., 1997).

In vitro, generation of colonies from aplastic anemia bone marrow can be stimulated by growth factors, in particular by stem-cell factor (SCF) (Bagnara et al.,
1992; Gibson et al., 1994; Wodnar Filipowicz et al., 1992), granulocyte/
macrophage colony-stimulating factor (GM-CSF) (Bacigalupo et al., 1991; Gibson
et al., 1994; Scopes et al., 1996), interleukin-3 (IL-3) (Gibson et al., 1994; Scopes et
al., 1996) and G-CSF (Scopes et al., 1996). Flt3 ligand (flt3L) was less effective than
SCF at stimulating colony-forming cells from patients with aplastic anemia
(Wodnar Filipowicz et al., 1997). The cloning efficiency of sorted aplastic anemia
CD34$^+$ cells could be restored by G-CSF alone or in combination with IL-3, GM-

CSF or SCF. Multiple comparisons showed that, of these cytokines, G-CSF had by far the greatest effect on colony growth from separated aplastic anemia CD34$^+$ cells (Scopes et al., 1996). The hemopoietic defect in aplastic anemia might be partially overcome, at least in vitro, by appropriate cytokine stimuli, in particular G-CSF-containing cocktails (Scopes et al., 1996).

Serum/plasma levels and production of endogenous growth factors in aplastic anemia

Serum/plasma levels of most hemopoietic growth factors (G-CSF, GM-CSF, IL-6, erythropoietin, thrombopoietin, flt-3 ligand) are elevated in aplastic anemia (Das et al., 1992; Kojima et al., 1995, 1996, 1997b; Marsh et al., 1996; Schrezenmeier et al., 1993, 1994, 1995; Shinohara et al., 1995; Watari et al., 1989; Wodnar Filipowicz et al., 1996). It has been shown that serum G-CSF, erythropoietin and thrombopoietin levels correlate inversely with the degree of neutropenia, anemia or thrombocytopenia, respectively (Kojima et al., 1995, 1996, 1997a,b; Schrezenmeier et al., 1994, 1998). Thus there is no evidence to suggest that aplastic anemia is caused by a deficiency of any known hemopoietic growth factor. One remarkable exception is stem cell factor which is not elevated in serum of aplastic anemia patients (Kojima et al., 1997a; Nimer et al., 1994a; Wodnar Filipowicz et al., 1993).

In vitro, the production of G-CSF, GM-CSF and interleukin-6 (IL-6) by bone marrow stroma cells from aplastic anemia patients is increased (Kojima et al., 1992a), while the mRNA expression of these factors in stroma cells and of IL-1 and SCF appears to be normal or increased (Hirayama et al., 1993; Krieger et al., 1995; Stark et al., 1993). In contrast to the normal IL-1 mRNA expression in bone marrow stroma cultures, production of IL-1 by monocytes is reduced in aplastic anemia (Gascon and Scala, 1988; Nakao et al., 1989). Production of G-CSF in long-term marrow cultures of normal bone marrow can be stimulated by exogenous IL-1. In contrast, only about half of the aplastic anemia patients showed an increase of G-CSF production in long-term marrow cultures whereas G-CSF levels actually decreased in response to IL-1 (Migliaccio et al., 1992). It is not clear whether low IL-1 production and, in some cases, the unresponsiveness to IL-1 contribute to marrow failure in some patients with aplastic anemia.

Clinical trials of hemopoietic growth factors in aplastic anemia

Many hemopoietic growth factors have been used to treat aplastic anemia, both as single agents and in combination with immunosuppression. The growth factors studied in detail to date are G-CSF, GM-CSF and erythropoietin (EPO). There is less experience of interleukin-1 (IL-1), IL-3, IL-6, and SCF. So far, no data are available on the clinical effects of Flt-3 ligand, thrombopoietin and interleukin-11 in aplastic anemia.

Granulocyte colony-stimulating factor

G-CSF stimulates cells of neutrophil lineage to proliferate, differentiate, and activate (Welte et al., 1996). In addition, G-CSF has modulatory effects on T-cell function (Hirokawa et al., 1995; Iizuka et al., 1997; Pan et al., 1995) and tumor necrosis factor-α production (Kitabayashi et al., 1995). All these effects might be important for the clinical efficacy of G-CSF in aplastic anemia.

G-CSF was used in several pilot studies either alone or in combination with androgens, to treat aplastic anemia (Dufour et al., 1998; Fukutoku et al., 1994; Imashuku et al., 1994; Kojima and Matsuyama, 1994; Kojima et al., 1991; Shimizu et al., 1996; Sonoda et al., 1992, 1993) (Table 11.1). The neutrophil counts improved significantly in more than 80% of patients (Table 11.1). The neutrophil response was delayed in many cases and counts returned to baseline levels on cessation of G-CSF treatment (Kojima et al., 1991; Sonoda et al., 1993). Patients who retained residual marrow function had the best neutrophil responses. However, neutrophil responses were reported even for patients with very severe aplastic anemia and a neutrophil count of less than $0.05 \times 10^9/l$ (Kojima and Matsuyama, 1994). In some of these patients bacterial or fungal infections present at the start of the study were resolved during G-CSF treatment (Kojima and Matsuyama, 1994). Even after prolonged periods of treatment, less than 20% of patients gained a bi- or trilineage response to G-CSF treatment (see Table 11.1).

Several pilot trials used a combination of immunosuppression with ATG and/or cyclosporin A (CSA) and G-CSF (Bacigalupo et al., 1995; Führer et al., 1998; Ippoliti et al., 1995; Kojima et al., 1990; Lefrere et al., 1986; Shichino et al., 1996; Weide et al., 1993). The vast majority of patients responded with an increased neutrophil count and about 80% of patients experienced a trilineage response. In the pilot study of the Aplastic Anemia Working Party of the European Group for Blood and Marrow Transplantation (EBMT) 40 patients were treated with a combination of ATG, cyclosporin A and G-CSF (5 μg/kg per day, days 1–90) (Bacigalupo et al., 1995). Eighty-two percent of these patients achieved trilineage hemopoietic reconstitution and became transfusion independent at a median interval of 115 days from treatment. Median follow-up for surviving patients was 428 days and actuarial survival was 92% (Bacigalupo et al., 1995). This pilot study was continued and a total of 108 patients were treated. An update confirmed the high response rate (76% of previously untreated patients), with an unusually high proportion of complete responses (45%) and excellent survival (92% at 3 years) (A. Bacigalupo, personal communication).

These encouraging data formed the basis for prospective randomized trials: the Aplastic Anemia Working Party of the EBMT conducted a trial comparing ATG and cyclosporin A with or without G-CSF (5 µg/kg per day; days 1–90). The Japanese study group compared different combinations of G-CSF and immuno-suppressive agents. In a trial of the German Aplastic Anemia Study Group 111 patients were randomized to receive either standard treatment with ATG plus cyclosporin A or treatment with cyclosporin A plus G-CSF (5 µg/kg per day, days 1–90) (Raghavachar et al., 1998b). Preliminary analysis revealed a significantly higher response rate on day 112 in the standard treatment group compared to the cyclosporin A/G-CSF group (54.7% versus 39.5%). Including second treatments, the best response rated were 72.1% and 40.5% in each treatment arm (Raghavachar et al., 1998b). The rate of infections requiring intravenous antibio-tic treatment was low and comparable in both groups (Raghavachar et al., 1998b).

In summary, G-CSF effectively increases neutrophil counts in the vast majority of patients with aplastic anemia. The data available so far do not prove that G-CSF on its own can induce sustained trilineage remission. Therefore, the EBMT Aplastic Anemia Working Party has discouraged the use of G-CSF as a single agent in patients with newly diagnosed aplastic anemia (Marsh et al., 1994). Preliminary results of combinations of G-CSF with immunosuppression are promising in terms of response, the incidence of infection, and survival (Bacigalupo et al., 1995; Shichino et al., 1996). Although the survival in the EBMT pilot study is seemingly superior to that in other published trials of immunosup-pressive treatment without hemopoietic growth factors careful interpretation is warranted. The improved treatment results over the 1990s might be due to a number of factors (see Chapters 8–10 in this volume). Therefore prospective ran-domized trials are required to clarify the definitive impact of G-CSF on the response rate to standard immunosuppression and to analyze whether the increased neutrophil count translates into a reduction of infections and improved survival. It remains to be determined whether the immunomodulatory effect of G-CSF is relevant for its clinical efficacy in the treatment of aplastic anemia.

G-CSF has also been used to mobilize progenitor cells for autologous stem-cell transplantation (Bacigalupo et al., 1993b; Koza et al., 1997) or for allogeneic stem-cell transplantation in aplastic anemia. The use of G-CSF-mobilized peripheral-blood stem cells might be a feasible treatment option, particularly for patients with primary graft failure after bone marrow transplantation in aplastic anemia (Redei et al., 1997; Zecca et al., 1996).

G-CSF was very well tolerated in the treatment of aplastic anemia, even with prolonged periods of application. In most patients there were no signs of toxic-ity attributable to G-CSF (Bacigalupo et al., 1995; Kojima and Matsuyama, 1994; Kojima et al., 1991; Sonoda et al., 1992, 1993). Few patients complained of tran-sient, mild bone pain (Sonoda et al., 1993). A few patients developed Sweet's

Table 11.1. Published reports on G-CSF treatment of patients with aplastic anemia

Growth factor(s) alone

No. of patients	Severity	Pretreatment yes/no	G-CSF Dose	Route	Concomitant treatment	Response ANC	Response Other lineages	Reference
20	6 vSAA 11 SAA 3 nSAA	15/5	400 μg/m² per day 800 μg/m² per day	i.v. i.v.	No	12/20 2/5	No response No response	Kojima et al., 1991
5	4 SAA 1 nSAA	5/0	250–500 μg/day 75–300 μg/day	i.v. s.c.	No	5/5*	2/5 RBC↑	Sonoda et al., 1992
27	3 vSAA 16 SAA 8 nSAA	21/5	100–400 μg/day 250–1500 μg/day	s.c. i.v.	No	2/3* vSAA 24/24* SAA/nSAA	10/27 RBC↑ 3/27 platelets↑	Sonoda et al., 1993
45	24 SAA# 21 nSAA	n.r.	400–1000 μg/m² 100–200 μg/m² per day	i.v. s.c.	No	43/45**	7/45 bi- or trilineage response	Imashuku et al., 1994
10	10 vSAA	0/10	400–2000 μg/m² per day	i.v.	No	6/10	No response	Kojima and Matsuyama, 1994

Growth factor(s) in combination with immunosuppression

No. of patients	Severity	Pretreatment yes/no	G-CSF Dose	Route	Concomitant treatment	Response ANC	Response Other lineages	Reference
4	4 vSAA	4/0	400–1200 μg/kg per day	i.v.	Cyclosporin A	4/4	2/4 trilineage response	Kojima et al., 1990
2	1 vSAA 1 SAA	2/0	5 μg/kg per day	s.c.	Cyclosporin A	2/2	2/2 trilineage response	Bertrand et al., 1991

		#						
1	1 SAA	1/0	10 µg/kg per day	s.c.	EPO 8000 U/kg b.i.w.; Cyclosporin A	1/1	1/1 trilineage response	Weide et al., 1993
40	21 vSAA 19 vSAA	0/40	5 µg/kg per day	s.c.	ATG Cyclosporin A	n.r.	33/40 trilineage response	Bacigalupo et al., 1995
1	1 SAA	0/1	300 µg per day	s.c.	Cyclosporin A	1/1	1/1 trilineage response	Ippoliti et al., 1995
5	3 vSAA 2 nSAA	0/5	5 µg/kg per day	i.v.	ATG Cyclosporin A	5/5**	4/5 trilineage response	Shichino et al., 1996

Notes:

No. of vSAA cases not reported.

* Increase of neutrophils by ≥500 µl above baseline.

** Assessment by investigator, no detailed information in publication.

† Increase compared to pretreatment values.

ANC = absolute neutrophil count; ATG = antithymocyte globulin; b.i.w. = twice a week; EPO = erythropoietin; G-CSF = granulocyte colony-stimulating factor; i.v. = intravenously; n.r. = not reported; nSAA = nonsevere aplastic anemia; RBC = red blood cells; s.c. = subcutaneously; vSAA = very severe aplastic anemia.

syndrome (Fukutoku et al., 1994; Shimizu et al., 1996). Apart from a slight increase in the serum alkaline phosphatase level, no other significant changes in serum chemistry were noted during G-CSF treatment (Kojima and Matsuyama, 1994; Kojima et al., 1991; Sonoda et al., 1993).

The development of late clonal complications after G-CSF treatment, particularly in children, causes great concern (Führer et al., 1998; Hashino et al., 1996; Imashuku et al., 1995; Kojima et al., 1992b; Ohara et al., 1997; Ohsaka et al., 1995; Yamazaki et al., 1997; Yasuda et al., 1994). So far, the studies of the EBMT Severe Aplastic Anemia Working Party and the German Aplastic Anemia Study Group have not reported any increased incidence of late clonal disorders (Bacigalupo et al., 1995; Raghavachar et al., 1998b) (A. Bacigalupo, A. Raghavachar; personal communication). It is striking that the majority of patients who developed secondary myelodysplastic syndrome (MDS) or acute myeloid leukemia (AML) after G-CSF treatment for their aplastic anemia had monosomy 7 (Hashino et al., 1996; Imashuku et al., 1995; Kojima et al., 1992b; Ohara et al., 1997; Ohsaka et al., 1995; Yasuda et al., 1994). A relationship between aplastic anemia and clonal disorders of hemopoiesis has long been recognized (reviewed in Chapter 6, Table 6.1, this volume). The retrospective analysis of patients treated without hemopoietic growth factors demonstrates that long-term survivors have a 5–15% risk of developing MDS or AML. A minority of patients with aplastic anemia show clonal cytogenetic abnormalities at diagnosis (Appelbaum et al., 1987; Mikhailova et al., 1996), and there is evidence of clonal hemopoiesis, assessed by X-inactivation analysis, in some 13% of patients with aplastic anemia (Raghavachar et al., 1995) (see Chapter 6). Therefore, clonal disorders that develop after growth factor treatment might just reflect the natural course of the disease, or might also be due to the failure to obtain cytogenetics prior to treatment. So far, there is no convincing evidence that treatment with G-CSF or other growth factors increases the risk of cytogenetic abnormalities and malignant clonal disorders in aplastic anemia. Cytogenetic evaluation both at diagnosis and during follow-up is recommended for aplastic anemia patients treated with growth factors.

Granulocyte/macrophage colony-stimulating factor (GM-CSF)

GM-CSF induces the growth and differentiation of both multilineage hemopoietic progenitor cells and committed progenitor cells of the granulocyte and macrophage lineages (Grant and Heel, 1992). It enhances the function of mature neutrophils, eosinophils, monocytes, and macrophages.

GM-CSF was used in phase I and II studies, mainly for patients refractory to other treatment modalities (see Table 11.2) (Antin et al., 1988; Champlin et al., 1989; Guinan et al., 1990; Khan et al., 1995; Kurzrock et al., 1992; Nissen et al., 1988; Potter et al., 1990; Raghavachar et al., 1992; Takahashi et al., 1993a,b;

Vadhan–Raj et al., 1988). GM-CSF treatment was associated with a high proportion of myeloid responses (about two-thirds of patients) that were transient in most cases. Improved haemoglobin levels and increased platelet counts were observed only rarely (less than 10% of patients). Doses used ranged from 5 μg/m^2 body surface area to 500 μg/m^2 and a clear dose/response relationship could not be established. Even very low doses of GM-CSF (alone or in combination with erythropoietin) are efficacious (Kurzrock et al., 1992).

A randomized controlled trial comparing GM-CSF treatment (3 μg/kg per day over 90 days) with observation also demonstrated that GM-CSF treatment increases neutrophil and eosinophil counts, but does not affect the platelet count or hemoglobin level (Schuster et al., 1990). In this trial GM-CSF-treated patients experienced fewer major infections during the 90-day treatment period (Schuster et al., 1990).

A randomized clinical trial confirmed that recombinant GM-CSF following ATG treatment increases the granulocyte count compared with placebo (Gordon–Smith et al., 1991). In this randomized trial, as well as in nonrandomized phase II trials, it was seen that patients with the most severe aplasia responded least well to GM-CSF (Champlin et al., 1989; Gordon–Smith et al., 1991; Nissen et al., 1988). Patients who received recombinant GM-CSF had fewer febrile days and appeared to respond more rapidly to ATG than the group treated with placebo (Gordon–Smith et al., 1991). However, there was no difference in response to treatment and survival at 1 year (Gordon–Smith et al., 1991).

Though in some patients preexisting infections resolved during GM-CSF treatment (Nissen et al., 1988; Raghavachar et al., 1992), other patients acquired infections during GM-CSF treatment (Champlin et al., 1989; Gordon–Smith et al., 1991; Takahashi et al., 1993b; Vadhan–Raj et al., 1988) and preexisting infections were not cured, but were even aggravated by a capillary leak syndrome (Raghavachar et al., 1992) that was probably caused by GM-CSF (Arning et al., 1991; Emminger et al., 1990; Webb and Bundtzen, 1993).

The frequency and severity of adverse events seem to depend on preexisting infections and glycosylation of GM-CSF (Dorr, 1993; Grant and Heel, 1992; Raghavachar et al., 1992). GM-CSF was well tolerated by patients who did not have infections. Adverse events consisted of headache, myalgia, bone pain and low-grade fever (Antin et al., 1988; Doney et al., 1993; Guinan et al., 1990; Raghavachar et al., 1992; Schuster et al., 1990). GM-CSF can cause hypoalbuminemia (Kaczmarski and Mufti, 1990; Raghavachar et al., 1992; Takahashi et al., 1991, 1993). GM-CSF was less well tolerated by patients with preexisting infections (Arning et al., 1991; Emminger et al., 1990; Raghavachar et al., 1992).

In the clinical studies glycosylated GM-CSF expressed in yeast or mammalian cells (Antin et al., 1988; Champlin et al., 1989; Doney et al., 1993; Gordon–Smith

Table 11.2. Published reports on GM-CSF treatment of patients with aplastic anemia§

No. of patients	Pretreatment Severity	Pretreatment yes/no	GM-CSF Dose	GM-CSF Duration	GM-CSF Route	Other AA treatment (concomitantly or sequentially)	Response PMN	Mono	Eos	Hb/Hk	Plat.	Multilineage	Reference
Growth factor alone													
7	1 nSAA 2 SAA 4 vSAA	6/1	15–480 µg/m²	7–14 days	i.v. 1–12 h	—	6	6	0	6°	0	0	Antin et al., 1988
4	4 nSAA	4/0	4–32 µg/kg	14 days	i.v./s.c.	—	1	0	0	0	0	0	Nissen et al., 1988
10	3 nSAA 5 SAA 2 vSAA	8/2	120–500 µg/m²	14 days (2 cycles)	i.v.	—	9	10	10	1	1	0	Vadhan-Raj et al., 1988
13	4 nSAA 7 SAA 2 vSAA	13/0	4–64 µg/kg	28 days	i.v.	—	10/11	10/11	10/11	1/11	1/11	1	Champlin et al., 1989
9	n.r.	8/1	8–32 µg/kg	28 days	i.v. cont.	—	6/8	n.r.	n.r.	1/8	1/8	1	Guinan et al., 1990
21	1 nSAA 8 SAA 12 vSAA	17/4	125–250 µg/m²	14–28 days	i.v./s.c.	—	12***	5	9****	±	±	0	Raghavachar et al., 1992
37	8 nSAA 29 SAA*	n.r.	60–250 µg/m²	28 days	s.c.	—	↑	±	↑	±	±	1	Takahashi et al., 1993b
10	1 nSAA 9 SAA*	n.r.	10 µg/kg	14–56 days	s.c.	—	n.r.	n.r.	n.r.	0	0	0	Khan et al., 1995

GM-CSF in combination with erythropoietin

No.	Diagnosis	Responders	GM-CSF dose	Duration	Route	Combination							Reference
13	8/5		5–20 µg/m² per day	0.5–18 mo	s.c.	Erythropoietin (4000 U/day; s.c. 4/12 pts.)	5	↑	↑	1	2	1	Kurzrock et al. 1992
1	nSAA		250–500 µg/m²			6000 U/dose t.i.w.		n.r.	↑	↑°°	±	↑°°	Takahashi et al., 1993*a*

Growth factors in combination with immunosuppression

No.	Diagnosis	Responders	GM-CSF dose	Duration	Route	Combination							Reference
13	n.r.		300 µg/m²	28 days	i.v./s.c.	ATG, steroids	↑	↑	↑	±	±	7##	Gordon-Smith et al. 1991
17	3 nSAA, 14 SAA*	1/16	240 µg/m²	14 days	i.v., 2 hrs	ATG: 11 pts.; None: 6 pts.	4	n.r.	n.r.	4	4	4** / 2	Doney et al., 1993
7	4 SAA, 3 vSAA	0/7	5–10 µg/kg	long term+	s.c.	ATG, CSA	7	n.r.	n.r.	5	5	5	Hord et al., 1995

Notes:

§ Some case reports are not listed in the table (Potter et al., 1990; Lopez Karpovitch et al., 1992).

* Includes SAA and vSAA.

** Responders after IS treatment, 2 of these showed transient increase of ANC to GM-CSF alone.

*** Increase by ≥0.5 g/l above baseline.

**** Eosinophils >1.5 g/l.

± No change.

↑ Increase of counts in the GM-CSF-treated group compared to placebo groups or pretreatment level in GM-CSF-treated patients.

° Temporary improvement in reticulocyte count.

°° Response occurred after addition of erythropoietin to GM-CSF and was transient.

2/9 patients in the placebo group achieved multilineage response.

+ Until neutrophil recovery and transfusion independence.

ANC = absolute neutrophil count; eos = eosinophils; GM-CSF = granulocyte/macrophage colony-stimulating factor; IS = immunosuppressive treatment; n.r. = not reported; mono = monocytes; nSAA = nonsevere AA; plat. = platelets; PMN = neutrophils; SAA = severe AA; vSAA = very severe AA.

et al., 1991; Guinan et al., 1990; Hord et al., 1995; Khan et al., 1995; Vadhan–Raj et al., 1988) and *Escherichia-coli*-expressed unglycosylated GM-CSF (Raghavachar et al., 1992; Takahashi et al., 1993b) were used. Glycosylation of GM-CSF affects its pharmacokinetics, biological activity, and immunogenicity. Comparison of published trials showed that the frequency of adverse events was higher in patients treated with *E. coli*-derived GM-CSF (Dorr, 1993).

Erythropoietin

Erythropoietin (EPO) is a glycoprotein that stimulates erythropoietic progenitor cells. The endogenous EPO level is elevated in aplastic anemia (Krantz, 1991) and the EPO response to anemia is normal. Therefore, the rationale behind using EPO to treat patients with aplastic anemia is that pharmacological doses of EPO may stimulate residual erythropoiesis, even in patients whose endogenous levels are elevated. EPO can enhance the mobilizing capacity of G-CSF (Olivieri et al., 1995). Since some investigators hypothesize that the mobilization and reseeding of progenitor cells might be a prerequisite for hemopoietic recovery in aplastic anemia (Bacigalupo et al., 1993b), EPO could also act through its synergistic activity on the mobilizing capacity of other growth factors.

EPO was used in different schedules with doses up to 24,000 U/m^2 per day for several weeks (see Table 11.3a) (Bernell, 1996; Hanada et al., 1986; Urabe et al., 1993; Yoshida et al., 1993). An increase of hemoglobin levels and/or a reduction of red cell transfusion requirements were seen in about one-third of patients, but no reproducible effect on the other lineages could be demonstrated.

Since a multilineage response in patients treated with G-CSF or EPO alone is uncommon, several investigators combined EPO and G-CSF (see Table 11.3b) (Bessho et al., 1994, 1997; Imamura et al., 1995; Yonekura et al., 1997). In most of the patients responses were restricted to neutrophils and erythrocytes with trilineage responses occurring in a minority of patients. One of these studies compared different doses of EPO [0, 200, 400 U/kg three times a week (t.i.w.), and reported that the highest erythroid response rate (37%) was in the group of patients who received 400 U/kg t.i.w.

Combinations of G-CSF and EPO with immunosuppression produced encouraging results (Hinterberger et al., 1988; Nawata et al., 1994; Osterwalder et al., 1988; Weide et al., 1993). However, since all these trials were performed without a control group it is not possible to estimate the importance of the various components of the multimodal treatment.

EPO given alone or in combination with G-CSF was very well tolerated (Bessho et al., 1997; Hirashima et al., 1991; Imamura et al., 1995; Yoshida et al., 1993). Hypertension was observed in only a few patients (Bessho et al., 1997). Antibody formation was not observed (Bessho et al., 1994; Hirashima et al., 1991).

Table 11.3a. Published reports on treatment of patients with aplastic anemia with erythropoietin

No. of patients	Severity	Pretreatment yes/no	Erythropoietin		Concomitant treatment	Response		Reference
			Dose	Route		RBC	Other lineages	
4	2 nSAA 2 SAA	1/3	50 U/kg t.i.w.	i.v.	—	1	0	Bessho et al., 1990
29	13 nSAA 16 SAA	20/9	3000 U/day 24,000 U/day	s.c.*	—	10		Urabe et al., 1993
7	3 nSAA 4 SAA	7/0	6000–24,000 U t.i.w.	i.v.	—	3	1 platelet[↑]	Yoshida et al., 1993

Notes:

* 3/29 patients received EPO intravenously because of thrombocytopenia.

[↑] Increase of count in erythropoietin-treated group.

Table 11.3b. Published reports on treatment of patients with aplastic anemia with erythropoietin and G-CSF

No. of patients	Severity	Pretreatment yes/no	Dose		Concomitant treatment	Response				Reference
			G-CSF	Erythropoietin		ANC	RBC	Platelets	Multilineage	
Growth factors										
10	3 nSAA 4 SAA 3 vSAA	5/5	5–20 µg/kg/t.i.w. s.c.	120–240 U/kg t.i.w. s.c.	IS/androgens in 4 pts.	9	6	4	6	Bessho et al., 1994
28	14 nSAA 13 SAA	10/18	400–1200 µg/m² per day	100–400 IU/kg per day	—	25	12		6	Imamura et al., 1995
110	61 nSAA 49 SAA*	n.r. —	5 µg/kg per day lenograstim i.v. or 400 µg/m² per day i.v. filgrastim if ANC<1000/µl	no EPO (n=31) 200 IU/kg t.i.w. (n=41) 400 IU/kg t.i.w. (n=38)		↑ ↑ ↑	4/31 ↑ 6/41 ↑ 14/38 ↑			Bessho et al., 1997
20	8 nSAA 12 SAA	0/20	50–800 µg/m² i.v. or 50–100 µg/m² s.c.	2000–8000 U/m² t.i.w. i.v.	—	20	9	5	2	Yonekura et al., 1997
Growth factors in combination with immunosuppression										
7	7 SAA*	7/0	12 µg/kg per day t.i.w.	100 U/kg t.i.w.	Cyclosporin	5	5	5	5	Wickramanayake et al., 1993
1	1 SAA	1/0	10 µg/kg per day	8000 U/kg t.i.w.	Cyclosporin	1	1	1	1	Weide et al., 1993
1	1 vSAA	0/1	15 µg/kg per day	100 U/kg t.i.w.	Cyclosporin	1	1	1	1	Nawata et al., 1994

Notes:

* Includes SAA and vSAA.

ANC = absolute neutrophil count; G-CSF = granulocyte colony-stimulating factor; IS = immunosuppressive treatment; nSAA = nonsevere aplastic anemia; RBC = red blood cells; vSAA = very severe aplastic anemia.

Interleukin-3 (IL-3)

IL-3 regulates early hemopoiesis and stimulates the proliferation and differentiation of early hemopoietic progenitor cells and lineage-committed precursors (Eder et al., 1997). It synergizes with other hemopoietic growth factors.

In vitro, the production of IL-3 from stromal cells in long-term marrow cultures is reduced in aplastic anemia compared to normal bone marrow (Gibson et al., 1995). Addition of GM-CSF and IL-3 increased the output of clonogeneic cells in long-term marrow cultures of aplastic anemia bone marrow. However, this occurred mainly in patients with less severe disease (Gibson et al., 1994). Production of IL-3 from stimulated blood mononuclear cells is reduced in aplastic anemia patients compared to controls (Kawano et al., 1992).

The clinical trials in aplastic anemia conducted with IL-3 are listed in Table 11.4 (Bargetzi et al., 1995; Ganser et al., 1990; Gillio et al., 1991; Kurzrock et al., 1991; Nimer et al., 1994b; Raghavachar et al., 1996). In trials using IL-3 alone, a transient and dose-dependent increase of neutrophil counts occurred in about half of the patients, whereas a multilineage response occurred only occasionally ($<10\%$ of patients) (Bargetzi et al., 1995; Ganser et al., 1990; Gillio et al., 1991; Kurzrock et al., 1991; Nimer et al., 1994b).

In a phase I/II study IL-3 (250 $\mu g/m^2$, until day 90) was administered in combination with ATG and cyclosporin A in 13 patients with aplastic anemia who were refractory to, or relapsed after, previous immunosuppressive therapy (Raghavachar et al., 1996). Three of eight patients with refractory aplastic anemia and four patients with relapsed aplastic anemia responded to the combined treatment within 4 months. There was evidence of an IL-3-dependent response in two patients. Two patients developed acute myeloid leukemia 4 and 22 months after cessation of IL-3 (Raghavachar et al., 1996).

Since IL-3 exerts a synergistic activity with other growth factors in vivo (Gibson et al., 1992) and in vitro (Donahue et al., 1988; Geissler et al., 1992b), combinations of IL-3 and GM-CSF or G-CSF were used in single cases. The case reports suggest that IL-3 pretreatment might sensitize progenitor cells to subsequent or concomitant treatment with late-acting cytokines such as GM-CSF (Herrmann et al., 1990) or G-CSF (Geissler et al., 1992a; Schleuning et al., 1994). However, these observations have to be confirmed in a larger group of patients.

Occurrence of IL-3 side-effects seems to be dose dependent. Headache, musculoskeletal pain, chills, fever, erythema at the injection site, nausea, vomiting, diarrhea, edema, weight gain, chest pain, and dyspnea have been observed in aplastic anemia patients treated with IL-3 (Bargetzi et al., 1995; Ganser et al., 1990; Gillio et al., 1991; Kurzrock et al., 1991; Nimer et al., 1994b). In the trial combining IL-3 with immunosuppression only a few patients experienced these adverse events, although the IL-3 application period was substantially longer than in other trials (Raghavachar et al., 1996). In one case fatal vascular

Table 11.4. Recombinant human interleukin-3 aplastic anemia[§]

No. of patients	Severity	Dosage	Duration (days)	Route	Concomitant treatment	Response				Reference
						PMN	Retics	Plt.	BM-Cellularity	
Growth factor alone										
9	1 vSAA 6 SAA 2 nSAA	250–500 µg/m² per day	15	s.c. daily	—	8	4	1	3/7	Ganser et al., 1990
8	n.r.	0.15–10 µg/kg per day	14–264	s.c.		2	2	2	n.r.	Gillio et al., 1991
8	n.r.	30–1000 µg/m² per day	28	i.v. (4 hrs)	—	1	1	1	1	Kurzrock et al., 1991
7	n.r.	0.5–10 µg/kg per day	21	s.c.	—	1	1	–	2/7	Nimer et al., 1994*b*
15	15 SAA*	1.0–16 µg/kg per day	21	i.v.	—	9	0[#]	0	n.r.	Bargetzi et al., 1995
Growth factor in combination with immunosuppression										
13	4 vSAA 6 SAA 3 nSAA	250 µg/m² per day	90	s.c. daily	ATG CSA	9	—	8	n.r.	Raghavachar et al., 1996

Notes:

[§] Case reports are disregarded.

* Includes SAA and vSAA.

[#] Assessed by hemoglobin levels and transfusion requirement.

ATG = antithymocyte globulin; BM = bone marrow; CSA = cyclosporin A; nSAA = nonsevere aplastic anemia; Plt. = platelets; PMN = polymorphonuclear cells; Retics = reticulocytes; vSAA = very severe aplastic anemia.

leak syndrome and reactive erythrophagocytosis was reported (Hurwitz et al., 1996). Side-effects might be caused by the IL-3-mediated release of secondary cytokines such as IL-6, tumor necrosis factor-α and interferon-γ (Nachbaur et al., 1993). The IL-3-mediated induction of inhibitory cytokines (e.g., tumor necrosis factor-α) may counteract the stimulatory activity of IL-3 (Seipelt et al., 1993). Comedication with immunosuppressive drugs might modulate the IL-3-induced cytokine release, thus mitigating IL-3-related adverse events.

Interleukin-1 (IL-1)

IL-1 is a pleiotropic cytokine that stimulates the secretion of other cytokines and hemopoietic growth factors (e.g., G-CSF, GM-CSF, M-CSF, IL-3), may induce early progenitor cells to enter the cell cycle, induces the synthesis of hepatic acute-phase protein, and modulates the expression of cell surface proteins (Dinarello, 1994).

The production of IL-1 by monocytes from patients with aplastic anemia is significantly depressed (Gascon and Scala, 1988; Nakao et al., 1989). The addition of IL-1 to standard long-term marrow cultures from aplastic anemia patients normalized the reduced production of G-CSF, IL-6 and leukemia-inhibitory factor (Holmberg et al., 1994).

Two clinical trials failed to demonstrate that IL-1 improved peripheral blood counts, when given either as a single agent (Walsh et al., 1992) or in combination with immunosuppressive treatment (Doney et al., 1996) (see Table 11.5a). IL-1 was well tolerated. Side-effects included fever, rigors, headache, fatigue, nausea, and transient hypotension (Doney et al., 1996; Walsh et al., 1992).

Interleukin-6 (IL-6)

IL-6 is also a pleiotropic cytokine with multiple effects on different target cells including hemopoiesis (Lotz, 1995). In vitro, IL-6 has been shown to promote the maturation of megakaryocytes, and IL-6 (Ishibashi et al., 1989b) plays a synergistic role with IL-3 in the proliferation of early hemopoietic progenitor cells (Ikebuchi et al., 1987; Leary et al., 1988). Animal models show that IL-6 is a potent thrombopoietic factor in vivo (Asano et al., 1990; Hill et al., 1990; Ishibashi et al., 1989a,b; Mayer et al., 1991; Stahl et al., 1991).

Since IL-6 has thrombopoietic activity, a phase II study with $E.\ coli$-derived IL-6 (0.5–5.0 μg/kg per day for two periods of 28 days) was performed, using 11 patients with aplastic anemia who had not responded to or had relapsed after, immunosuppressive treatment (Table 11.5b; Schrezenmeier et al., 1995). Only one patient had a sustained increase in her platelet count. IL-6 caused the preexisting anemia to deteriorate in most of the patients, and in some patients a decline of leukocyte numbers was observed after a prolonged

Table 11.5a. Published reports on treatment of patients with aplastic anemia with interleukin-1 (IL-1)

No. of patients	Severity	Pretreatment yes/no	IL-1 Dose	Route	Concomitant treatment	ANC	Mono	Eos	RBC	Plat.	Multilineage	Reference
4	4 SAA	4/0	0.03–0.1 µg/kg	i.v.	—	0	0	0	0	0	0	Walsh et al., 1992
6	6 SAA	n.r.	0.1–0.3 µg/m^2	i.v.	ATG (5) or cyclosporin (1) + androgens	0	0	0	0	0	2*	Doney et al., 1996

Notes:

* Minimal improvement according to published criteria (Doney et al., 1993).

ANC = absolute neutrophil count; Eos = eosinophils; Mono = monocytes; RBC = red blood cells.

Table 11.5b. Published reports on treatment of patients with aplastic anemia with IL-6

No. of patients	Severity	Pretreatment yes/no	IL-1 Dose	Route	Concomitant treatment	ANC	Mono	Eos	RBC	Plat.	Multilineage	Reference
11	3 nSAA 8 SAA/FA*	11/0	0.5–5.0 µg/kg	s.c.	—	±	±	±	↓	↑	↑	Schrezenmeier et al., 1995

Notes:

* Fanconi's anemia.

± No change.

↑ Increase of counts in the GM-CSF-treated group compared to placebo groups or pretreatment level in GM-CSF-treated patients.

↓ Decrease.

period of treatment. This study was discontinued prematurely on account of its toxicity to hemopoiesis. Other adverse events included fever, headache, arthralgia, tachycardia, and hypertension (Schrezenmeier et al., 1995). These results suggest that recombinant human IL-6 (rhIL-6) given alone at dose levels up to 5 μg/kg per day for 28 days does not improve thrombocytopenia in the majority of AA patients. Further clinical trials could be carried out to investigate whether combining IL-6 with other hemopoietic growth factors and sequential application improves thrombocytopenia in patients with bone marrow failure. In vitro, IL-6 demonstrates synergistic effects on hemopoiesis with a number of factors including GM-CSF (Caracciolo et al., 1989), M-CSF (Bot et al., 1989) and in particular IL-3 (Ikebuchi et al., 1987; Leary et al., 1988; Okano et al., 1989). Preclinical models have demonstrated that rhIL-3 potentiates the thrombopoietic effect of rhIL-6 (Geissler et al., 1992b).

Before long, other thrombopoietic factors might be used to treat aplastic anemia. Thrombopoietin, which has been purified and cloned recently, shows promise as an alternative for the treatment of thrombocytopenia (de Sauvage et al., 1994; Fanucchi et al., 1997; Kaushansky et al., 1994; Levin, 1997; Lok et al., 1994). Interleukin-11 is another cytokine with thrombopoietic activity that has been shown to reduce chemotherapy-induced thrombocytopenia (Du and Williams, 1994; Gordon et al., 1996). No data on the effects of thrombopoietin or interleukin-11 in patients with aplastic anemia are available to date.

Stem-cell factor (SCF)

SCF is the natural ligand for the proto-oncogene c-*kit* that acts on hemopoietic progenitor cells. While SCF alone exerts little colony-stimulating activity on hemopoietic progenitor cells, SCF acts synergistically with other growth factors such as IL-3, G-CSF, GM-CSF or EPO, and enhances the proliferation of both early and lineage-committed progenitor cells (Broudy, 1997). It also enhances the growth of mast cells and stimulates the release of mediators from mast cells (Broudy, 1997).

SCF levels are not elevated in patients with aplastic anemia (Kojima et al., 1997a; Nimer et al., 1994a; Wodnar Filipowicz et al., 1993). This contrasts with the levels of other hemopoietic growth factors, which are highly elevated. One study suggests that higher SCF levels could be associated with a better outcome in terms of survival and transfusion requirement (Wodnar Filipowicz et al., 1993). SCF in combination with other growth factors can enhance the growth of hemopoietic progenitor cells in aplastic anemia patients (Bacigalupo et al., 1993a; Bagnara et al., 1992; Wodnar Filipowicz et al., 1992). In vitro, the release of soluble SCF from marrow stromal cells and the expression of SCF mRNA is the same in aplastic anemia and control (Kojima et al., 1997a; Krieger et al., 1995). Low levels of SCF were measured in poorly growing aplastic anemia stroma cell cultures.

Stroma cell growth is defective in most patients with aplastic anemia, but is enhanced by addition of SCF in combination with other factors (Krieger et al., 1995).

The data from these in vitro studies suggest that endogenous SCF levels in aplastic anemia are low, and that optimal stimulation of stromal cells and progenitor cells from patients with aplastic anemia is obtained by growth factor combinations that contain SCF. In a dose-finding study, 39 patients with aplastic anemia who had failed to respond to prior ATG or ALG treatment were treated with SCF (5–50 μg/kg t.i.w.) or SCF plus G-CSF (Kurzrock et al., 1998). A trilineage response occurred in 35% of patients who were treated with $\geqslant$25 μg/kg SCF t.i.w. and G-CSF (10 μg/kg per day). Neutrophil responses occurred in the majority of patients (86%) receiving SCF plus G-CSF. SCF was generally well tolerated. Mild to moderate erythema at the injection site was seen in 74% of patients and systemic allergic-like reactions occurred in three patients (Kurzrock et al., 1998).

Conclusion

Published evidence does not support the use of currently available hemopoietic growth factors as first-line treatment other than in a clinical trial. There is no evidence that growth factors alone can cure aplastic anemia. In most patients with aplastic anemia treatment with G-CSF, GM-CSF or IL-3 will lead to a transient increase of neutrophil counts and in patients treated with EPO a rise in the hemoglobin level is observed. However, the probability of inducing a sustained bi- or trilineage response by treating with hemopoietic growth factors alone is very low, in particular for patients with very severe disease. Treating newly diagnosed patients with growth factors could even be harmful because treatment with immunosuppression or stem-cell transplantation is delayed (Marsh et al., 1994). There are promising results from the studies looking at combining growth factors with immunosuppressive treatment or combining different hemopoietic growth factors. However, despite almost a decade of growth factor studies in aplastic anemia it is still not clear whether growth factors change the course of the disease and improve the long-term outcome of these patients. The answers to many open questions can only be given by well-designed prospective randomized trials. The next generation of trials will focus on using hemopoietic growth factors as adjuvant treatment in combination with immunosuppression, and on using growth factors as supportive treatment in aplastic anemia. Combinations of early-acting (e.g., SCF, flt-3 ligand) and late-acting hemopoietic growth factors might be beneficial and should be assessed in controlled clinical trials. Use of growth-factor-mobilized peripheral-blood stem cells for autologous stem-cell rescue after escalated immunosuppressive treatment (Brodsky et al., 1996) or for allogeneic stem-cell transplantation might introduce further applications of growth factors in the treatment of aplastic anemia.

It is essential that future studies evaluate not only the effect of growth factors on hemopoietic recovery, but also the long-term course of aplastic anemia, including the evolution of late clonal disorders.

References

Adachi, S., Kubota, M., Matsubara, K., Wakazono, Y., Hirota, H., Kuwakado, K., Akiyama, Y. and Mikawa, H. (1993) Role of protein kinase C in neutrophil survival enhanced by granulocyte colony-stimulating factor. *Experimental Hematology*, **21**, 1709–13.

Antin, J. H., Smith, B. R., Holmes, W. and Rosenthal, D. S. (1988) Phase I/II study of recombinant human granulocyte-macrophage colony-stimulating factor in aplastic anemia and myelodysplastic syndrome. *Blood*, **72**, 705–13.

Appelbaum, F. R., Barrall, J., Storb, R., Ramberg, R., Doney, K., Sale, G. E. and Thomas, E. D. (1987) Clonal cytogenetic abnormalities in patients with otherwise typical aplastic anemia. *Experimental Hematology*, **15**, 1134–9.

Arning, M., Kliche, K. O. and Schneider, W. (1991) GM-CSF therapy and capillary-leak syndrome [letter; comment]. *Annals of Hematology*, **62**, 83.

Asano, S., Okano, A., Ozawa, K., Nakahata, T., Ishibashi, T., Koike, K., Kimura, H., Tanioka, Y., Shibuya, A., Hirano, T., Kishimoto, T., Takaku, F. and Akiyama, Y. (1990) In vivo effects of recombinant human interleukin-6 in primates: stimulated production of platelets. *Blood*, **75**, 1602–5.

Bacigalupo, A., Piaggio, G., Figari, O., Tong, J., Sogno, G., Tedone, E., Sette, A., Ratto, M. R., Caciagli, P., Badolati, G. et al. (1991) Response of CFU-GM to increasing doses of rhGM-CSF in patients with aplastic anemia. *Experimental Hematology*, **19**, 829–32.

Bacigalupo, A., Piaggio, G., Podesta, M., Raffo, M. R., Tedone, E., Sogno, G., Benvenuto, F., Figari, O., Grassia, L., Bagnara, G. P. et al. (1993*a*) In vitro effect of stem cell factor on colony growth from acquired severe aplastic anemia. *Stem Cells Dayton*, **11** [Suppl. 2], 175–9.

Bacigalupo, A., Piaggio, G., Podesta, M., Van Lint, M. T., Valbonesi, M., Lercari, G., Mori, P. G., Pasino, M., Franchini, E., Rivabella, L. et al. (1993*b*) Collection of peripheral blood hemopoietic progenitors (PBHP) from patients with severe aplastic anemia (SAA) after prolonged administration of granulocyte colony-stimulating factor. *Blood*, **82**, 1410–14.

Bacigalupo, A., Broccia, G., Corda, G., Arcese, W., Carotenuto, M., Gallamini, A., Locatelli, F., Mori, P. G., Saracco, P., Todeschini, G. et al. (1995) Antilymphocyte globulin, cyclosporin, and granulocyte colony- stimulating factor in patients with acquired severe aplastic anemia (SAA): a pilot study of the EBMT SAA Working Party. *Blood*, **85**, 1348–53.

Bagnara, G. P., Strippoli, P., Bonsi, L., Brizzi, M. F., Avanzi, G. C., Timeus, F., Ramenghi, U., Piaggio, G., Tong, J., Podesta, M. et al. (1992) Effect of stem cell factor on colony growth from acquired and constitutional (Fanconi) aplastic anemia. *Blood*, **80**, 382–7.

Barbano, G. C., Schenone, A., Roncella, S., Ghio, R., Corcione, A., Mori, P. G., Ferrarini, M. and Pistoia, V. (1988) Anti-lymphocyte globulin stimulates normal human T cells to proliferate and to release lymphokines in vitro. A study at the clonal level. *Blood*, **72**, 956–63.

Bargetzi, M. J., Gluckman, E., Tichelli, A., Devergie, A., Esperou, H., Kabata, J., Wodnar Filipowicz, A., Nissen, C., Speck, B. and Gratwohl, A. (1995) Recombinant human interleukin-3 in refractory severe aplastic anaemia: a phase I/II trial. *British Journal of Haematology*, **91**, 306–12.

Bernell, P. (1996) Aplastic anaemia with a trilineage response to erythropoietin therapy. *Journal of Internal Medicine*, **239**, 79–81.

Bertrand, Y., Amri, F., Capdeville, R., French, M. and Philippe, N. (1990) The successful treatment of two cases of severe aplastic anemia with granulocyte colony-stimulating factor and cyclosporine A. *British Journal of Haematology*, **79**, 648–9.

Bessho, M., Jinnai, I., Matsuda, A., Saito, M. and Hirashima K. (1990) Improvement of anemia by recombinant erythropoietin in patients with myelodysplastic syndromes and aplastic anemia. *International Journal of Cell Cloning*, **8**, 445.

Bessho, M., Jinnai, I., Hirashima, K., Saito, M., Murohashi, I., Ino, H., Tsuji, M., Fukuda, M., Maruyama, M., Kusumoto, S. et al. (1994) Trilineage recovery by combination therapy with recombinant human granulocyte colony-stimulating factor and erythropoietin in patients with aplastic anemia and refractory anemia. *Stem Cells Dayton*, **12**, 604–15.

Bessho, M., Hirashima, K., Asano, S., Ikeda, Y., Ogawa, N., Tomonaga, M., Toyama, K., Nakahata, T., Nomura, T., Mizoguchi, H., Yoshida, Y., Niitsu, Y. and Kohgo, Y. (1997) Treatment of the anemia of aplastic anemia patients with recombinant human erythropoietin in combination with granulocyte colony-stimulating factor: a multicenter randomized controlled study. Multicenter Study Group. *European Journal of Haematology*, **58**, 265–72.

Bot, F. J., van Eijk, L., Broeders, L., Aarden, L. A. and Löwenberg, B. (1989) Interleukin-6 synergizes with M-CSF in the formation of macrophage colonies from purified human marrow progenitor cells. *Blood*, **73**, 435–7.

Brodsky, R. A., Sensenbrenner, L. L. and Jones, R. J. (1996) Complete remission in severe aplastic anemia after high-dose cyclophosphamide without bone marrow transplantation. *Blood*, **87**, 491–4.

Broudy, V. C. (1997) Stem cell factor and hemopoiesis. *Blood*, **90**, 1345–64.

Caracciolo, D., Clark, S. C. and Rovera, G. (1989) Human interleukin-6 supports granulocyte differentiation of hemopoietic progenitor cells and acts synergistically with GM-CSF. *Blood*, **73**, 666–70.

Champlin, R. E., Nimer, S. D., Ireland, P., Oette, D. H. and Golde, D. W. (1989) Treatment of refractory aplastic anemia with recombinant human granulocyte-macrophage-colony-stimulating factor. *Blood*, **73**, 694–9.

Das, R. E., Milne, A., Rowley, M., Smith, E. C. and Cotes, P. M. (1992) Serum immunoreactive erythropoietin in patients with idiopathic aplastic and Fanconi's anaemias. *British Journal of Haematology*, **82**, 601–7.

de Sauvage, F. J., Hass, P. E., Spencer, S. D., Malloy, B. E., Gurney, A. L., Spencer, S. A., Darbonne, W. C., Henzel, W. J., Wong, S. C., Kuang, W. J., Oles, K. J., Hultgren, B., Solberg, L. A., Goedell, D. V., Eaton, D. L. et al. (1994) Stimulation of megakaryocytopoiesis and thrombopoiesis by the c-Mpl ligand [see comments]. *Nature*, **369**, 533–8.

Dinarello, C. A. (1994) The biological properties of interleukin-1. *European Cytokine Network*, **5**, 517–31.

Donahue, R. E., Seehra, J., Metzger, M., Lefebvre, D., Rock, B., Carbone, S., Nathan, D. G., Garnick, M., Sehgal, P. K., Laston, D. et al. (1988) Human IL-3 and GM-CSF act synergistically in stimulating hemopoiesis in primates. *Science*, **241**, 1820–3.

Doney, K., Storb, R., Appelbaum, F. R., Buckner, C. D., Sanders, J., Singer, J. and Hansen, J. A. (1993) Recombinant granulocyte-macrophage colony stimulating factor followed by immunosuppressive therapy for aplastic anaemia. *British Journal of Haematology*, **85**, 182–4.

Doney, K., Storb, R., Lilleby, K. and Appelbaum, F. R. (1996) Recombinant interleukin-1 followed by immunosuppressive therapy for aplastic anemia [letter]. *American Journal of Hematology*, **52**, 61–2.

Dorr, R. T. (1993) Clinical properties of yeast-derived versus Escherichia coli-derived granulocyte-macrophage colony-stimulating factor. *Clinical Therapeutics*, **15**, 19–29.

Du, X. X. and Williams, D. A. (1994) Interleukin-11: a multifunctional growth factor derived from the hemopoietic microenvironment. *Blood*, **83**, 2023–30.

Dufour, C., Maher, J., Murray, N., Manning, M., Dokal, I., Luzzatto, L. and Roberts, I. A. (1998) An unusual case of familial aplastic anaemia: in vitro and in vivo evidence for a multipotent progenitor responsive to G-CSF [letter]. *European Journal of Haematology*, **60**, 209–12.

Eder, M., Geissler, G. and Ganser, A. (1997) IL-3 in the clinic. *Stem Cells*, **15**, 327–33.

Emminger, W., Emminger Schmidmeier, W., Peters, C., Susani, M., Hawliczek, R., Hocker, P. and Gadner, H. (1990) Capillary leak syndrome during low dose granulocyte-macrophage colony-stimulating factor (rh GM-CSF) treatment of a patient in a continuous febrile state [see comments]. *Blut*, **61**, 219–21.

Fanucchi, M., Glaspy, J., Crawford, J., Garst, J., Figlin, R., Sheridan, W., Menchaca, D., Tomita, D., Ozer, H. and Harker, L. (1997) Effects of polyethylene glycol-conjugated recombinant human megakaryocyte growth and development factor on platelet counts after chemotherapy for lung cancer [see comments]. *New England Journal of Medicine*, **336**, 404–9.

Fukutoku, M., Shimizu, S., Ogawa, Y., Takeshita, S., Masaki, Y., Arai, T., Hirose, Y., Sugai, S., Konda, S. and Takiguchi, T. (1994) Sweet's syndrome during therapy with granulocyte colony-stimulating factor in a patient with aplastic anaemia. *British Journal of Haematology*, **86**, 645–8.

Führer, M., Rampf, U., Ebell, W., Friedrich, W., Gadner, H., Haas, R., Janka, G., Niemeyer, C., Zeidler, C. and Bender-Götze, C. (1998) Immunosuppressive therapy and BMT for aplastic anemia in children: results of the German/Austrian SAA94 study [Abstract]. *Bone Marrow Transplant*, **21**, S45.

Ganser, A., Lindemann, A., Seipelt, G., Ottmann, O. G., Eder, M., Falk, S., Herrmann, F., Kaltwasser, J. P., Meusers, P., Klausmann, M., Frisch, J., Schulz, G., Mertelsmann, R. and Hoelzer, D. (1990) Effects of recombinant human interleukin-3 in aplastic anemia. *Blood*, **76**, 1287–92.

Gascon, P. and Scala, G. (1988) Decreased interleukin-1 production in aplastic anemia. *American Journal of Medicine*, **85**, 668–74.

Geissler, K., Forstinger, C., Kalhs, P., Knobl, P., Kier, P., Kyrle, P. and Lechner, K. (1992*a*) Effect of interleukin-3 on responsiveness to granulocyte-colony-stimulating factor in severe aplastic anemia. *Annals of Internal Medicine*, **117**, 223–5.

Geissler, K., Valent, P., Bettelheim, P., Sillaber, C., Wagner, B., Kyrle, P., Hinterberger, W., Lechner, K., Liehl, E. and Mayer, P. (1992*b*) In vivo synergism of recombinant human interleukin-3 and recombinant human interleukin-6 on thrombopoiesis in primates. *Blood*, **79**, 1155–60.

Gibson, F. M., Bagnara, M., Ioannidou, E. and Gordon–Smith, E. C. (1992) Interaction of granulocyte-macrophage colony-stimulating factor and interleukin 3 in human long-term bone marrow culture. *Experimental Hematology*, **20**, 235–40.

Gibson, F. M., Scopes, J., Daly, S., Ball, S. E. and Gordon–Smith, E. C. (1994) In vitro response of normal and aplastic anemia bone marrow to mast cell growth factor and in combination with granulocyte-macrophage colony-stimulating factor and interleukin-3. *Experimental Hematology*, **22**, 302–12.

Gibson, F. M., Scopes, J., Daly, S., Ball, S. and Gordon–Smith, E. C. (1995) Haemopoietic growth factor production by normal and aplastic anaemia stroma in long-term bone marrow culture. *British Journal of Haematology*, **91**, 551–61.

Gillio, A. P., Castro Malaspina, H., Gasparetto, C., Small, T. N., Childs, B., Reilly, L. K., Young, D., Oldham, F., Nadler, P., Moore, M. A. and O'Reilly, R. J. (1991) Human recombinant interleukin-3 treatment in patients with myelodysplastic syndrome and aplastic anemia [Abstract]. *Blood*, **78** [Suppl. 1], 95a.

Gordon, M. S., McCaskill Stevens, W. J., Battiato, L. A., Loewy, J., Loesch, D., Breeden, E., Hoffman, R., Beach, K. J., Kuca, B., Kaye, J. and Sledge, G. W. Jr. (1996) A phase I trial of recombinant human interleukin-11 (neumega rhIL-11 growth factor) in women with breast cancer receiving chemotherapy. *Blood*, **87**, 3615–24.

Gordon–Smith, E. C., Yandle, A., Milne, A., Speck, B., Marmont, A., Willemze, R. and Kolb, H. (1991) Randomised placebo controlled study of RH-GM-CSF following ALG in the treatment of aplastic anaemia. *Bone Marrow Transplant*, **7** [Suppl. 2], 78–80.

Grant, S. M. and Heel, R. C. (1992) Recombinant granulocyte-macrophage colony-stimulating factor (rGM-CSF) A review of its pharmacological properties and prospective role in the management of myelosuppression. *Drugs*, **43**, 516–60.

Guinan, E. C., Sieff, C. A., Oette, D. H. and Nathan, D. G. (1990) A phase I/II trial of recombinant granulocyte-macrophage colony-stimulating factor for children with aplastic anemia. *Blood*, **76**, 1077–82.

Hanada, T., Aoki, Y., Ninomiya, H. and Abe, T. (1986) T cell-mediated inhibition of haematopoiesis in aplastic anaemia: serial assay of inhibitory activities of T cells to autologous CFU-E during immunosuppressive therapy. *British Journal of Haematology*, **63**, 69–74.

Hashino, S., Imamura, M., Tanaka, J., Kobayashi, S., Musashi, M., Kasai, M. and Asaka, M. (1996) Transformation of severe aplastic anemia into acute myeloblastic leukemia with monosomy 7. *Annals of Hematology*, **72**, 337–9.

Herrmann, F., Lindemann, A., Raghavachar, A., Heimpel, H. and Mertelsmann, R. (1990) In vivo recruitment of GM-CSF-response myelopoietic progenitor cells by interleukin-3 in aplastic anemia. *Leukemia*, **4**, 671–2.

Hill, R. J., Warren, M. K. and Levin, J. (1990) Stimulation of thrombopoiesis in mice by human recombinant interleukin 6. *Journal of Clinical Investigation*, **85**, 1242–7.

Hinterberger, W., Adolf, G., Aichinger, G., Dudczak, R., Geissler, K., Hocker, P., Huber, C., Kalhs, P., Knapp, W., Koller, U. et al. (1988) Further evidence for lymphokine overproduction in severe aplastic anemia. *Blood*, **72**, 266–72.

Hirashima, K., Bessho, M. and Jinnai, I. (1991) Improvement in anemia by recombinant human erythropoietin in patients with myelodysplastic syndrome and aplastic anemia. *Contributions to Nephrology*, **88**, 254–65.

Hirayama, Y., Kohgo, Y., Matsunaga, T., Ohi, S., Sakamaki, S. and Niitsu, Y. (1993) Cytokine mRNA expression of bone marrow stromal cells from patients with aplastic anaemia and myelodysplastic syndrome. *British Journal of Haematology*, **85**, 676–83.

Hirokawa, M., Kitabayashi, A., Niitsu, H., Takatsu, H. and Miura, A. B. (1995) Modulation of allogeneic immune responses by filgrastim (recombinant human granulocyte colony-stimulating factor) in bone marrow transplantation. *International Journal of Hematology*, **62**, 235–41.

Holmberg, L. A., Seidel, K., Leisenring, W. and Torok–Storb, B. (1994) Aplastic anemia: analysis of stromal cell function in long-term marrow cultures. *Blood*, **84**, 3685–90.

Hord, J. D., Gay, J. C., Whitlock, J. A., Janco, R. L., Edwards, J. R., Greer, J. P. and Lukens, J. N. (1995) Long-term granulocyte-macrophage colony-stimulating factor and immunosuppression in the treatment of acquired severe aplastic anemia. *Journal of Pediatric Hematology/Oncology*, **17**, 140–4.

Hurwitz, N., Probst, A., Zufferey, G., Tichelli, A., Pless, M., Kappos, L., Speck, B. and Gratwohl, A. (1996) Fatal vascular leak syndrome with extensive hemorrhage, peripheral neuropathy and reactive erythrophagocytosis: an unusual complication of recombinant IL-3 therapy. *Leukemia and Lymphoma*, **20**, 337–40.

Iizuka, K., Kaneko, H., Yamada, T., Kimura, H., Kokai, Y. and Fujimoto, J. (1997) Host F1 mice pretreated with granulocyte colony-stimulating factor accept parental bone marrow grafts in hybrid resistance system. *Blood*, **89**, 1446–51.

Ikebuchi, K., Wong, G. G., Clark, S. C., Ihle, J. N., Hirai, Y. and Ogawa, M. (1987) Interleukin 6 enhancement of interleukin 3-dependent proliferation of multipotential hemopoietic progenitors. *Proceedings of the National Academy of Sciences of the USA*, **84**, 9035–9.

Imamura, M., Kobayashi, M., Kobayashi, S., Yoshida, K., Mikuni, C., Ishikawa, Y., Matsumoto, S., Sakamaki, S., Niitsu, Y., Hinoda, Y. et al. (1995) Combination therapy with recombinant human granulocyte colony-stimulating factor and erythropoietin in aplastic anemia. *American Journal of Hematology*, **48**, 29–33.

Imashuku, S., Akiyama, Y., Nakajima, F., Hibi, S., Oguni, T. and Koike, M. (1994) Multilineage response to G-CSF in paediatric aplastic anaemia [letter; comment] [see comments]. *Lancet*, **344**, 1236–7.

Imashuku, S., Hibi, S., Kataoka Morimoto, Y., Yoshihara, T., Ikushima, S., Morioka, Y. and Todo, S. (1995) Myelodysplasia and acute myeloid leukaemia in cases of aplastic anaemia and congenital neutropenia following G-CSF administration. *British Journal of Haematology*, **89**, 188–90.

Ippoliti, G., Invernizzi, R., Negri, M., Incardona, S. and Ascari, E. (1995) Response to cyclosporin A and rhG-CSF in a case of aplastic anemia. *Haematologica*, **80**, 230–3.

Ishibashi, T., Kimura, H., Shikama, Y., Uchida, T., Kariyone, S., Hirano, T., Kishimoto, T., Takatsuki, F. and Akiyama, Y. (1989*a*) Interleukin-6 is a potent thrombopoietic factor in vivo in mice. *Blood*, **74**, 1241–4.

Ishibashi, T., Kimura, H., Uchida, T., Kariyone, S., Friese, P. and Burstein, S. A. (1989*b*) Human interleukin 6 is a direct promoter of maturation of megakaryocytes in vitro. *Proceedings of the National Academy of Science of the USA*, **86**, 5953–7.

Kaczmarski, R. S. and Mufti, G. J. (1990) Hypoalbuminaemia after prolonged treatment with recombinant granulocyte macrophage colony stimulating factor. *British Medical Journal*, **301**, 1312–13.

Kaushansky, K., Lok, S., Holly, R. D., Broudy, V. C., Lin, N., Bailey, M. C., Forstrom, J. W., Buddle, M. M., Oort, P. J., Hagen, F. S., Roth, G. J., Papayannopoulou, T., Foster, D. C. et al. (1994) Promotion of megakaryocyte progenitor expansion and differentiation by the c-Mpl ligand thrombopoietin [see comments]. *Nature*, **369**, 568–71.

Kawano, Y., Nissen, C., Gratwohl, A. and Speck, B. (1988) Immunostimulatory effects of different antilymphocyte globulin preparations: a possible clue to their clinical effect. *British Journal of Haematology*, **68**, 115–19.

Kawano, Y., Takaue, Y., Hirao, A., Watanabe, T., Abe, T., Shimizu, T., Sato, J., Saito, S., Kitamura, T., Takaku, F. et al. (1992) Production of interleukin 3 and granulocyte-macrophage colony-stimulating factor from stimulated blood mononuclear cells in patients with aplastic anemia. *Experimental Hematology*, **20**, 1125–8.

Khan, M. A., Hameed, A., Tahir, M., Gandapur, A. J., Rehman H., Durrani, F. M. and Ahmad, A. (1995) Haemopoietic growth factor GM-CSF for aplastic anaemia in children [letter]. *Lancet*, **345**, 199.

Kitabayashi, A., Hirokawa, M., Hatano, Y., Lee, M., Kuroki, J., Niitsu, H. and Miura, A. B. (1995) Granulocyte colony-stimulating factor downregulates allogeneic immune responses by posttranscriptional inhibition of tumor necrosis factor-alpha production. *Blood*, **86**, 2220–7.

Kojima, S. and Matsuyama, T. (1994) Stimulation of granulopoiesis by high-dose recombinant human granulocyte colony-stimulating factor in children with aplastic anemia and very severe neutropenia. *Blood*, **83**, 1474–8.

Kojima, S., Fukuda, M., Miyajima, Y. and Matsuyama, T. (1990) Cyclosporine and recombinant granulocyte colony-stimulating factor in severe aplastic anemia [letter]. *New England Journal of Medicine*, **323**, 920–1.

Kojima, S., Fukuda, M., Miyajima, Y., Matsuyama, T. and Horibe, K. (1991) Treatment of aplastic anemia in children with recombinant human granulocyte colony-stimulating factor. *Blood*, **77**, 937–41.

Kojima, S., Matsuyama, T. and Kodera, Y. (1992*a*) Hemopoietic growth factors released by marrow stromal cells from patients with aplastic anemia. *Blood*, **79**, 2256–61.

Kojima, S., Tsuchida, M. and Matsuyama, T. (1992*b*) Myelodysplasia and leukemia after treatment of aplastic anemia with G-CSF [letter]. *New England Journal of Medicine*, **326**, 1294–5.

Kojima, S., Matsuyama, T. and Kodera, Y. (1995) Circulating erythropoietin in patients with acquired aplastic anaemia. *Acta Haematologica*, **94**, 117–22.

Kojima, S., Matsuyama, T., Kodera, Y., Nishihira, H., Ueda, K., Shimbo, T. and Nakahata, T. (1996) Measurement of endogenous plasma granulocyte colony-stimulating factor in patients with aquired aplastic anemia by a sensitive chemiluminescent immunoassay. *Blood*, **87**, 1303–8.

Kojima, S., Matsuyama, T. and Kodera, Y. (1997*a*) Plasma levels and production of soluble stem cell factor by marrow stromal cells in patients with aplastic anaemia. *British Journal of Haematology*, **99**, 440–6.

Kojima, S., Matsuyama, T., Kodera, Y., Tahara, T. and Kato, T. (1997*b*) Measurement of endogenous plasma thrombopoietin in patients with acquired aplastic anaemia by a sensitive enzyme-linked immunosorbent assay. *British Journal of Haematology*, **97**, 538–43.

Koza, V., Svojgrova, M., Jindra, P. and Cetkovsky, P. (1997) Collection of peripheral blood hemopoietic progenitors (PBHP) from some patients with severe aplastic anemia (SAA) and subsequent autologous transplantation [Abstract]. *Bone Marrow Transplant*, **19** [Suppl. 1], S90.

Krantz, S. B. (1991) Erythropoietin. *Blood*, **77**, 419–34.

Krieger, M. S., Nissen, C. and Wodnar Filipowicz, A. (1995) Stem-cell factor in aplastic anemia: in vitro expression in bone marrow stroma and fibroblast cultures. *European Journal of Haematology*, **54**, 262–9.

Kurzrock, R., Talpaz, M., Estrov, Z., Rosenblum, M. G. and Gutterman, J. U. (1991) Phase I study of recombinant human interleukin-3 in patients with bone marrow failure. *Journal of Clinical Oncology*, **9**, 1241–50.

Kurzrock, R., Talpaz, M. and Gutterman, J. U. (1992) Very low doses of GM-CSF administered alone or with erythropoietin in aplastic anemia. *American Journal of Medicine*, **93**, 41–8.

Kurzrock, R., Gratwohl, A., Paquette, R., Wyres, M., Okamoto, D. and Young, N. (1998) Trilineage responses seen with stem cell factor (STEMGEN; SCF) and Filgrastim (G-CSF) treatment in aplastic anemia patients [Abstract]. *British Journal of Haematology*, **102**, 2.

Leary, A. G., Ikebuchi, K., Hirai, Y., Wong, G. G., Yang, Y. C., Clark, S. C. and Ogawa, M. (1988) Synergism between interleukin-6 and interleukin-3 in supporting proliferation of human hemopoietic stem cells: comparison with interleukin-1 alpha. *Blood*, **71**, 1759–63.

Lefrere, J. J., Courouce, A. M., Girot, R., Bertrand, Y. and Soulier, J. P. (1986) Six cases of hereditary spherocytosis revealed by human parvovirus infection. *British Journal of Haematology*, **62**, 653–8.

Levin, J. (1997) Thrombopoietin – clinically realized? [editorial; comment]. *New England Journal of Medicine*, **336**, 434–6.

Lok, S., Kaushansky, K., Holly, R. D., Kuijper, J. L., Lofton Day, C. E., Oort, P. J., Grant, F. J., Heipel, M. D., Burkhead, S. K., Kramer, J. M., Bell, L. A., Sprecher, C. A., Blumberg, H., Johnson, R., Prunkard, D., Ching, A. F. T., Mathewes, S. L., Bailey, M. C., Forstrom, J. W., Buddle, M. M., Osborn, S. G., Evans, S. J., Sheppard, P. O., Presnell, S. R., O'Hara, P. J., Hagen, F. S., Roth, G. J., Foster, D. C. et al. (1994) Cloning and expression of murine thrombopoietin cDNA and stimulation of platelet production in vivo [see comments]. *Nature*, **369**, 565–8.

Lopez Karpovitch, X., Ulloa Aguirre, A., von Eiff, C., Hurtado Monroy, R. and Alanis, A. (1992) Treatment of methimazole-induced severe aplastic anemia with recombinant human granulocyte-monocyte colony-stimulating factor and glucocorticosteroids. *Acta Haematologica*, **87**, 148–50.

Lotz, M. (1995) Interleukin-6: a comprehensive review. *Cancer Treatment Research*, **80**, 209–33.

Maciejewski, J., Selleri, C., Anderson, S. and Young, N. S. (1995a) Fas antigen expression on CD34+ human marrow cells is induced by interferon gamma and tumor necrosis factor alpha and potentiates cytokine-mediated hemopoietic suppression in vitro. *Blood*, **85**, 3183–90.

Maciejewski, J. P., Selleri, C., Sato, T., Anderson, S. and Young, N. S. (1995b) Increased expression of Fas antigen on bone marrow CD34+ cells of patients with aplastic anaemia. *British Journal of Haematology*, **91**, 245–52.

Marsh, J. C., Socié, G., Schrezenmeier, H., Tichelli, A., Gluckman, E., Ljungman, P., McCann, S. R., Raghavachar, A., Marín, P., Hows, J. M. et al. (1994) Haemopoietic growth factors in aplastic anaemia: a cautionary note. European Bone Marrow Transplant Working Party for Severe Aplastic Anaemia. *Lancet*, **344**, 172–3.

Marsh, J. C., Gibson, F. M., Prue, R. L., Bowen, A., Dunn, V. T., Hornkohl, A. C., Nichol, J. L. and Gordon–Smith, E. C. (1996) Serum thrombopoietin levels in patients with aplastic anaemia. *British Journal of Haematology*, **95**, 605–10.

Mayer, P., Geissler, K., Valent, P., Ceska, M., Bettelheim, P. and Liehl, E. (1991) Recombinant human interleukin 6 is a potent inducer of the acute phase response and elevates the blood platelets in nonhuman primates. *Experimental Hematology*, **19**, 688–96.

Migliaccio, A. R., Migliaccio, G., Adamson, J. W. and Torok–Storb, B. (1992) Production of granulocyte colony-stimulating factor and granulocyte/macrophage-colony-stimulating factor after interleukin-1 stimulation of marrow stromal cell cultures from normal or aplastic anemia donors. *Journal of Cell Physiology*, **152**, 199–206.

Mikhailova, N., Sessarego, M., Fugazza, G., Caimo, A., De Filippi, S., Van Lint, M. T., Bregante, S., Valeriani, A., Mordini, N., Lamparelli, T., Gualandi, F., Occhini, D. and Bacigalupo, A. (1996) Cytogenetic abnormalities in patients with severe aplastic anemia. *Haematologica*, **81**, 418–22.

Nachbaur, D., Gratwohl, A., Herold, M., Tichelli, A., Slanicka, M., Nissen, C., Niederwieser, D. and Speck, B. (1993) Cytokine serum levels during treatment with high-dose recombinant human IL-3 in a patient with severe aplastic anemia. *Annals of Hematology*, **66**, 71–5.

Nakao, S., Matsushima, K. and Young, N. (1989) Decreased interleukin 1 production in aplastic anaemia. *British Journal of Haematology*, **71**, 431–6.

Nawata, J., Toyoda, Y., Nisihira, H., Honda, K., Kigasawa, H. and Nagao, T. (1994) Haematological improvement by long-term administration of recombinant human granulocyte-colony stimulating factor and recombinant human erythropoietin in a patient with severe aplastic anaemia. *European Journal of Pediatrics*, **153**, 325–7.

Nimer, S. D., Golde, D. W., Kwan, K., Lee, K., Clark, S. and Champlin, R. (1991) In vitro production of granulocyte-macrophage colony-stimulating factor in aplastic anemia: possible mechanisms of action of antithymocyte globulin. *Blood*, **78**, 163–8.

Nimer, S. D., Leung, D. H., Wolin, M. J. and Golde, D. W. (1994a) Serum stem cell factor levels in patients with aplastic anemia. *International Journal of Hematology*, **60**, 185–9.

Nimer, S. D., Paquette, R. L., Ireland, P., Resta, D., Young, D. and Golde, D. W. (1994b) A phase I/II study of interleukin-3 in patients with aplastic anemia and myelodysplasia. *Experimental Hematology*, **22**, 875–80.

Nissen, C., Tichelli, A., Gratwohl, A., Speck, B., Milne, A., Gordon–Smith, E. C. and Schaedelin, J. (1988) Failure of recombinant human granulocyte-macrophage colony-stimulating factor therapy in aplastic anemia patients with very severe neutropenia. *Blood*, **72**, 2045–7.

Ohara, A., Kojima, S., Hamajima, N., Tsuchida, M., Imashuku, S., Ohta, S., Sasaki, H., Okamura, J., Sugita, K., Kigasawa, H., Kiriyama, Y., Akatsuka, J. and Tsukimoto, I. (1997) Myelodysplastic syndrome and acute myelogenous leukemia as a late clonal complication in children with acquired aplastic anemia. *Blood*, **90**, 1009–13.

Ohsaka, A., Sugahara, Y., Imai, Y. and Kikuchi, M. (1995) Evolution of severe aplastic anemia to myelodysplasia with monosomy 7 following granulocyte colony-stimulating factor, erythropoietin and high-dose methylprednisolone combination therapy [see comments]. *Internal Medicine*, **34**, 892–5.

Okano, A., Suzuki, C., Takatsuki, F., Akiyama, Y., Koike, K., Ozawa, K., Hirano, T., Kishimoto, T., Nakahata, T. and Asano, S. (1989) In vitro expansion of the murine pluripotent hemopoietic stem cell population in response to interleukin 3 and interleukin 6. Application to bone marrow transplantation. *Transplantation*, **48**, 495–8.

Olivieri, A., Offidani, M., Cantori, I., Ciniero, L., Ombrosi, L., Masia, M. C., Brunori, M., Montroni, M. and Leoni, P. (1995) Addition of erythropoietin to granulocyte colony-stimulating factor after priming chemotherapy enhances hemopoietic progenitor mobilization. *Bone Marrow Transplant*, **16**, 765–70.

Osterwalder, B., Gratwohl, A., Reusser, P., Tichelli, A. and Speck, B. (1988) Hematological support in patients undergoing allogeneic bone marrow transplantation. *Recent Results in Cancer Research*, **108**, 44–52.

Pan, L., Delmonte, J. Jr., Jalonen, C. K. and Ferrara, J. L. (1995) Pretreatment of donor mice with granulocyte colony-stimulating factor polarizes donor T lymphocytes toward type-2 cytokine production and reduces severity of experimental graft-versus-host disease. *Blood*, **86**, 4422–9.

Philpott, N. J., Scopes, J., Marsh, J. C., Gordon–Smith, E. C. and Gibson, F. M. (1995) Increased apoptosis in aplastic anemia bone marrow progenitor cells: possible pathophysiologic significance. *Experimental Hematology*, **23**, 1642–8.

Philpott, N. J., Prue, R. L., Marsh, J. C., Gordon–Smith, E. C. and Gibson, F. M. (1997) G-CSF-mobilized CD34 peripheral blood stem cells are significantly less apoptotic than unstimulated peripheral blood CD34 cells: role of G-CSF as survival factor. *British Journal of Haematology*, **97**, 146–52.

Potter, M. N., Mott, M. G. and Oakhill, A. (1990) The successful treatment of a case of very severe aplastic anaemia with granulocyte-macrophage colony stimulating factor and anti-lymphocyte globulin. *British Journal of Haematology*, **75**, 618–19.

Raghavachar, A., Hinterberger, W., Kaltwasser, J. P., Höffken, K., Herrmann, F., Freund, M., Platzer, E., Frisch, J., Heimpel, H. and Frickhofen, N. (1992) Recombinant human granulocyte-macrophage colony-stimulating factor in aplastic anemia: a phase I/II trial with emphasis on very severe neutropenia and active infection. In *Cytokines in hemopoiesis, oncology, and AIDS II*, ed. M. Freund, H. Link, R. E. Schmidt and K. Welte, pp. 1–555. Berlin: Springer-Verlag.

Raghavachar, A., Janssen, J. W., Schrezenmeier, H., Wagner, B., Bartram, C. R., Schulz, A. S., Hein, C., Cowling, G., Mubarik, A., Testa, N. G. et al. (1995) Clonal hemopoiesis as defined by polymorphic X-linked loci occurs infrequently in aplastic anemia. *Blood*, **86**, 2938–47.

Raghavachar, A., Ganser, A., Freund, M., Heimpel, H., Herrmann, F. and Schrezenmeier, H. (1996) Long-term interleukin-3 and intensive immunosuppression in the treatment of aplastic anemia. *Cytokines and Molecular Therapy*, 215–23.

Raghavachar, A., Bacigalupo, A. and Schrezenmeier, H. (1998a) Use of filgrastim (r-metHuG-CSF) in aplastic anemia. In *Filgrastim (r-metHuG-CSF) in clinical practice*, ed. G. Morstyn, T. M. Dexter and M. A. Foote, pp. 1–533. New York: Marcel Dekker.

Raghavachar, A., Kolbe, K., Höffken, K., Seipelt, G., Burk, M., Geissler, R. G., Pasold, R., Zwingers, T. and Schrezenmeier, H. (1998*b*) Standard immunosuppression is superior to cyclosporine/filgrastim in severe aplastic anemia [Abstract]. *British Journal of Haematology*, **102**, 154.

Redei, I., Waller, E. K., Holland, H. K., Devine, S. M. and Wingard, J. R. (1997) Successful engraftment after primary graft failure in aplastic anemia using G-CSF mobilized peripheral stem cell transfusions. *Bone Marrow Transplant*, **19**, 175–7.

Schleuning, M., Thomssen, C., Kolb, H. J., Sauer, H. J. and Wilmanns, W. (1994) Treatment of refractory severe aplastic anemia with granulocyte colony stimulating factor and interleukin 3 [letter]. *American Journal of Hematology*, **46**, 250–1.

Schrezenmeier, H., Raghavachar, A. and Heimpel, H. (1993) Granulocyte-macrophage colony-stimulating factor in the sera of patients with aplastic anemia. *The Clinical Investigator*, **71**, 102–8.

Schrezenmeier, H., Noe, G., Raghavachar, A., Rich, I. N., Heimpel, H. and Kubanek, B. (1994) Serum erythropoietin and serum transferrin receptor levels in aplastic anaemia. *British Journal of Haematology*, **88**, 286–94.

Schrezenmeier, H., Marsh, J. C. W., Stromeyer, P., Müller, H., Heimpel, H., Gordon–Smith, E. C. and Raghavachar, A. (1995) A phase I/II trial of recombinant human interleukin-6 in patients with aplastic anaemia. *British Journal of Haematology*, **90**, 283–92.

Schrezenmeier, H., Griesshammer, M., Hornkohl, A., Nichol, J. L., Hecht, T., Heimpel, H., Kubanek, B. and Raghavachar, A. (1998) Thrombopoietin serum levels in patients with aplastic anaemia: correlation with platelet count and persistent elevation in remission. *British Journal of Haematology*, **100**, 571–6.

Schuster, M. W., Liu, E. T., Solberg, L. A., Stadtmauer, E., Bennett, J. M. and Israel, R. J. (1990) Granulocyte-macrophage colony-stimulating factor (GM-CSF) for aplastic anemia. Preliminary results of a multicenter randomized controlled trial [Abstract]. *Blood*, **76** [Suppl. 1], 47a.

Scopes, J., Daly, S., Ball, S. E., McGuckin, C. P., Gordon–Smith, E. C. and Gibson, F. M. (1995) The effect of human flt-3 ligand on committed progenitor cell production from normal, aplastic anaemia and Diamond-Blackfan anaemia bone marrow. *British Journal of Haematology*, **91**, 544–50.

Scopes, J., Daly, S., Atkinson, R., Ball, S. E., Gordon–Smith, E. C. and Gibson, F. M. (1996) Aplastic anemia: evidence for dysfunctional bone marrow progenitor cells and the corrective effect of granulocyte colony-stimulating factor in vitro. *Blood*, **87**, 3179–85.

Seipelt, G., Ganser, A., Duranceyk, H., Maurer, A., Ottmann, O. G. and Hoelzer, D. (1993) Induction of TNF-alpha in patients with myelodysplastic syndromes undergoing treatment with interleukin-3. *British Journal of Haematology*, **84**, 749–51.

Shichino, H., Mugishima, H., Takamura, M., Shimada, T., Suzuki, T., Chin, M., Harada, K., Ryo, S. and Kojima, S. (1996) Treatment of aplastic anemia with antithymocyte globulin, cyclosporin A, methylprednisolone, danazol and recombinant human granulocyte-colony stimulating factor. *Acta Paediatrica Japonica*, **38**, 644–7.

Shimizu, T., Yoshida, I., Eguchi, H., Takahashi, K., Inada, H. and Kato, H. (1996) Sweet syndrome in a child with aplastic anemia receiving recombinant granulocyte colony-stimulating factor. *Journal of Pediatric Hematology/Oncology*, **18**, 282–4.

Shinohara, K., Oeda, E., Nomiyama, J., Inoue, H., Kamei, S., Tajiri, M., Ichikawa, T., Kuwaki, T. and Tachibana, K. (1995) The levels of granulocyte colony-stimulating factor in the plasma of the bone marrow aspirate in various hematological disorders. *Stem Cells Dayton*, **13**, 421–7.

Sonoda, Y., Yashige, H., Fujii, H., Tsuda, S., Maekawa, T., Misawa, S. and Abe, T. (1992) Bilineage response in refractory aplastic anemia patients following long-term administration of recombinant human granulocyte colony-stimulating factor. *European Journal of Haematology*, **48**, 41–8.

Sonoda, Y., Ohno, Y., Fujii, H., Takahashi, T., Nakayama, S., Haruyama, H., Nasu, K., Shimazaki, C., Hara, H., Kanamaru, A. et al. (1993) Multilineage response in aplastic anemia patients following long-term administration of filgrastim (recombinant human granulocyte colony stimulating factor) *Stem Cells Dayton*, **11**, 543–54.

Stahl, C. P., Zucker Franklin, D., Evatt, B. L. and Winton, E. F. (1991) Effects of human interleukin-6 on megakaryocyte development and thrombocytopoiesis in primates. *Blood*, **78**, 1467–75.

Stark, R., Andre, C., Thierry, D., Cherel, M., Galibert, F. and Gluckman, E. (1993) The expression of cytokine and cytokine receptor genes in long-term bone marrow culture in congenital and acquired bone marrow hypoplasias. *British Journal of Haematology*, **83**, 560–6.

Takahashi, M., Nikkuni, K., Moriyama, Y. and Shibata, A. (1991) GM-CSF-mediated impairment of liver to synthesize albumin, cholinesterase, and cholesterol. *American Journal of Hematology*, **36**, 213–14.

Takahashi, M., Aoki, A., Mito, M., Nikkuni, K., Ohtsuka, T., Saitoh, H., Moriyama, Y. and Shibata, A. (1993*a*) Combination therapy with rhGM-CSF and rhEpo for two patients with refractory anemia and aplastic anemia. *Hematology and Pathology*, **7**, 153–8.

Takahashi, M., Yoshida, Y., Kaku, K., Masaoka, T., Moriyama, Y., Nakanishi, S., Kaneko, T., Shibata, A. and Miwa, S. (1993*b*) Phase II study of recombinant human granulocyte-macrophage colony-stimulating-factor in myelodysplastic syndrome and aplastic anemia. *Acta Haematologica*, **89**, 189–94.

Taniguchi, Y., Frickhofen, N., Raghavachar, A., Digel, W. and Heimpel, H. (1990) Antilymphocyte immunoglobulins stimulate peripheral blood lymphocytes to proliferate and release lymphokines. *European Journal of Haematology*, **44**, 244–51.

Tong, J., Bacigalupo, A., Piaggio, G., Figari, O., Sogno, G. and Marmont, A. (1991) In vitro response of T cells from aplastic anemia patients to antilymphocyte globulin and phytohemagglutinin: colony-stimulating activity and lymphokine production. *Experimental Hematology*, **19**, 312–16.

Torok Storb, B., Doney, K., Brown, S. L. and Prentice, R. L. (1984) Correlation of two in vitro tests with clinical response to immunosuppressive therapy in 54 patients with severe aplastic anemia. *Blood*, **63**, 349–55.

Urabe, A., Mizoguchi, H., Takaku, F., Miyazaki, T., Yachi, A., Niitsu, Y., Miura, Y., Mutoh, Y., Fujioka, S., Nomura, T. et al. (1993) [Effects of rHuEPO on aplastic anemia: results of a phase II clinical study]. *Japanese Journal of Clinical Hematology*, **34**, 1002–10.

Vadhan–Raj, S., Buescher, S., Broxmeyer, H. E., LeMaistre, A., Lepe Zuniga, J. L., Ventura, G., Jeha, S., Horwitz, L. J., Trujillo, J. M., Gillis, S., Hittelman, W. N. and Gutterman, J. U. (1988) Stimulation of myelopoiesis in patients with aplastic anemia by recombinant human granulocyte-macrophage colony-stimulating factor [published erratum appears in *New England Journal of Medicine* 1989, **320**, 329]. *New England Journal of Medicine*, **319**, 1628–34.

Walsh, C. E., Liu, J. M., Anderson, S. M., Rossio, J. L., Nienhuis, A. W. and Young, N. S. (1992) A trial of recombinant human interleukin-1 in patients with severe refractory aplastic anaemia. *British Journal of Haematology*, **80**, 106–10.

Watari, K., Asano, S., Shirafuji, N., Kodo, H., Ozawa, K., Takaku, F. and Kamachi, S. (1989) Serum granulocyte colony-stimulating factor levels in healthy volunteers and patients with various disorders as estimated by enzyme immunoassay. *Blood*, **73**, 117–22.

Webb, D. I. and Bundtzen, J. L. (1993) The effect of granulocyte-macrophage colony stimulating factor on paroxysmal nocturnal hemoglobinuria: a case report. *Alaska Medicine*, **35**, 216–17, 224.

Weide, R., Lyttelton, M., Samson, D., Gorg, C., Koppler, H., Pfluger, K. H. and Havemann, K. (1993) Sustained trilineage response in a patient with ALG-resistant severe aplastic anaemia after treatment with G-CSF, erythropoietin and cyclosporin A: association of recovery with marked elevation of serum alkaline phosphatase. *British Journal of Haematology*, **85**, 608–10.

Welte, K., Gabrilove, J., Bronchud, M. H., Platzer, E. and Morstyn, G. (1996) Filgrastim (r-metHuG-CSF): the first 10 years. *Blood*, **88**, 1907–29.

Wickramanayake, P. D., Katav, I., Mantovani, L., Sieg, K., Schulz, A., Ackerman, M. and Diehl, V. (1993) Succesful treatment of refractory severe aplastic anemia (SAA) with recombinant human granulocyte colony stimulating factor (G-CSF, filgrastim), recombinant human erythropoietin (EPO) and cyclosporin A (CSA) [Abstract]. *Blood*, **82** [Suppl. 1], 91a.

Wodnar Filipowicz, A., Tichelli, A., Zsebo, K. M., Speck, B. and Nissen, C. (1992) Stem cell factor stimulates the in vitro growth of bone marrow cells from aplastic anemia patients. *Blood*, **79**, 3196–202.

Wodnar Filipowicz, A., Yancik, S., Moser, Y., dalle Carbonare, V., Gratwohl, A., Tichelli, A., Speck, B. and Nissen, C. (1993) Levels of soluble stem cell factor in serum of patients with aplastic anemia. *Blood*, **81**, 3259–64.

Wodnar Filipowicz, A., Lyman, S. D., Gratwohl, A., Tichelli, A., Speck, B. and Nissen, C. (1996) Flt3 ligand level reflects hemopoietic progenitor cell function in aplastic anemia and chemotherapy-induced bone marrow aplasia. *Blood*, **88**, 4493–9.

Wodnar Filipowicz, A., Chklovskaia, E., Manz, C. Y., Lyman, S. D. and Nissen, C. (1997) Effect of flt3 ligand on in vitro growth and expansion of colony-forming bone marrow cells from patients with aplastic anemia. *Experimental Hematology*, **25**, 573–81.

Yamazaki, E., Kanamori, H., Taguchi, J., Harano, H., Mohri, H. and Okubo, T. (1997) The evidence of clonal evolution with monosomy 7 in aplastic anemia following granulocyte colony-stimulating factor using the polymerase chain reaction. *Blood Cells, Molecules and Diseases*, **23**, 213–18.

Yasuda, M., Shiokawa, S., Yamaguchi, M., Suenaga, Y., Wada, T., Nonaka, S. and Nobunaga, M. (1994) Trilineage response to rhG-CSF with subsequent clonal hemopoiesis in a patient with severe bone marrow aplasia. *Leukemia Lymphoma*, **14**, 347–51.

Yonekura, S., Kawada, H., Watanabe, S., Masumoto, A., Ogawa, Y., Fukuda, R., Nishihira, H., Matsuyama, S., Katoh, S., Mouri, H., Motomura, S., Shionoya, S. and Hotta, T. (1997). Hematologic response in patients with aplastic anemia after long-term administration of recombinant human granulocyte colony-stimulating factor and erythropoietin. *Clinical Therapeutics*, **19**, 1394–1407.

Yoshida, Y., Anzai, N., Kawabata, H., Kohsaka, Y. and Okuma, M. (1993) Serial changes in endogenous erythropoietin levels in patients with myelodysplastic syndromes and aplastic anemia undergoing erythropoietin treatment. *Annals of Hematology*, **66**, 175–80.

Zecca, M., Perotti, C., Marradi, P., Montagna, D., Giorgiani, G., Balter, R., Prete, L. and Locatelli, F. (1996) Recombinant human G-CSF-mobilized peripheral blood stem cells for second allogeneic transplant after bone marrow graft rejection in children. *British Journal of Haematology*, **92**, 432–4.

12

HLA-identical sibling bone marrow transplantation to treat severe aplastic anemia

Shaun R. McCann

St James's Hospital, Dublin

Jakob R. Passweg

Kantonsspital Basel, Basel

Rainer Storb and
H. Joachim Deeg

University of Washington

Introduction

Severe aplastic anemia (SAA) is defined by a marrow cellularity of $<25\%$ and at least two of the following: (1) a neutrophil count $<0.5\times10^9/l$; (2) a platelet count $<20\times10^9/l$; and (3) a reticulocyte count $<20\times10^9/l$ (SAA Working Party consensus conference). Very severe AA is defined by a neutrophil count of $<0.2\times10^9/l$.

SAA is rare and in most patients the etiology is unknown (idiopathic SAA). Acquired SAA may be linked to ionizing radiation, chemicals (e.g., benzene), chemotherapeutic agents (International Agranulocytosis and Aplastic Anaemia Study, 1987; Yardley-Jones et al., 1991) or drugs that cause idiosyncratic marrow injury (e.g., gold, chloramphenicol, phenylbutazone and others). Occasionally SAA is associated with viral diseases such as nonA, nonB, nonC hepatitis, parvovirus (pure red cell aplasia) or Epstein–Barr virus and autoimmune disorders such as eosinophilic fasciitis (Fonseca and Tefferi, 1997).

The pathophysiology of SAA is incompletely understood and it is possible that there are various etiologies ultimately presenting as marrow failure. Defective hemopoietic stem cells, a defective marrow microenvironment, impairment of cellular interactions and immunological suppression of marrow function may be involved (Jandl, 1996). A role for autoimmune mechanisms is suggested by the therapeutic response to immunosuppressive treatment (Hathaway et al., 1967; Parkman et al., 1974), and by autologous recovery of marrow function following attempted allogeneic bone marrow transplantation or cyclophosphamide treatment without marrow infusion. Although up to 50% of syngeneic marrow infusions engraft without prior immunosuppression, supporting the hypothesis of a stem-cell defect, the other 50% require the host to be immunosuppressed prior to successful engraftment, indicating that immune mechanisms may operate at least in some patients.

When treated with supportive care, including blood transfusions and antibiotics, only 25–30% of patients with SAA survive for 2 years (Camitta et al., 1979). More than 50% are expected to die within 6 months of diagnosis without specific therapy (Camitta et al., 1983). Effective therapy for SAA consists of either immunosuppressive therapy with agents such as antithymocyte globulin (ATG) and cyclosporin or bone marrow transplantation (BMT). The outcome for patients in the 1990s who do not receive specific treatment is unknown.

HLA-identical sibling transplants

Most transplants for SAA performed to date have been from HLA-identical sibling donors. Successful allogeneic BMT is dependent on a stem-cell product of sufficient quality to guarantee stable engraftment. In preparation for an allogeneic HLA-identical sibling BMT, recipients are conditioned with intensive immunosuppressive regimens to prevent graft rejection. Immunosuppressive agents include cyclophosphamide given either alone at 50 mg/kg per day on four successive days or combined with ATG. Alternatively, cyclophosphamide (60 mg/kg per day for 2 days) is combined with total body irradiation (300–1200 cGy) or limited field irradiation, such as total lymphoid irradiation or thoracoabdominal irradiation (450–750 cGy). Generally, pretransplant conditioning regimens for patients with SAA are of lower intensity than for patients with malignant disease. Posttransplant complications include graft failure, acute and chronic graft-versus-host disease (GVHD), interstitial pneumonitis, infections, and late complications such as infertility, growth impairment and secondary malignancies that influence the quality of life and the probability of survival.

Survival, current results, and trends over time

During the 1970s survival rates among patients receiving transplants from an HLA-genotypically identical donor were commonly 40–50% compared to 60–90% in recent years (Bortin and Rimm, 1981; Storb et al., 1994) (see Table 12.1). Results obtained at the Fred Hutchinson Cancer Research Center (FHCRC) are illustrated in Figure 12.1. A recent comprehensive analysis of results with 1305 HLA-identical sibling transplants reported to the International Bone Marrow Transplant Registry (IBMTR) showed that survival had increased from $48 \pm 7\%$ in 1976–80 to $66 \pm 6\%$ in 1988–92 (Figure 12.2). The incidence of grades II–IV acute GVHD decreased from 39% in 1976–80 to 19% in 1988–92 (Passweg et al., 1997) and overall improvement appeared

Table 12.1. HLA-identical marrow transplants for severe aplastic anemia (SAA)

Transplant team (Ref)	Year of transplant	No. of patients	Age (years) range (median)	Conditioning regimen*	GVHD prophylaxis**	Rejection (%)***	Incidence of GVHD % Acute	Incidence of GVHD % Chronic	Survival (%)	Follow-up (years), range (median)
UCLA (Feig et al., 1983)	1977–81	46	2–44 (19)	CY + 300 cGy TBI	MTX	2	70	NA	63	0.75–4.5 (2)
Boston (Smith et al., 1985)	1977–84	40	2–35 (17)	PAPAPA-CY	MTX	10	53	>35	61	<0.8–11 (5)
FHCRC (Sanders et al., 1986)	1971–81	81	2–17 (13)	CY	MTX	18	30	30	71	10–20
FHCRC (Anasetti et al., 1986; Storb et al., 1980)	1972–84	50	3–32 (17)	CY	MTX	10	23	37	82	1–12 (7)
Minneapolis (McGlave et al., 1987; Ramsay et al., 1983)	1977–86	58	2–45 (18)	CY + 750 cGy TLI	MTX, MTX + ATG + PSE	5	38	12–54	70	<0.05–8
EBMT (Bacigalupo et al., 1988b)	1981–88	218	1–50	CY ± TLI, TAI or TBI	MTX or CSP	NA	NA	NA	63	<1–6
FHCRC (Anasetti et al., 1988; Storb et al., 1982)*	1976–81	42	1–49 (20)	CY	MTX	14	36	60	67	7–11
London (Hows et al., 1989)	1979–85	49	3–47 (22)	CY	CSP	17	50	37	69	1.8–7.8 (5.8)
IBMTR (Champlin et al., 1989)	1978–86	625	–	CY / CY + TLI or TAI / CY + TBI	MTX or CSP	20 / 9 / 5	NA	NA	NA	NA
UCLA (Champlin et al., 1990)	1984–88	29	0.7–41 (19)	CY + 300 cGy TLI	MTX + CSP	23	22	NA	78	0.6–5 (2)
EBMT (Locasciulli et al., 1990)	1970–88	171	1–15	CY ± TLI, TAI, or TBI	MTX or CSP	NA	NA	NA	63	0.08–15 (4.5)
FHCRC (Storb et al., 1991; Storb et al., 1992)	1981–90	35	1–18 (10)	CY	MTX + CSP	24	15	30	94	1–10.5 (5)
Paris (Gluckman et al., 1991)	1980–89	107	5–46 (19)	CY + 600 cGy TAI	MTX, CSP, or MTX + CSP	3	32	55	62	1–10 (3.75)
IBMTR (Gluckman et al., 1992)	1980–87	595	1–<40	CY ± TLI, TAI, or TBI	MTX, CSP, or MTX + CSP	10	40	45	63	>2–>7

Study	Years	N	Age range (median)	Conditioning	GVHD prophylaxis					Follow-up range (median)
FHCRC (Storb et al., 1992)	1988–91	29	2–46 (24)	CY + ATG	MTX + CSP	3	15	30	93	0.5–3.5 (2)
FHCRC (Storb et al., 1997a; Storb et al., 1994b)	1988–93	39	2–52 (24.5)	CY + ATG	MTX + CSP	5	15	34	92	3.2–8.2 (5.2)
Vancouver (Cuthbert et al., 1995)	1982–92	16	2–40 (15)	CY ± ATG ± TBI	MTX, MTX + CSP	6	36	31	75	2.1–11 (6)
Memorial Sloan-Kettering (Castro-Malaspina et al., 1994)	1983–90	23	2.5–32 (13)	CY + TLI	CSP + PSE, MTX + CSP; others	14	27	18	60	3.2–10.4 (5.7)
Hamburg (Horstmann et al., 1995)	1990–93	9	7–30 (25)	CY + ATG	MTX + CSP	0	0	0	87	1.6–3.1 (2.5)
Children's Hospital of Philadelphia (Bunin et al., 1996)	1989–94	11	1.5–16 (3)	CY + ATG	CSP	0	NA	0	100	0.6–4.6 (2.2)
Hopkins (May et al., 1993)	1984–91	24	4–53 (21)	CY	CSP	29	5	0	79	NA
Helsinki (Makipernaa et al., 1995)	1974–92	11	0.6–17.3 (9.3)	CY ± TLI	Various	9	NA	0	73	2–19
UCLA/Sloan-Kettering/MD Anderson (Paquette et al., 1995)	1977–88	55	NA	CY ± TBI or ± TLI	MTX, MTX + CSP	9	45	38	52	(6)
Japan (Azuma et al., 1997)	1993–96	10	1.5–14 (8)	CY + ATG	MTX + CSP	0	0	10	100	0.6–3.4
IBMTR (Passweg et al., 1997)	1976–80	186	2–56 (19)	CY, CY + TBI, CY + LFR	Various	20	39	37	48	(6)
	1981–87	648	1–57 (20)	CY, CY + TBI, CY + LFR	Various	11	37	47	61	(6)
	1988–92	471	1–51 (20)	CY, CY + LFR, CY + ATG	Various	16	19	32	66	(5)

Notes:

* ATG = antithymocyte globulin; CY = cyclophosphamide; LFR = limited field irradiation (either TLI or TAI); PAPAPA = alternating procarbazine and antithymocyte globulin; TAI = thoracoabdominal irradiation; TBI = total body irradiation; TLI = total lymphoid irradiation. – = Data not reported.

** CSP = cyclosporin; MTX = methotrexate; PSE = prednisone.

*** Graft failure with first transplant.

In all series the majority of patients were previously transfused except those designated with an asterisk (*).

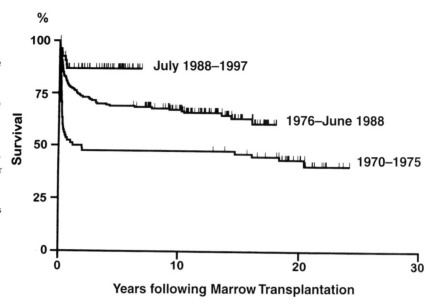

Figure 12.1. Marrow grafts from HLA-identical family members after cyclophosphamide at FHCRC. Overall survival by transplant year (1970–75, $n=63$; 1976 to June 1988, $n=212$; July 1988 to 1997, $n=55$). The combination of methotrexate and cyclosporin has been used for prophylaxis against graft-versus-host disease in some patients since 1981 and in all patients since 1985. Most patients transplanted since July 1988 were conditioned with cyclophosphamide and antithymoycte globulin without supplemental buffy coat cell infusions. Tick marks indicate surviving patients as of April 1997.

to be related to the use of cyclosporin for GVHD prophylaxis. Similar improvement in pediatric patients over time was also reported by the EBMT group (Locasciulli et al., 1990) (Figure 12.3). Among previously transfused patients, aged 2–52 years (median 24.5), undergoing allogeneic BMT at the FHCRC between 1988 and 1993, receiving conditioning with cyclophosphamide plus ATG and GVHD prophylaxis with methotrexate and cyclosporin, 5% experienced graft failure, 15% acute GVHD (no grade-IV GVHD), 34% chronic GVHD (Storb et al., 1997a) and 92% were alive at 3–8.2 years (median 5.2) (Figures 12.4 and 12.5). Three other reports showed survival probabilities of 85% and higher in patients conditioned with cyclophosphamide plus ATG (Azuma et al., 1997; Bunin et al., 1996; Hortsmann et al., 1995). Survival in patients conditioned with cyclophosphamide and irradiation has been reported to be 60–78% (Castro–Malaspina et al., 1994; Champlin et al., 1990). Pediatric patients (less than 19 years of age) generally fared better than adult patients with survival rates of 94–100% as reported in four studies (Azuma et al., 1997; Bunin et al., 1996; Storb et al., 1991, 1992). Two additional studies showed 73% and 63% survival of pediatric patients, respectively (Locasciulli et al., 1990; Makipernaa et al., 1995).

Several factors have been consistently associated with survival in analyses involving different patient cohorts. In a recent survey of 562 patients receiving HLA-identical sibling transplants worldwide between 1990 and 1995 and reported to the IBMTR, the most important factors influencing survival in multivariate analysis were: (1) transfusion history, with patients receiving multiple transfusions faring significantly worse than those receiving fewer transfusions prior to transplant (Figure 12.6A,B), (2) patient age, and (3) pretransplant Karnofsky performance score favoring young age and good performance status. Overall 5-year

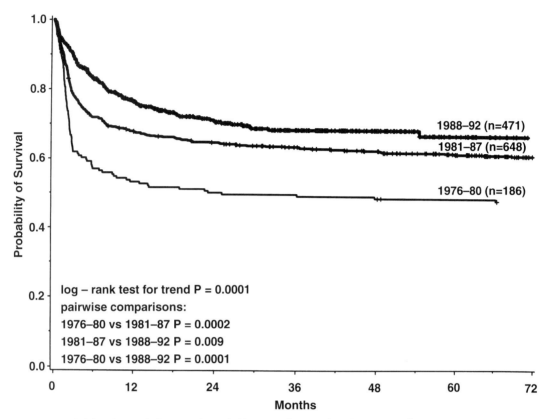

Figure 12.2. Probability of survival after HLA-identical sibling transplantation for aplastic anemia for patient cohorts transplanted in 1976–80, 1981–87 and 1988–92 and reported to the International Bone Marrow Transplant Registry (IBMTR). (Adapted from Passweg et al. 1997.)

survival in this cohort was 69±5%. In the 1990s 95% of patients received GVHD prophylaxis with cyclosporin alone, in combination with methotrexate or other drugs. The pretransplant conditioning regimen included cyclophosphamide alone (54%) cyclophosphamide plus ATG (19%), and cyclophosphamide plus either total body irradiation or total lymphoid irradiation (24%), and there appeared to be no significant association between the pretransplant conditioning regimen and survival. Therefore, patients considered for BMT should be referred to the transplant center as rapidly as possible after diagnosis, and before multiple transfusions are given and infections have resulted in a decreased performance score.

Engraftment

Primary graft failure (without any evidence of hemopoietic engraftment) and secondary graft failure (following transient establishment of donor hemopoiesis)

Figure 12.3. Probability of survival after HLA-identical sibling transplant by transplant year. A – 1970–80; B – 1981–83; C – 1984–88. (Adapted from Locasciulli et al., 1990.)

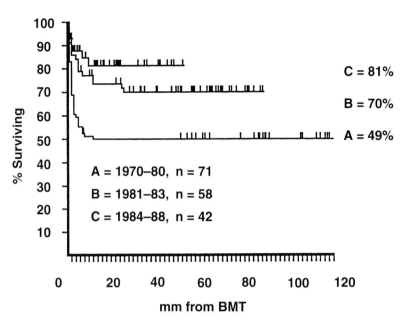

Figure 12.4. Cumulative incidences of graft rejection (A) and acute graft-versus-host disease (GVHD) (B) in patients with severe aplastic anemia given HLA-identical marrow transplants and GVHD prophylaxis with methotrexate and cyclosporin. Shown are data from 39 historical patients conditioned with cyclophosphamide (CY) alone, 63% of whom were given donor buffy coat infusions, and 39 patients conditioned with CY and anti-thymocyte globulin (ATG). P values for rejection and acute GVHD calculated by log-rank test were 0. 96 and 0. 64, respectively. (Adapted from Storb et al., 1994.)

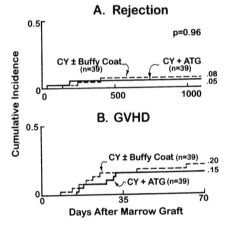

were relatively common in the early 1970s, and were reported in 35% of cases at the FHCRC (Storb et al., 1992), and in 32% of patients transplanted before 1980 (McCann et al., 1994) by the EBMT Group (Figure 12.7A,B). The probability of primary or secondary graft failure in patients transplanted after 1990 and reported to the IBMTR is $15 \pm 4\%$, 5 years following BMT. It is difficult to ascertain if late graft failure, i.e., pancytopenia and marrow hypoplasia following an initial period of hemopoietic engraftment, is truly caused by rejection of the donor marrow or by a relapse of the initial disease. The observation that graft failure/rejection following BMT for SAA is more frequent than experienced following BMT for hemopoietic malignancies supports the possibility that immune

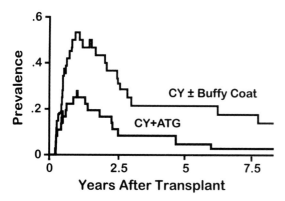

Figure 12.5. The prevalence of chronic GVHD among patients described in Figure 12.4. There was a statistically significant lower incidence of chronic GVHD among patients conditioned with CY and ATG compared to those who received CY for conditioning with or without buffy coat infusions. $P=0.01$ by the log-rank test. (Adapted from Storb et al., 1997a.)

mcchanisms are important in the etiology of SAA and its recurrence after transplant.

As stated previously, prior blood transfusion is a major risk factor for survival following BMT for SAA. Sensitization to antigens expressed by the BMT donor and the transfusion donor is a likely mechanism of graft rejection. Clinical and experimental data indicate that leukocytes contained in the transfusion product, in particular dendritic cells, are responsible for sensitization (Kalhs et al., 1995; Storb and Deeg, 1986). Thus, depleting blood products of leukocytes is recommended for patients who are candidates for transplantation (Schuening et al., 1993).Gamma irradiation of blood products is also recommended to prevent third-party GVHD.

The dose of mononuclear cells infused is very important in SAA. A retrospective analysis showed that the number of marrow cells infused is inversely correlated with the incidence of graft failure in patients conditioned with cyclophosphamide at the FHCRC (Storb et al., 1977). Attempts to increase the number of hemopoietic stem cells transplanted by infusing viable donor buffy coat cells in addition to marrow were successful in reducing the incidence of graft failure, but were associated with an increased incidence of de novo chronic GVHD (Niederwieser et al., 1988, Storb et al., 1982). Buffy coat infusions have since been abandoned, but efforts should still be directed at maximizing the number of marrow cells infused by harvesting $\geqslant 3.5 \times 10^8$ cells/kg (Deeg et al., 1986; Niederwieser et al., 1988).

Increasing the intensity of the conditioning regimen with combinations of cyclophosphamide plus total body irradiation or limited field irradiation have also been effective in reducing the incidence of rejection, but radiation-based regimens increase the incidence of secondary malignancy and cause problems with growth, development, and fertility (Deeg and Socié, 1998; Deeg et al., 1996b; Sanders et al., 1996).

A regimen combining cyclophosphamide and ATG was developed to rescue patients rejecting their first graft after conditioning with cyclophosphamide

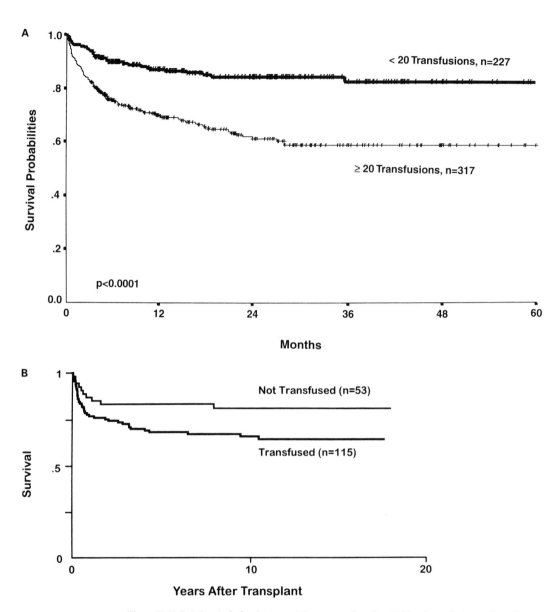

Figure 12.6A,B. A, Survival of patients receiving more or less than 20 blood transfusions prior to bone marrow transplantation (with kind permission of IBMTR). B, The effect of pretransplant transfusion on actuarial survival. Untransfused patients have a significantly superior survival ($P=0.04$). (Adapted from Doney et al., 1997.)

alone (Storb et al., 1974*a,b*; Weiden et al., 1976). At the FHCRC, 50% of recipients of second transplants became long-term survivors (Storb et al., 1994) and survival after a second BMT has increased to 83% by introducing further refinements to this approach (Stucki et al., 1997).

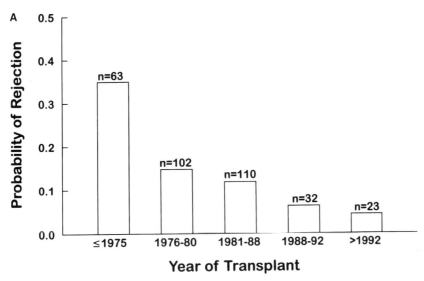

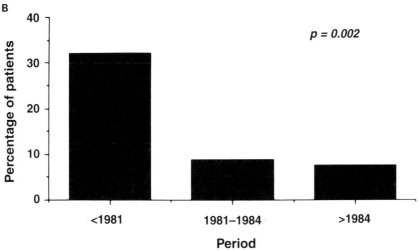

Figure 12.7A,B. A, Graft rejection after HLA-identical sibling transplants carried out at the FHCRC. All patients were conditioned with cyclophosphamide-containing regimens. Numbers indicate the numbers of patients transplanted during a given time interval. The data are current as of May 1997. B, Percentage of patients in Europe (EBMT) experiencing graft rejection from 1976 to 1990. (Adapted from McCann et al., 1994.)

Cyclophosphamide and ATG were also used as a conditioning regimen for patients receiving first transplants at the FHCRC beginning in 1988 (Storb et al., 1994). Analysis of the outcome for 39 patients compared to 39 historical controls receiving cyclophosphamide alone (24 of whom had been given donor buffy coat) reveals similar incidences of graft rejection and acute GVHD, but survival of patients conditioned with cyclophosphamide and ATG was significantly better (Figure 12.8) owing to less chronic GVHD (Figure 12.4). These results, obtained by studying patients treated with cyclophosphamide and ATG, have since been confirmed in a study of a larger number of patients (Storb et al., 1997*a*). However, analysis of IBMTR data did not show that cyclophosphamide plus ATG increased survival compared to cyclophosphamide alone, but the number of patients

Figure 12.8.
Kaplan–Meier estimates
of survival in the two
patient groups
described in Figure 12.4.
There was a statistically
significant higher rate of
survival among patients
conditioned with cyclo-
phosphamide (CY) and
ATG versus those who
received CY with or
without buffy coat infu-
sions (*P*=0.02). *P* values
were calculated using
the log-rank test. The
data are current as of
January 1997. (Adapted
from Storb et al., 1997*a*.)

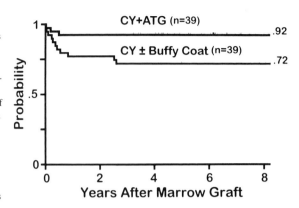

receiving cyclophosphamide plus ATG was small (Passweg et al., 1997). The IBMTR is currently conducting a prospective, randomized trial comparing pretransplant conditioning with cyclophosphamide and ATG versus cyclophosphamide alone.

There is evidence that posttransplant immunosuppression, aimed at controlling GVHD, may also suppress the host-versus-graft (HVG) reaction, i.e., help to suppress graft rejection. Early studies of a canine model of marrow transplantation showed that postgrafting methotrexate had a graft-facilitating effect (Deeg et al., 1987; Thomas et al., 1963). Preclinical studies showed methotrexate plus cyclosporin to be superior to cyclosporin alone both for controlling GVHD and suppressing HVG reactions (Storb et al., 1997*b*). A retrospective analysis of clinical data by the EBMT group suggests that using cyclosporin as prophylaxis against GVHD decreased the rejection rate as compared to methotrexate (McCann et al., 1994). A randomized prospective study from the FHCRC failed to show a difference in rejection incidence (Storb et al., 1986, 1992) among patients given long-term methotrexate and 'short methotrexate' (days 1, 3, 6, and 11) combined with cyclosporin. Recent results suggest that a combination of mycophenolate mofetil plus cyclosporin achieves even better control of HVG reactions than methotrexate plus cyclosporin (Storb et al., 1997*a*). Thus, posttransplant GVHD prophylactic regimens may affect the interpretation of the efficacy of a given conditioning regimen in decreasing the risk of graft rejection. Anecdotal reports suggest that the antiCD3 antibody BC3 plus high-dose corticosteroids (Bjerke et al., 1995), a regimen including Campath-1G, the use of peripheral-blood stem cells mobilized by granulocyte-colony stimulating factor (G-CSF) without reconditioning (Redei et al., 1997), or the use of rabbit ATG (Yoshida et al., 1994) may be useful in overcoming graft failure.

The most frequently used GVHD prophylaxis currently is cyclosporin plus methotrexate and, to prevent late graft failure, cyclosporin is continued for at least a year after the transplant in many centers. There is no established standard treatment for patients experiencing graft failure. Retransplantations using a

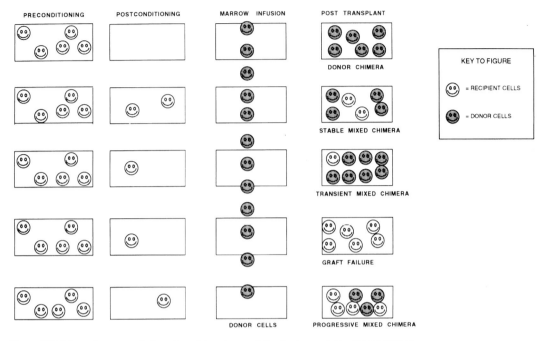

Figure 12.9. Schematic representation of possible outcomes following bonemarrow transplantation. The chimeric status of recipients is depicted by representations of the relative proportions of donor and host hemopoietic cells. (Adapted from McCann & Lawler, 1993, *Bone Marrow Transplantation*, **11**, 91–4.)

conditioning regimen of higher intensity (i.e., with radiation, additional drugs) is most commonly recommended.

Hemopoietic chimerism

The goal of allogeneic BMT for SAA has been to establish complete donor hemopoiesis, i.e., donor chimerism. The ideal result is illustrated in Figure 12.9 where host hemopoietic cells are completely destroyed following conditioning and are subsequently replaced by donor stem cells. The survival of recipient hemopoietic cells following BMT for SAA may have different connotations compared with a similar result following BMT for leukemia. In the leukemic recipient mixed hemopoietic chimerism, i.e., the persistence of host cells following BMT, may increase the risk of leukemic relapse whereas in SAA the possibility is that residual host cells may influence the possibility of graft rejection. It is also possible that the preservation of recipient cells may have a beneficial effect on the development of GVHD.

There are few serial studies, using sensitive techniques, of large numbers of patients transplanted for SAA which address the above questions. Major problems facing investigators are choosing which technique to use and deciding at what time intervals following BMT the patients should be studied. Techniques that depend on karyotypic analysis are hampered by the small number of metaphases, especially in the early postBMT phase, and are usually only applicable to sex-mismatched transplants. DNA-based technologies which include analysis of variable-number tandem repeats (VNTR) or PCR-based strategies using highly polymorphic short tandem repeats (STR) have the advantage of being sensitive, robust and applicable to archival material, but do not necessarily evaluate viable cellular material, nor do they give any indication as to cell lineage. Persistent host DNA may reflect recipient stromal or dendritic cells rather than viable hemopoietic cells.

Early studies from the FHCRC, using karyotyping, indicated a 60% incidence of mixed chimerism but two-thirds of these patients eventually converted to complete donor type hemopoiesis and the remainder rejected their grafts, indicating the importance of serial studies (Hill et al., 1986) and the influence of persistent mixed hemopoietic chimerism on graft rejection. A follow-up study [116 patients transplanted from sex-mismatched HLA-identical siblings and using karyotyping and fluorescence in situ hybridization (FISH)] indicated a 54% incidence of mixed chimerism with a graft rejection rate of 14%, whereas the incidence of graft rejection among donor chimeras was 9% (Huss et al., 1996). However, there were striking differences between patients receiving single-agent (methotrexate or cyclosporin) GVHD prophylaxis and those given methotrexate plus cyclosporin. For patients who received a single agent, mixed chimerism was associated with a lower incidence of acute GVHD and a better overall survival (64%) than for patients who were complete donor chimeras (43% survival) (Huss et al., 1996). No such difference was observed among patients who received methotrexate plus cyclosporin for GVHD prophylaxis.

Using a highly sensitive technique which relies on the amplification of short tandem repeats (STRs) of material taken from archival blood or bone marrow slides (Lawler et al., 1991), the EBMT recently completed a study of 91 patients from 15 centers. Complete donor chimerism was seen in 40%, transient mixed chimerism in 18%, stable mixed chimerism in 20% and progressive mixed chimerism (progressive rise in host cells to >20%) in 19% of recipients. In the first three groups graft rejection was observed in 2% of patients whereas in the group exhibiting progressive mixed chimerism the graft rejection rate was 76%. There was an inverse correlation between the detection of host cells and the occurrence of acute GVHD and progressive mixed chimerism was a bad prognostic indicator of survival (Lawler et al., 1995). Seven patients lost their grafts during the time of cyclosporin withdrawal (Figure 12.10), suggesting that careful monitoring of chimeric status is important at this critical juncture.

The conditioning therapy undoubtedly influences the pattern of chimerism postBMT, with radiation-based regimens being associated with complete donor chimerism (Gluckman et al., 1992). However the high incidence of secondary malignancies following radiation has made this approach unacceptable in the

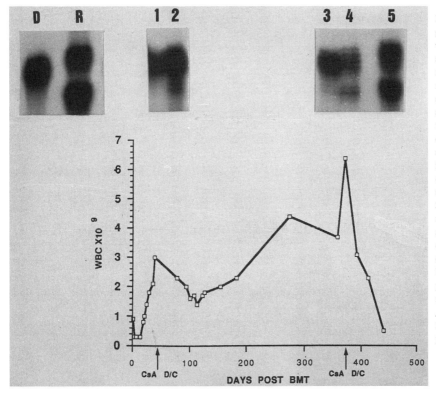

Figure 12.10. Example of graft rejection following withdrawal of cyclosporin (CsA). Donor and recipient alleles (polymerase chain reaction of short tandem repeats) are polymorphic and the emergence of recipient bands can be clearly seen on two occasions, firstly when the patient discontinued cyclosporin at approximately 3 months after bone marrow transplantation and secondly when cyclosporin was discontinued 1 year after bone marrow transplantation. (With permission of the *British Journal of Haematology*, Lawler et al., 1999, in press.)

majority of centers. A recent study (Hamblin et al., 1996) showed that pretreatment with in vivo Campath-1G confers a low incidence of GVDH but a high incidence of mixed chimerism, tipping the balance towards graft rejection.

A comparative randomized study is currently being conducted by the EBMT to assess the degree of chimerism and graft rejection in patients receiving cyclosporin or cyclosporin plus methotrexate as prophylaxis for prevention of GVHD.

Acute GVHD

Despite the use of prophylaxis, GVHD continues to be a problem and has a strong adverse effect on survival. Early data from the FHCRC showed an actuarial probability of survival at 11 years of 45% for patients with grade II–IV acute GVHD compared to 80% among patients with minimal or no acute GVHD (Storb et al., 1983*a*). Similarly, an analysis of IBMTR data showed a 5-year actuarial probability of survival of 31% for patients with grades II–IV acute GVHD compared to 80% for patients with no or mild GVHD (Gluckman et al., 1992). The probability of grade II–IV acute GVHD at 100 days posttransplant was $18 \pm 3\%$ in patients transplanted after 1990 and reported to the IBMTR.

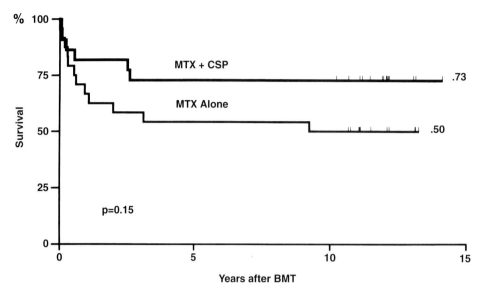

Figure 12.11. Survival of patients given grafts from HLA-identical siblings after conditioning with cyclophosphamide. Shown are the updated results of a randomized prospective trial comparing methotrexate (*n*=24) alone versus methotrexate and cyclosporin (*n*=22) for prophylaxis against graft-versus-host disease (Storb et al., 1986). Most of the patients enrolled in the trial were adults because of Food and Drug Administration restrictions for the use of cyclosporin. The death at 9 years was from HIV infection. Tick marks indicate survival as of April 1996.

In early studies GVHD prophylaxis was with methotrexate whereas cyclosporin became available in 1978. Several retrospective analyses concluded that survival was increased for patients given cyclosporin compared to historical controls given methotrexate (Bacigalupo et al., 1988*a*, *b*; Gordon–Smith et al., 1987; Hows et al., 1985, 1989; Passweg et al., 1997). However, the results of several controlled prospective randomized trials showed no significant differences in the incidence of acute GVHD or in survival between patients given cyclosporin and those given methotrexate (Ringden et al., 1986; Storb et al., 1983*b*, 1988).

A randomized prospective study has shown that a combination of cyclosporin and prednisone (PS) is only marginally better than cyclosporin alone in preventing acute GVHD, and is associated with more chronic GVHD (Storb et al., 1990). Another study found a combination of methotrexate, cyclosporin and PS more effective than cyclosporin and PS in preventing acute GVHD (Chao et al., 1993).

Studies of canine models led to the combination of a short course of methotrexate (on days 1, 3, 6, and 11 after transplant) and daily cyclosporin (Deeg et al., 1982, 1984) being introduced. A randomized trial from the FHCRC showed a significant reduction in the incidence and severity of acute GVHD in 22 patients given this combination compared to 24 patients receiving methotrexate alone (Storb et al., 1986). Survival was higher for patients who received the combination of drugs (Figure 12.11). In a retrospective analysis of 595 patients with SAA reported to the IBMTR who received a matched sibling BMT, patients who received either cyclosporin alone or cyclosporin plus methotrexate compared to methotrexate alone had a significantly improved survival of 69% versus 56% respectively (Gluckman et al., 1992). Importantly, no grade-IV acute GVHD was seen in patients given methotrexate plus cyclosporin. The reduction in acute GVHD resulted in improved survival, most prominently among pediatric patients (Storb et al., 1991). At least one retrospective analysis suggested that compliance with the prescribed doses of methotrexate and cyclosporin was important for the control of GVHD (Nash et al., 1992).

Chronic GVHD

Chronic GVHD continues to be a major complication of BMT for SAA. In a few small series of pediatric patients, the incidence varied from 0 to 25% (Azuma et al., 1997; Bunin et al., 1996; Makipernaa et al., 1995; Sanders et al., 1994); however, an incidence as high as 40–60% was observed in other series that included adult patients and patients who had received buffy coat infusions (Anasetti et al., 1988; Passweg et al., 1997). In most recent series of matched sibling transplants the incidence of chronic GVHD was around 30% (Cuthbert et al., 1995; Passweg et al., 1997; Storb et al., 1991) (see Table 12.1). In patients transplanted after 1990 and reported to the IBMTR (median age: 20 years) the probability of chronic GVHD of any grade at 5 years was $26 \pm 5\%$.

A history of acute GVHD, older patient age, and the use of donor buffy coat infusions are associated with an increased risk of chronic GVHD (Atkinson et al., 1990; Storb et al., 1983a,b). In addition, Gluckman et al. (1991) have suggested that radiation given as part of the conditioning regimen increases the risk of chronic GVHD.

Chronic GVHD causes considerable morbidity, and requires prolonged immunosuppressive therapy in many patients (Sullivan et al., 1991). One-third of affected patients may die, often from infectious complications. PS, cyclosporin, azathioprine, cyclophosphamide, procarbazine, and thalidomide have been used either alone or in combination to treat chronic GVHD.

Figure 12.12 shows that the cumulative mortality after diagnosis of chronic GVHD did not change significantly over four different time periods among patients transplanted at the FHCRC. Clearly, improvements in the prevention and treatment of chronic GVHD are needed.

Interstitial pneumonitis

In an analysis of IBMTR data on 547 patients with SAA receiving HLA-identical marrow grafts, the incidence of interstitial pneumonitis was 17% (Weiner et al., 1989). Pneumonitis was associated with cytomegalovirus (CMV) infection in 37%

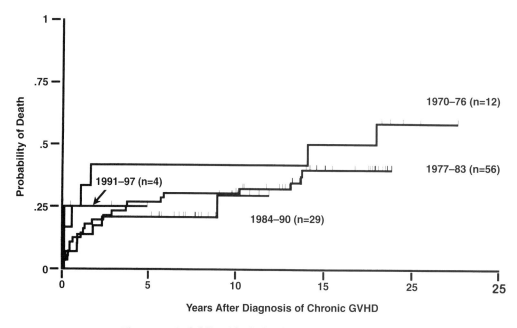

Figure 12.12. Probability of death after diagnosis of chronic graft-versus-host disease following HLA-identical marrow grafts conditioned with cyclophosphamide in FHCRC over four different time periods. Tick marks indicate census times. The data are current as of September 1997.

of cases, with other organisms in 22%, and in 41% of cases no organism was identified. The case fatality rate was 64%. Four factors were associated with the development of interstitial pneumonitis: (1) the use of methotrexate rather than cyclosporin for GVHD prophylaxis; (2) moderate to severe acute GVHD; (3) total body irradiation compared to cyclophosphamide in the preparative regimen; and (4) increased patient age. By comparison, the overall incidence of interstitial pneumonitis among 329 patients transplanted at the FHCRC over a 21-year period was 16% (Storb et al., 1992). It was associated with CMV in 44%, other organisms in 37%, and in 19% no etiology could be determined. As in the IBMTR analysis, total body irradiation and the presence of acute GVHD were significant risk factors. However, no adverse influences of patient age and of methotrexate prophylaxis were noted. A recent study of idiopathic lung disease after transplantation showed that patients with SAA receiving cyclophosphamide conditioning had a significantly lower incidence (less than 5%) than those transplanted for malignant disease preconditioned with total body irradiation or busulphan-containing regimens (Kantrow et al., 1997). The case fatality rates reported in this study and an earlier FHCRC study, both of which contained large numbers of patients with malignant diseases, were 71–74% (Crawford and Hackman, 1993; Kantrow et al., 1997). In the cohort of recently transplanted SAA patients (1990 and later) the probability of interstitial pneumonia at one year posttransplant was reported to be $8 \pm 2\%$.

Late complications

A recent study of the long-term outcome for 212 patients transplanted for SAA at the FHCRC shows that, among patients receiving transplants from HLA-identical siblings who survive at least 2 years and who were conditioned with cyclophosphamide, the presence of GVHD influences survival. Twenty-year survival was 89% for those without chronic GVHD and 69% for those with chronic GVHD. A total of 17 patients died between 2.5 and 20.4 years after transplant (13 had chronic GVHD while 4 did not) (Deeg et al., 1996a). Among the 13 patients with chronic GVHD, two died of human immunodeficiency virus (HIV) disease, five died of pulmonary failure (one from pulmonary complications of dyskeratosis congenita), three died of septicemia, and three of squamous cell carcinoma (see below). Among the four patients without chronic GVHD, one committed suicide, one died in an automobile accident, one died of HIV disease and one died of pulmonary complications from dyskeratosis congenita. Most of the surviving patients returned to a fully functional life (Deeg et al., 1996a).

In children prepared for transplantation without the use of irradiation, growth and development is normal, unless they develop chronic GVHD. Radiation exposure may result in growth impairment (Beatty et al., 1987) and endocrine dysfunction (Hinterberger–Fischer et al., 1991; Jacobs and Dubovsky, 1981; Sanders et al., 1988, Sanders and the Seattle Marrow Transplant Team, 1991; Schmidt et al., 1987). After conditioning with cyclophosphamide alone, gonadal function generally returns to normal, at least in younger individuals (up to 25 years of age), and many successful pregnancies have been reported (Sanders et al., 1996).

In a recent study of secondary malignancies in patients with SAA transplanted at the FHCRC and the Hôpital Saint Louis in Paris, the projected risk of developing a malignancy 20 years after transplantation was 14%, ninefold higher than in the general population (Deeg et al., 1996b). Overall, 18 of 621 patients developed malignancies. Five of these were lymphoid malignancies which occurred at a median of 3 months, and 13 were solid tumors, generally squamous cell carcinoma, which occurred at a median of 99 months after transplant. Significant risk factors included the use of azathioprine to treat chronic GVHD, older age, and use of irradiation in the conditioning regimen (Deeg et al., 1996b). The current recommendation is, therefore, to avoid irradiation in preparation for transplantation whenever possible.

The influence of SAA etiology on outcome

Patients with hepatitis-associated SAA, Fanconi's anemia, and dyskeratosis congenita have been successfully treated with BMT. As for hepatitis-associated SAA, there were concerns that hepatic impairment might lead to increased liver damage from cyclophosphamide or that the damaged liver might not be able to activate cyclophosphamide. However, these concerns have not been sustained (Feig et al., 1983; Witherspoon et al., 1984). Marrow grafts were almost uniformly successful, and patient survival was in excess of 80% (Witherspoon et al., 1984). Similarly an EBMT study found that the graft rejection rate in the posthepatitis SAA group was significantly lower than in the group with idiopathic SAA (McCann et al., 1994).

Syngeneic transplants

Patients with an identical twin donor were the first to receive BMTs for SAA. Six of the 12 patients treated in Seattle showed complete and sustained marrow recovery after marrow infusion without prior conditioning. The other six patients failed to show sustained recovery, and a second marrow infusion was successfully given in five of six patients after conditioning with 200 mg/kg of cyclophosphamide. Three patients died, one with graft failure, one from multi-organ failure due to complications of diabetes mellitus, and one died 10 years post-transplant with acute myeloid leukemia. Nine of 12 patients are alive with follow-up ranging from 1.5 to 30 years (Storb et al., 1992). Forty syngeneic transplants were reported to the IBMTR. Twenty-three patients received marrow without conditioning and eight of these had a full hematological recovery; the other 15 received second transplants after conditioning. Twelve of 17 patients whose initial BMT was preceded by conditioning had full hematological recovery; four died from various causes within 20 days of transplant. One patient failed to show hemopoietic recovery and was given a second successful transplant after reconditioning. Ten-year survival was 87% and 70% for patients without and with initial conditioning respectively (Hinterberger et al., 1997). Thus, results of syngeneic BMTs are consistent with the concept that some cases of SAA are due to a defect in hemopoietic stem cells, whereas others are likely to be mediated by immune mechanisms or are the result of unknown factors that can be overcome by conditioning with cyclophosphamide and a second marrow infusion (Thomas and Storb, 1984).

HLA-phenotypically identical donors

Of special interest are patients who lack an HLA-genotypically identical sibling donor but have a phenotypically matched donor within the family. A report on eight patients from the FHCRC who were conditioned for transplant with cyclophosphamide showed a survival of 100% at 3–16 years (Wagner et al., 1996). A similar report by the EBMT on 11 patients showed a survival of 64% (Locasciulli et al., 1991). It appears, therefore, that these patients should be conditioned and transplanted with regimens as used for HLA-identical sibling donors.

Conclusion

For almost three decades, patients with SAA have been treated successfully by HLA-identical BMT. Outcome has improved from about 45% survival in early studies to 65–90% in most recent trials. Improvement is due in part to a decreased incidence of graft rejection, resulting from more judicious use of transfusions before BMT, the removal of sensitizing leukocytes from transfusion products, and a decrease in the incidence and severity of acute GVHD achieved through better GVHD prophylaxis, e.g., the use of methotrexate plus cyclosporin. Morbidity and mortality from chronic GVHD remain a problem. Radiation-based regimens should be avoided in HLA-identical recipients to minimize the likelihood of inducing posttransplant malignancies and the deleterious effect on fertility, growth, and development. Monitoring of chimeric status prior to discontinuation of cyclosporin may be useful in preventing late graft failure.

References

Anasetti, C., Doney, K., Storb, R. et al. (1986) Marrow transplantation for severe aplastic anemia. Long-term outcome in fifty 'untransfused' patients. *Annals of Internal Medicine*, **104**, 461–6.

Anasetti, C., Storb, R., Longton, G., Witherspoon, R., Doney, K., Sullivan, K. M. and Thomas, E. D. (1988) Donor buffy coat infusion after marrow transplantation for aplastic anaemia (Letter to the Editor) *Blood*, **72**, 1099–100.

Atkinson, K., Horowitz, M. M., Gale, R. P., van Bekkum, D. W., Gluckman, E., Good, R. A., Jacobsen, N., Kolb, H., Rimm, A. A, Ringden, O., Rozman, C., Sobocinski, K. A., Zwaan, F. E. and Bortin, M. M. (1990) Risk factors for chronic graft-versus-host disease after HLA-identical sibling bone marrow transplantation. *Blood*, **75**, 2459–64.

Azuma, E., Kojima, S., Kato, K., Matsuyama, T., Yamada, Y., Kondo, N., Sawada, H., Hanada, M., Shibata, T., Tabata, N., Watanabe, M., Shimono, Y., Deguchi, T., Umemoto, M., Higashikawa, M., Kawasaki, H., Komada, Y. and Sakurai, M. (1997) Conditioning with cyclophosphamide/antithymocyte globulin for allogeneic bone marrow transplantation from HLA-identical matched siblings in children with severe aplastic anaemia. *Bone Marrow Transplantation*, **19**, 1085–7.

Bacigalupo, A., Hows, J., Gluckman, E., Nissen, C., Marsh, J., Van Lint, M. T., Congiu, M., De Planque, M. M., Ernst, P., McCann, S., Vitale, V., Frickhofen, N., Wursch, A., Marmont, A. M., Gordon–Smith, E. C. and for the EBMT Working Party on Severe Aplastic Anaemia (1988*a*) Bone marrow transplantation (BMT) versus immunosuppression for the treatment of severe aplastic anaemia (SAA): a report of the EBMT SAA Working Party. *British Journal of Haematology*, **70**, 177–82.

Bacigalupo, A., Van Lint, M. T., Congiu, M. and Marmont, A. M (1988*b*) Bone marrow transplantation (BMT) for severe aplastic anaemia (SAA) in Europe: a report of the EBMT-SAA Working Party. *Bone Marrow Transplantation*, **3**, 44–5.

Beatty, P. G., Di Bartolomeo, P., Storb, R., Clift, R. A., Buckner, C. D., Sullivan, K. M., Doney, K., Appelbaum, F. R., Anasetti, C., Witherspoon, R., Sanders, J., Stewart, P., Martin, P. J., Ciancarelli, M., Hansen, J. A. and Thomas, E. D (1987) Treatment of aplastic anaemia with marrow grafts from related donors other than HLA genotypically-matched sibling. *Clinical Transplantation*, **1**, 117–24.

Bjerke, J. W., Lorenz, J., Martin, P. J., Storb, R., Hansen, J. A. and Anasetti, C. (1995) Treatment of graft failure with anti-CD3 antibody, glucocorticoids and infusion of donor haematopoietic cells [Abstract]. *Blood*, **86**, 107a, #415.

Bortin, M. M. and Rimm, A. A. (1981) Treatment of 144 patients with severe aplastic anaemia using immunosuppression and allogeneic marrow transplantation. A report from the International Bone Marrow Registry. *Transplantation Proceedings*, **13**, 227–33.

Bunin, N., Leahey, A., Kamani, N. and August, C. (1996) Bone marrow transplantation in paediatric patients with severe aplastic anaemia: cyclophosphamide and anti-thymocyte globulin conditioning followed by recombinant human granulocyte-macrophage colony stimulating factor. *Journal of Pediatric Hematology/Oncology*, **18**, 68–71.

Camitta, B. M., Thomas, E. D., Nathan, D. G., Gale, R. P., Kopecky, K. J., Rappeport, J. M., Santos, G., Gordon–Smith, E. C. and Storb, R. (1979) A prospective study of androgens and bone marrow transplantation for treatment of severe aplastic anaemia. *Blood*, **53**, 504–14.

Camitta, B., O'Reilly, R. J., Sensenbrenner, L., Rappeport, J., Champlin, R., Doney, K., August, C., Hoffmann, R. G., Kirkpatrick, D., Stuart, R., Santos, G., Parkman, Gale, R. P., Storb, R. and Nathan, D. (1983) Anti-thoracic duct lymphocyte globulin therapy of severe aplastic anaemia. *Blood*, **62**, 883–8.

Castro–Malaspina, H., Childs, B., Laver, J., Shank, B., Brochstein, J., Gillio, A., Flomenberg, N., Young, J., Boulad, F., Black, P., Kernan, N., Fuks, Z. and O'Reilly, R. (1994) Hyperfractioned total lymphoid irradiation and cyclophosphamide for preparation of previously transfused patients undergoing HLA-identical marrow transplantation for severe aplastic anaemia. *International Journal of Radiation Oncology, Biology, Physics*, **29**, 847–54.

Champlin, R. E., Horowitz, M. M., van Bekkum, D. W., Camitta, B. M., Elfenbein, G. E., Gale, R. P., Gluckman. E., Good. R. A., Rimm, A. A., Rozman, C., Speck. B. and Bortin, M. M. (1989) Graft failure following bone marrow transplantation for severe aplastic anemia : risk factors and treatment results. *Blood*, **73**, 606–13.

Champlin, R. E., Ho, W. G., Nimer, S. D., Gajewski, J. G., Selch, M., Burnison, M., Holley, G., Yam, P., Petz, L., Winston, D. J. and Feig, S. A. (1990) Bone marrow transplantation for severe aplastic anaemia. Effect of a preparative regimen of cyclophosphamide-low-dose total-lymphoid irradiation and posttransplant cyclosporine-methotrexate therapy. *Transplantation*, **49**, 720–4.

Chao, N. J., Schmidt, G. M., Niland, J. C., Amylon, M. D., Dagis, A. C., Long, G. D., Nademanee, A. P., Negrin, R. S., O'Donnell, M. R., Parker, P. M., Smith, E. P., Snyder, D. S., Stein, A. S., Wong, R. M., Blume, K. G. and Forman, S. J. (1993) Cyclosporine, methotrexate, and prednisone compared with cyclosporine and prednisone for prophylaxis of acute graft-versus-host disease. *New England Journal of Medicine*, **329**, 1225–30.

Crawford, S. W. and Hackman, R. C. (1993) Clinical course of idiopathic pneumonia after bone marrow transplantation. *American Review of Respiratory Disease*, **147**, 1393–400.

Cuthbert, R. J., Shepherd, J. D., Nantel, S. H., Barnett, M. J., Reece, D. E., Klingemann, H. G., Chan, K. W., Spineli, J. J., Sutherland, H. J. and Phillips, G. L. (1995) Allogeneic bone marrow transplantation for severe aplastic anaemia: the Vancouver experience. *Clinical and Investigative Medicine*, **18**, 122–30.

Deeg, H. J. and Socié, G. (1998) Malignancies after hemopoietic stem cell transplantation: many questions, some answers. *Blood*, **91**, 1833–44.

Deeg, H. J., Storb, R., Weiden, P. L., Raff, R. F., Sale, G. E., Atkinson, K., Graham, T. C. and Thomas, E. D. (1982) Cyclosporin A and methotrexate in canine marrow transplantation: engraftment, graft-versus-host-disease, and induction of tolerance. *Transplantation*, **34**, 30–5.

Deeg, H. J., Storb, R., Appelbaum, F. R., Kennedy, M. S., Graham, T. C. and Thomas, E. D. (1984) Combined immunosuppression with cyclosporin and methotrexate in dogs given bone marrow grafts from DLA-haploidentical littermates. *Transplantation*, **37**, 62–5.

Deeg, H. J., Self, S., Storb, R., Doney, K., Appelbaum, F. R., Witherspoon, R. P., Sullivan, K. M., Sheehan, K., Sanders, J., Mickelson, E. and Thomas, E. D. (1986) Decreased incidence of marrow graft rejection in patients with severe aplastic anaemia. Changing impact of risk factors. *Blood*, **68**, 1363–8.

Deeg, H. J., Sale, G. E., Storb, R., Graham, T. C., Schuening, F., Appelbaum, F. R. and Thomas, E. D. (1987) Engraftment of DLA-nonidentical bone marrow facilitated by recipient treatment with anti-class II monoclonal antibody and methotrexate. *Transplantation*, **44**, 340–5.

Deeg, H. J., Leisenring, W., Nims, J., Flowers, M., Witherspoon, R. P., Storb, R. and Sullivan, K. M. (1996*a*) Long-term outcome and quality of life after marrow transplantation for severe aplastic anaemia [Abstract]. *Blood*, **88**, 643a, #2560.

Deeg, H. J., Socié G., Schoch, G., Henry–Amar, M., Witherspoon, R. P., Devergie, A., Sullivan, K. M., Gluckman, E. and Storb, R. (1996*b*) Malignancies after marrow transplantation for aplastic anaemia and Fanconi anaemia: a joint Seattle and Paris analysis of results in 700 patients. *Blood*, **87**, 386–92.

Doney, K., Leisenring, W., Storb, R., Appelbaum, F. R. and for the Seattle Bone Marrow Transplant Team (1997) Primary treatment of acquired aplastic anaemia: outcomes with bone marrow transplantation and immunosuppressive therapy. *Annals of Internal Medicine*, **126**, 107–15.

Feig, S. A., Champlin, R., Arenson, E., Yale, C., Ho, W., Tesler, A. and Gale, R. P. (1983) Improved survival following bone marrow transplantation for aplastic anaemia. *British Journal of Haematology*, **54**, 509–17.

Fonseca, R. and Tefferi, A. (1997) Practical aspects in the diagnosis and management of aplastic anemia. *American Journal of the Medical Sciences*, **313**, 159–69.

Gluckman, E., Socié, G., Devergie, A., Bourdeau–Esperou, H., Traineau, R. and Cosset, J. M. (1991) Bone marrow transplantation in 107 patients with severe aplastic anaemia using cyclophosphamide and thoraco-abdominal irradiation for conditioning: long-term follow-up. *Blood*, **78**, 2451–5.

Gluckman, E., Horowitz, M. M., Champlin, R. E., Hows, J. M., Bacigalupo, A., Biggs, J. C., Camitta, B. M., Gale, R. P., Gordon–Smith, E. C., Marmont, A. M., Masaoka, T., Ramsay, N. K. C., Rimm, A. A., Rozman, C., Sobocinsk, K. A., Speck, B. and Bortin, M. M. (1992) Bone marrow transplantation for severe aplastic anaemia: influence of conditioning and graft-versus-host disease prophylaxis regimens on outcome. *Blood*, **79**, 269–27.

Gordon–Smith, E. C., Howes, J., Bacigalupo, A., Gluckman, E., Van Lint, M. T., Congiu, A., James, D. C. O., Barrett, A. J., De Planque, M. M., Siimes, M. A., Toivanen, A., Ringden, O. and Marmont, A. M. (1987) Bone marrow transplantation for severe aplastic anaemia (SAA) from donors other than HLA identical siblings: a report of the EBMT working party. *Bone Marrow Transplantation*, **2**, 100.

Hamblin, M., Marsh, J. C. W., Lawler, M., McCann, S. R., Wickham, N., Dunlop, L., Ball, S., Davies, E. G., Hale, G., Waldmann, H., and Gordon–Smith, E. C. (1996) Campath-1G *in vivo* confers a low incidence of graft versus host disease associated with a high incidence of mixed chimaerism after bone marrow transplantation for severe aplastic anaemia using HLA–identical sibling donors. *Bone Marrow Transplantation*, **17**, 819–24.

Hathaway, W. E., Fulginiti, V. A., Pierce, C. W., Githens, J. H., Pearlman, D. S., Muschenheim, F. and Hammer, R. E. (1967) Graft-vs-host reaction following a single blood transfusion. *Journal of the American Medical Association*, **201**, 1015–20.

Hill, R. S., Petersen, F. B., Storb, R., Appelbaum, F. R., Doney, K., Dahlberg, S., Rambery, R. and Thomas, E. D. (1986) Mixed hematologic chimerism after allogeneic marrow transplant for severe aplastic anemia is associated with a higher risk of graft rejection and a lessened incidence of acute graft-versus-host disease. *Blood*, **67**, 811–16.

Hinterberger, W., Rowlings, P. A., Hinterberger–Fischer, M., Gibson, J., Jacobsen, N., Klein, J. P., Kolb, H. J., Stevens, D. A. Horowitz, M. M. and Gale, R. P. (1997) Results of transplanting bone marrow from genetically identical twins into patients with aplastic anaemia. *Annals of Internal Medicine*, **26**, 116–22.

Hinterberger–Fischer, M., Kier, P., Kalhs, M. P., Marosi, C., Geissler, K., Schwarzinger, I., Pabinger, I., Huber, J., Kolbabek, H., Koren, H., Müller, G., Hawliczek, R., Lechner, K., Hayek–Rosenmayr, A. and Hinterberger, W. (1991) Fertility, pregnancies and offspring complications after bone marrow transplantation. *Bone Marrow Transplantation*, **7**, 5–9.

Horstmann, M., Stockschlader, M., Kruger, W., Hoffknecht, M., Betker, R., Kabisch, H. and Zander, A. (1995) Cyclophosphamide/antithymocyte globulin conditioning with severe asplastic anaemia for marrow transplantation from HLA-identical siblings: preliminary results. *Annals of Hematology*, **71**, 77–81.

Hows, J., Palmer, S. and Gordon–Smith, E. C. (1985) Cyclosporine and graft failure following bone marrow transplantation for severe aplastic anemia. *British Journal of Haematology*, **60**, 611–17.

Hows, J. M., Marsh, J. C., Yin, J. L., Durrant, S., Swirsky, D., Worsley, A., Fairhead, S. M., Chipping, P. M., Palmer, S. and Gordon–Smith, E. C. (1989) Bone marrow transplantation for severe aplastic anaemia using cyclosporin: long-term follow-up. *Bone Marrow Transplantation*, **4**, 11–16.

Huss, R., Deeg, H. J., Gooley, T., Bryant, E., Leisenring, W., Clift, R., Buckner, C. D., Martin, P., Storb, R. and Appelbaum, F. R. (1996) Effect of mixed chimerism on graft-versus-host disease, disease recurrence, and survival after HLA-identical marrow transplantation for aplastic anemia or chronic myelogenous leukaemia. *Bone Marrow Transplantation*, **18**, 767–76.

International Agranulocytosis and Aplastic Anaemia Study. (1987) Incidence of aplastic anaemia: the relevance of diagnostic criteria. *Blood*, **70**, 1718–21.

Jacobs, P. and Dubovsky, D. W. (1981) Bone marrow transplantation followed by normal pregnancy. *American Journal of Hematology*, **11**, 209–12.

Jandl, J. H. (1996) Aplastic anemia. In *Blood textbook for hematology*, 2nd edn, ed. J. H. Jandl, pp. 201–50. Boston: Little, Brown and Company.

Kalhs, P., White, J. S., Gervassi, A., Storb, R. and Bean, M. A. (1995) In vitro recall of proliferative and cytolytic responses to minor histocompatibility antigens by dendritic cell enriched canine peripheral blood mononuclear cells. *Transplantation*, **59**, 112–18.

Kantrow, S. P., Hackman, R. C., Boeckh, M., Myerson, D. and Crawford, S. W. (1997) Idiopathic pneumonia syndrome: changing spectrum of lung injury after marrow transplantation. *Transplantation*, **63**, 1079–86.

Lawler, M., Humphries, P. and McCann, S. R. (1991) Evaluation of mixed chimerism by in vitro amplification of dinucleotide repeat sequences using the polymerase chain reaction. *Blood*, **77**, 2504–14.

Lawler, M., McCann, S. R., Gardiner, N., Marsh, J. C. W., Ljungman, P., Locasciulli, A., Socié, G., Marin, P., Gluckman, E., Frickhofen, H., Schrezenmeier, H., Hows, J., Raghavachar, A. and Bacigalupo, A. (1995) Mixed chimaerism predicts graft rejection following BMT for severe aplastic anaemia [Abstract]. *Bone Marrow Transplantation Supplement*, **15**, S64.

Loscasciulli, A., van,t Veer, L., Bacigalupo, A., Hows, J., Van Lint, M. T., Gluckman, E., Nissen, C., McCann, S., Vossen, J., Schrezenmeier, A., Hinterberger, W. and Marin, A. (1990) Treatment with marrow transplantation or immunosuppression of childhood acquired severe aplastic anemia: a report from the EBMT SAA Working Party. *Bone Marrow Transplantation*, **6**, 211–17.

Locasciulli, A., van,t Veer, L., Hows, J., Van Lint, M. T., Gluckman, E., Nissen, C., McCann, S., Vossen, J., Schrezenmeier, A., Hinterberger, W., Marin, P. and Bacigalupo, A. (1991) Bone marrow transplantation (BMT) in children with severe aplastic anaemia (SAA) from donors other than HLA–identical siblings, EBMT Working Party on Severe Aplastic Anemia. *Bone Marrow Transplantation*, **7** [Suppl. 3], 90–1.

Makipernaa, A., Saarinen, U. M. and Siimes, M. A. (1995) Allogeneic bone marrow transplantation in children: single institution experience from 1974 to 1992. *Acta Paediatrica*, **84**, 683–8.

May, W. S., Sensenbrenner, L. L., Burns, W. H., Ambinder, R., Carroll, M. P., Griffin, C. A., Jones, R. J., Miller, C. B., Mellits, E. D., Vogelsang, G. B., Wagner, J. E., Wingard, J. R., Yeager, A. and Santos, G. W. (1993) BMT for severe aplastic anemia using cyclosporine. *Bone Marrow Transplantation*, **11**, 459–64.

McCann, S. R., Bacigalupo, A., Gluckman, E., Hinterberger, W., Hows, J., Ljungman, P., Marin, P., Nissen, C., van,t Veer, K. E., Raghavachar, A., Socié, G., Frickhofen, N., Locasciulli, A. and Schrezenmeier, H. (1994) Graft rejection and second bone marrow transplants for acquired aplastic anaemia: a report from the Aplastic Anaemia Working Party of the European Bone Marrow Transplant Group. *Bone Marrow Transplantation*, **13**, 233–7.

McGlave, P. B., Haake, R., Miller, W., Kim, T., Kersey, J. and Ramsay, N. K. C. (1987). Therapy of severe aplastic anemia in young adults and children with allogeneic bone marrow transplantation. *Blood*, **70**, 1325–30.

Nash, R. A., Pepe, M. S., Storb, R., Longton, G., Pettinger, M., Anasetti, C., Appelbaum, F. R., Bowden, R., Deeg, H. J., Doney, K., Martin, P. J., Sullivan, K. M., Sanders, J. and Witherspoon, R. P. (1992) Acute graft-versus-host disease: analysis of risk factors after allogeneic marrow transplantation and prophylaxis with cyclosporin and methotrexate. *Blood*, **80**, 1838–45.

Niederwieser, D., Pepe, M., Storb, R., Loughran, T. P. Jr., Longton, G. and for the Seattle Marrow Transplant Team. (1988) Improvement in rejection, engraftment rate and survival without increase in graft-versus-host disease by high marrow cell dose in patients transplanted for aplastic anemia. *British Journal of Haematology*, **69**, 23–8.

Paquette, R. L., Tebyani, N., Frane, M., Ireland, P., Ho, W. G., Champlin, R. E. and Nimer, S. D. (1995) Long-term outcome of aplastic anemia in adults treated with antithymocyte globulin: comparison with bone marrow transplantation. *Blood*, **85**, 283–90.

Parkman, R., Mosier, D., Umansky, I., Cochran, W., Carpenter, C. B. and Rosen, F. S. (1974) Graft-versus-host disease after intrauterine and exchange transfusions for hemolytic disease of the newborn. *New England Journal of Medicine*, **290**, 359–63.

Passweg, J. R., Socié, G., Hinterberger, W., Bacigalupo, A., Biggs, J. C., Camitta, B. M., Champlin, R. E., Gale, R. P., Gluckman, E., Gordon–Smith, E. C., Hows, J. M., Klein, J. P., Nugent, M. L., Pasquini, R., Rowlings, P. A., Speck, B., Tichelli, A., Zhang, M. J., Horowitz, M. M. and Bortin, M. M. (1997) Bone marrow transplantation for severe aplastic anaemia: has outcome improved? *Blood*, **90**, 858–64.

Ramsay, N. K., Kim, T. H., McGlave, P., Goldman, A., Nesbit, M. E. Jr., Krivit, W., Woods, W. G. and Kersey, J. H. (1983) Total lymphoid irradiation and cyclophosphamide conditioning prior to bone marrow transplantation for patients with severe aplastic anemia. *Blood*, **62**, 622–6.

Redei, I., Waller, E. K., Holland, H. K., Devine, S. M. and Wingard, J. R. (1997) Successful engraftment after primary graft failure in aplastic anemia using G-CSF mobilized peripheral stem cell transfusions. *Bone Marrow Transplantation*, **19**, 175–77.

Ringden, O., Backman, L., Lonnqvist, B., Heimdahl, A., Lindholm, A., Bolme, P. and Gahrton, G. (1986) A randomized trial comparing use of cyclosporin and methotrexate for graft-versus-host disease prophylaxis in bone marrow transplant recipients with hematologic malignancy. *Bone Marrow Transplantation*, **1**, 41–51.

Sanders, J. E. and the Seattle Marrow Transplant Team. (1991) The impact of marrow transplant preparative regimens on subsequent growth and development. *Seminars in Hematology*, **28**, 244–9.

Sanders J. E., Whitehead, J., Storb, R., Buckner, C. D., Clift, R. A., Mickelson, E., Appelbaum, F. R., Bensinger, W. I., Stewart, P. S. and Doney, K. (1986) Bone marrow transplant experience for children with aplastic anemia. *Pediatrics*, **77**, 179–86.

Sanders, J. E., Buckner, C. D., Amos, D., Levy, E., Appelbaum, F. R., Doney, K., Storb, R., Sullivan, K. M., Witherspoon, R. P. and Thomas, E. D. (1988) Ovarian function following marrow transplantation for aplastic anemia or leukaemia. *Journal of Clinical Oncology*, **6**, 813–18.

Sanders, J. E., Storb, R., Anasetti, C., Deeg, H. J., Doney, K., Sullivan, K. M., Witherspoon, R. P. and Hansen, J. (1994) Marrow transplant experience for children with severe aplastic anemia. *American Journal of Pediatric Hematology Oncology*, **16**, 43–9.

Sanders, J. E., Hawley, J., Levy, W., Gooley, T., Buckner, C. D., Deeg, H. J., Doney, K., Storb, R., Sullivan, K., Witherspoon, R. and Appelbaum, F. R. (1996) Pregnancies following high-dose cyclophosphamide with or without high-dose busulphan or total-body irradiation and bone marrow transplantation. *Blood*, **87**, 3045–52.

Schmidt, H., Ehninger, G., Dopfer, R. and Waller, H. D. (1987) Pregnancy after bone marrow transplantation for severe aplastic anaemia. *Bone Marrow Transplantation*, **2**, 329–32.

Schuening, F., Bean, M. A., Deeg, H. J. and Storb, R. (1993) Prevention of graft failure in patients with aplastic anemia. *Bone Marrow Transplantation*, **12**, S48–S49.

Smith, B. R., Guinan, E. C., Parkman R., Ferrara J., Levey, R. H., Nathan, D. G. and Rappaport. J. M. (1985) Efficacy of a cyclophosphamide-procarbazine-antithymocyte serum regimen for prevention of graft rejection following bone marrow transplantation for transfused patients with aplastic anemia. *Transplantation*, **39**, 671–3.

Storb, R. and Deeg, H. J. (1986) Failure of allogeneic canine marrow grafts after total body irradiation: allogeneic 'resistance' vs transfusion induced sensitization. *Transplantation*, **42**, 571–80.

Storb, R., Floersheim, G. L., Weiden, P. L., Graham, T. C., Kolb, H. J., Lerner, K. G., Schroeder, M. L. and Thomas, E. D. (1974*a*) Effect of prior blood transfusions on marrow grafts: abrogation of sensitization by procarbazine and antithymocyte serum. *Journal of Immunology*, **112**, 1508–16.

Storb, R., Thomas, E. D., Buckner, C. D., Clift, R. A., Johnson, F. L., Fefer, A., Glucksberg, H., Giblett, E. R., Lerner, K. G. and Neiman, P. (1974*b*) Allogeneic marrow grafting for treatment of aplastic anemia. *Blood*, **43**, 157–80.

Storb, R., Prentice, R. L. and Thomas, E. D. (1977) Marrow transplantation for treatment of aplastic anemia. An analysis of factors associated with graft rejection. *New England Journal of Medicine*, **296**, 61–6.

Storb, R., Thomas, E. D., Buckner, C. D., Clift, R. A., Deeg, H. J., Feffer, A., Goodell, B. W., Sale, G. E., Sanders, J. E., Singer, J., Stewart, P. and Weiden, P. L. (1980) Marrow transplantation in thirty 'untransfused' patients with severe aplastic anemia. *Annals of Internal Medicine*, **92**, 30–6.

Storb, R., Doney, K. C., Thomas, E. D., Appelbaum, F., Buckner, C. D., Clift, R. A., Deeg, H. J., Goodell, B. W., Hackman, R., Hansen, J. A., Sanders, J., Sullivan, Weiden, P. L. and Witherspoon, R. P. (1982) Marrow transplantation with or without donor buffy coat cells for 65 transfused aplastic anemia patients. *Blood*, **59**, 236–46.

Storb, R., Prentice, R. L., Buckner, C. D., Clift, R. A., Appelbaum, F., Deeg, J., Doney, K., Hansen, J. A., Mason, M., Sanders, J. E., Singer, J., Sullivan, K. M., Witherspoon, R. P. and Thomas, E. D. (1983*a*) Graft-versus-host disease and survival in patients with aplastic anemia treated by marrow grafts from HLA-identical siblings. Beneficial effect of a protective environment. *New England Journal of Medicine*, **308**, 302–7.

Storb, R., Prentice, R. L., Sullivan, K. M., Shulman, H. M., Deeg, H. J., Doney, K C., Buckner, C. D., Clift, R. A., Witherspoon, R. P., Appelbaum, F. R., Sanders, J. E., Stewart, P. S. and Thomas, E. D. (1983*b*) Predictive factors in chronic graft-versus-host disease in patients with aplastic anemia treated by marrow transplantation from HLA-identical siblings. *Annals of Internal Medicine*, **98**, 461–6.

Storb, R., Deeg, H. J., Farewell, V., Doney, K., Appelbaum, F., Beatty, P., Bensinger, W., Buckner, C. D., Clift, R., Hansen, J., Hill, R., Longton, G., Lum, L., Martin, P., McGuffin, R., Sanders, J., Singer, J., Stewart, P., Sullivan, K., Witherspoon, R. and Thomas E. D. (1986) Marrow transplantation for severe aplastic anemia: methotrexate alone compared with a combination of methotrexate and cyclosporine for prevention of acute graft-versus-host disease. *Blood*, **68**, 119–25.

Storb, R., Deeg, H. J., Fisher, L. D., Appelbaum, F., Buckner, C. D., Bensinger, W., Clift, R., Doney, K., Irle, C., McGuffin, R., Martin, P., Sanders, J., Schoch, G., Singer, J., Stewart, P., Sullivan, K., Witherspoon, R. and Thomas, E. D. (1988) Cyclosporine vs methotrexate for graft-versus-host disease prevention in patients given marrow grafts for leukaemia: long-term follow-up of three controlled trials. *Blood*, **71**, 293–8.

Storb, R., Pepe, M., Anasetti, C., Appelbaum, F. R., Beatty, P., Doney, K., Martin, P., Stewart, P., Sullivan, K. M., Witherspoon, R., Bensinger, W., Buckner, C. D., Clift, R., Hansen, J., Longton, G., Loughran, T., Petersen, F. B., Slinger, J., Sanders, J. and Thomas E. D. (1990) What role for prednisone in prevention of acute graft-versus-host disease in patients undergoing marrow transplants? *Blood*, **76**, 1037–45.

Storb, R., Sanders, J. E., Pepe, M., Anasetti, C., Appelbaum, F. R., Buckner, C. D., Deeg, H. J., Doney, K., Hansen, J., Martin, P., Stewart, P., Sullivan, K. M., Thomas, E. D. and Witherspoon, R. P. (1991) Graft-versus-host disease prophylaxis with methotrexate/cyclosporin in children with severe aplastic anemia treated with cyclophosphamide and HLA-identical marrow grafts (Letter). *Blood*, **78**, 1144–5.

Storb, R., Longton, G., Anasetti, C., Appelbaum, F. R., Beatty, P., Bensinger, W., Crawford, S., Deeg, H. J., Doney, K., Fefer, A., Hansen, J., Loughran, T., Martin, P., Pepe, M., Petersen, F. B., Sanders, J. E., Singer, J., Stewart, P., Sullivan, K. M., Thomas, E. D. and Witherspoon, R. P. (1992) Changing trends in marrow transplantation for aplastic anemia [Review]. *Bone Marrow Transplantation*, **10**, 45–52.

Storb, R., Etzioni, R., Anasetti, C., Appelbaum, F. R., Buckner, C. D., Bensinger, E., Bryant, E., Clift, R., Deeg, H. J., Doney, K., Flowers, M., Hansen, J., Martin, P., Pepe, M., Sale, G., Sanders, J., Singer, J., Sullivan, K. M., Thomas, E. D. and Witherspoon, R. P. (1994) Cyclophosphamide combined with antithymocyte globulin in preparation for allogeneic marrow transplants in patients with aplastic anemia. *Blood*, **84**, 941–9.

Storb, R., Leisenring, W., Anasetti, C., Appelbaum, F. R., Buckner, C. D., Bensinger, W. I., Chauncey, T., Clift, R. A., Deeg, H. J., Doney, K. C., Flowers, M E. D., Hansen, J. A., Martin, P. J., Sanders, J. E., Sullivan, K. M. and Witherspoon, R. P. (1997*a*) Long-term follow up of allogeneic marrow transplants in patients with aplastic anemia conditioned by cyclophosphamide combined with antithymocyte globulin [Letter to Editor]. *Blood*, **89**, 3890–1.

Storb, R., Yu, C., Wagner, J. L., Deeg, H. J., Nash, R. A., Kiem, H.–P., Leisenring, W. and Shulman, H. (1997*b*) Stable mixed hemopoietic chimerism in DLA-identical littermate dogs given sublethal total body irradiation before and pharmacological immunosuppression after marrow transplantation. *Blood*, **89**, 3048–54.

Stucki, A., Leisenring, W., Sandmaier, B. M., Sanders, J., Anasetti C. and Storb, R. (1997) Increasing survival for severe aplastic anemia patients who undergo a second marrow transplant after rejection of the first graft [Abstract]. *Blood*, **90**, 550a, #2450.

Sullivan, K. M., Agura, E., Anasetti, C., Appelbaum, F. R., Badger, C., Bearman, S., Erickson, K., Flowers, M., Hansen, J. A., Loughran, T., Martin, P., Matthews, D., Petersdorf, E., Radich, J., Riddell, S., Rovira, D., Sanders, J., Schuening, F., Siadak, M., Storb, R. and Witherspoon, R. P. (1991) Chronic graft-versus-host disease and other late complications of bone marrow transplantation. *Seminars in Hematology*, **28**, 250–9.

Thomas, E. D. and Storb, R. (1984) Acquired severe aplastic anemia: progress and perplexity. *Blood*, **64**, 325–8.

Thomas, E. D., Kasakura, S., Cavins, J. A. and Ferrebee, J. W. (1963) Marrow transplants in lethally irradiated dogs: the effect of methotrexate on survival of the host and the homograft. *Transplantation*, **1**, 571–4.

Wagner, J. L., Deeg, H. J., Seidel, K., Anasetti, C., Doney, K., Sanders, J., Sullivan, K. M. and Storb, R. (1996) Bone marrow transplantation for severe aplastic anemia from genotypically HLA-nonidentical relatives: an update of the Seattle experience. *Transplantation*, **61**, 54–61.

Weiden, P. L., Storb, R., Slichter, S., Warren, R. P. and Sale, G. E. (1976) Effect of six weekly transfusions on canine marrow grafts: tests for sensitization and abrogation of sensitization by procarbazine and antithymocyte serum. *Journal of Immunology*, **117**, 143–50.

Weiner, R. S., Horowitz, M. M., Gale, R. P., Dicke, K. A., van Bekkum, D. W., Masaoka, T., Ramsay, N. K. C., Rimm, A. A., Rozman, C. and Bortin, M. M. (1989) Risk factors for interstitial pneumonia following bone marrow transplantation for severe aplastic anemia. *British Journal of Haematology*, **71**, 535–43.

Witherspoon, R. P., Storb, R., Shulman, H., Buckner, C. D., Deeg, H. J., Clift, R. A., Sanders, J. E., Doney, K., McDonald, G., Sullivan, K. M., Appelbaum, F. R. and Thomas, E. D. (1984) Marrow transplantation in hepatitis-associated aplastic anemia. *American Journal of Hematology*, **17**, 269–78.

Yardley–Jones, A., Anderson, D. and Parke, D. V. (1991) The toxicity of benzene and its metabolism and molecular pathology in human risk assessment [Review]. *British Journal of Industrial Medicine*, **48**, 437–44.

Yoshida, Y., Ishinoe, T., Dodo, M., Noukawa, M., Maeda, A., Oguma, S., Yajima, M., Yamamoto, K. and Okuma, M. (1994) Successful bone marrow transplantation with rabbit anti-human thymocyte globulin in aplastic anemia. Report of a case previously treated with equine anti-human lymphocyte globulin. *International Journal of Hematology*, **60**, 79–83.

13

Alternative donor bone marrow transplantation for severe acquired aplastic anemia

Jill Hows

Southmead Health Services, Bristol

Judith Veum Stone

Medical College of Wisconsin, Milwaukee

and

Bruce M. Camitta

Midwest Children's Cancer Center, Milwaukee

Introduction

Severe acquired aplastic anemia (SAA) is the first disease for which HLA-identical sibling bone marrow transplantation (ID-BMT) has been shown by a prospective study to be the preferred treatment (Camitta et al., 1976). In contrast the role of alternative donor BMT in the treatment of the 60–70% of patients with SAA who lack an HLA-identical sibling is not yet established. In this chapter we first briefly review factors that influence the outcome of ID-BMT. Secondly, we review published results of alternative donor BMT, highlighting major problems. Finally we present the results of an analysis of data from the International Bone Marrow Transplant Registry (IBMTR), the European Bone Marrow Transplant Group (EBMT) SAA Working Party, the Fred Hutchinson Cancer Research Center (FHCRC), and the International Marrow Unrelated Search and Transplant (IMUST) Study. From these data we make tentative recommendations for patient, donor and protocol selection for alternative donor BMT for SAA.

Prognostic factors for HLA-identical sibling BMT

ID-BMT results in a 90% probability of the long-term survival of minimally transfused patients (Storb et al., 1980). The probability of graft failure after ID-BMT increases with the number of pretransplant transfusions (Champlin et al., 1989). Data from the Seattle group suggest that a low dose of nucleated marrow cells and being male increase the risk of graft failure after ID-BMT (Storb et al., 1983*a*).

However, the IBMTR, in a retrospective analysis, could not confirm the effect of marrow cell dose (Champlin et al., 1989).

Most patients are multiply transfused before referral for ID-BMT. In the past decade both single-center and registry studies from Europe and North America have reported that more intensive transplant protocols allow satisfactory engraftment in transfused ID-BMT recipients. A small single-center study (Storb et al., 1994) showed that adding antithymocyte globulin (ATG) to pretransplant conditioning protocols gives a 92% probability of 3-year survival. The IBMTR is evaluating this observation in a prospective randomized study. The use of limited field irradiation (600cGy thoracoabdominal irradiation; Gluckman et al., 1991) or total body irradiation (750 cGy, McGlave et al., 1987) also enhances engraftment, but long-term survival is compromised by regimen-related toxicity (Gluckman et al., 1991).

Grade II–IV acute graft-versus-host disease (AGVHD) remains an important cause of morbidity and mortality after ID-BMT (Gluckman et al., 1992). Risk factors for AGVHD include increasing patient age (Storb et al., 1983b) and parous female donors (Flowers et al., 1990). The use of cyclosporin with or without methotrexate (MTX) for posttransplant immunosuppression leads to a small decrease in AGVHD and is associated with improved 5-year survival (Passweg et al., 1997). In summary, the results of ID-BMT for SAA have improved over recent years as a result of new BMT protocols and changes in supportive care, including improved antibiotic regimens and widespread use of leukocyte-poor blood products. As described below these developments have not had the same beneficial impact on BMT for SAA from allogeneic donors other than HLA-identical siblings.

Partially matched family donor BMT: early experience

Only 20–30% of patients with SAA in North America and Europe have an HLA-genotypically identical sibling. The probability of finding HLA-phenotypically matched family donors is only 1%. However, in the small number of such transplants reported for SAA, results are similar to those of ID-BMT (Bacigalupo et al., 1988a; Wagner et al., 1996). This suggests that when a patient's parents are first cousins or when the patient has at least one common HLA haplotype, an extended family donor search for a phenotypically matched family donor is worthwhile. A computer simulation program has been developed to predict the probability of a phenotypically matched donor in a patient's family (Schipper et al., 1996).

The probability of finding a one-antigen HLA-mismatched family donor in Europe and North America is 5–7% (Beatty et al., 1988). In early studies one-antigen-mismatched family donor BMT for SAA was performed late as salvage treatment, after the failure of immunosuppressive therapy. Most recipients were highly sensitized to HLA and non-HLA histocompatibility antigens through multiple blood transfusions and had a poor pretransplant performance status.

Not surprisingly, the results of BMT for these patients was poor. Death was caused by high rates of graft failure, severe AGVHD, and infection (Bacigalupo et al., 1988*a*; Hows et al., 1986; Wagner et al., 1996).

HLA-matched unrelated donor BMT: early experience

To extend the available donor pool, more than five million unrelated volunteer marrow donors have been recruited worldwide (BMDWW annual report 1997; http://bmdw.leidenuniv.nl./annrep/index.html). Despite the large number of potential donors, extensive HLA polymorphism makes finding a well-matched unrelated donor difficult. Linkage disequilibrium between HLA alleles leads to common and rare HLA phenotypes. The distribution of HLA phenotypes varies greatly between different ethnic groups. Therefore, the success of an unrelated donor search is highly dependent on the patient's HLA phenotype, and whether the patient has the same ethnic background as most registry donors. Since most registry donors are Caucasian, patients from this ethnic group have the best chance of finding a well-matched unrelated donor. The estimated probability of finding an unrelated donor for a Caucasian patient is 70%, but for other ethnic groups the probability is significantly lower (Hows et al., 1996). Logistic delays are inherent in finding suitable unrelated donors, so it is recommended that a preliminary unrelated donor search be carried out for patients who may become candidates for unrelated donor BMT at the time that immunosuppressive treatment starts.

The National Marrow Donor Program (NMDP) reported 31 unrelated donor BMT for SAA in patients of all ages. The 2-year survival was only 29% and several of the survivors still depended on transfusions (Kernan et al., 1993). Higher rates of engraftment and survival were reported by the Milwaukee group, who studied young patients treated with intensive conditioning (cyclophosphamide, cytosine arabinoside, total body irradiation and antithymocyte globulin), partial (1.5–2.0 log) T-cell depletion with monoclonal antibody $T_{10}B_9$, and cyclosporin (Margolis et al., 1996). In this study 30 patients were transplanted, 13 from donors matched for HLA-A, -B, and -DRB1, and 17 for whom one or more HLA antigens were mismatched. Transplantation was performed late, at a median of 14 months (range 4–72) after diagnosis. All but two patients were multiply transfused. The probability of survival at 2 years was 58% after HLA-phenotypically matched BMT and 50% after HLA-mismatched BMT.

Analysis of factors affecting outcome of alternative donor BMT

To date, the results of alternative donor BMT for adults with SAA are generally unsatisfactory. The improved results in younger patients reported from

Milwaukee require confirmation by other investigators. The factors influencing the outcome of alternative donor BMT for SAA are unclear and require urgent investigation so that appropriate patient and donor selection and transplant protocols can be recommended. To this end a large database has been assembled and analyzed with the collaboration of the IBMTR, the EBMT SAA working party, the FHCRC and the International Marrow Unrelated Search and Transplant (IMUST) Study Group. This retrospective analysis is presented below.

Patients and methods

Patient population

Altogether, 1469 patients with SAA who were transplanted between 1986 and 1995 from HLA-identical siblings, partially HLA-matched family donors or closely HLA-matched unrelated volunteers were available for analysis. Thirty-five patients were transplanted from unrelated donors at the FHCRC. The remaining 1434 patients were reported to the IBMTR, EBMT, or IMUST Study Group. A careful check was made for dual reporting and where overlap was detected the most complete dataset was used. One thousand one hundred and fifty-five patients received HLA-identical sibling donor transplants (ID-BMT) (all from the IBMTR database), 119 patients received transplants from allogeneic family donors other than HLA-identical siblings (ALTFAM-BMT) (all from the IBMTR database), and 195 patients received transplants from closely HLA-matched unrelated volunteers (UD-BMT). Pretransplant patient characteristics are shown in Table 13.1. Gender, preBMT Karnofsky score, and etiology of aplasia were similar for the three groups. Median patient ages were significantly lower in the UD-BMT (18 years) and ALTFAM-BMT (14 years) groups compared with the ID-BMT patients (20 years) ($P=0.0001$). The proportion of patients with preBMT polymorphonuclear cell numbers $\leqslant 0.2 \times 10^9/l$ was significantly higher in the ALTFAM-BMT group (62%) than in the ID-BMT (46%) and UD-BMT (47%) groups ($P=0.002$). The UD-BMT group had a significantly longer delay between diagnosis and BMT (median 12, range <1–245 months) than those receiving ID-BMT (median 2, range <1–258 months) or ALTFAM-BMT (median 4, range 1–367 months) ($P=<0.0001$). As expected, a prolonged time between diagnosis and BMT is associated with a high proportion of patients multiply transfused prior to BMT. UD-BMT recipients received the most transfusions before BMT (Table 13.1): 79% of UD-BMT recipients had received prior ATG, compared with 17% of ID-BMT recipients ($P=<0.001$).

Donor population and HLA matching

Table 13.2 shows donor characteristics, and the level of HLA matching for alternative donor BMT. HLA typing for HLA-A, -B, and -DR antigens was reported at

Table 13.1. Pretransplant characteristics of patients receiving allogeneic bone marrow transplants for severe aplastic anemia

Variable	ID sibling ($n = 1155$)	ALTFAM ($n = 119$)	Unrelated donor ($n = 195$)	Data missing*
Data source*				
FHCRC	0 (0)[a]	0 (0)	35 (18)	
IBMTR	1155 (100)	91 (76)	115 (59)	
Europe: EBMT	0 (0)	28 (24)	25 (13)	
: IMUST	0 (0)	0 (0)	20 (10)	
Patient				
Age (years): median (range)	20 (<1–55)	14 (<1–46)	18 (<1–54)	0
Gender: male	703 (61)	73 (61)	114 (59)	1
Karnofsky score <90	639 (56)	44 (48)	62 (42)	103
Disease etiology				
Idiopathic	963 (84)	95 (80)	117 (84)	59
Chemical/toxin	74 (6)	4 (3)	5 (4)	
Hepatitis	79 (7)	13 (11)	8 (6)	
Other	36 (3)	7 (6)	9 (7)	
Prior treatment				
Any specific treatment	584 (51)	72 (62)	118 (86)	66
Androgens	269 (23)	21 (24)	31 (27)	88
Corticosteroids	437 (38)	47 (54)	64 (57)	90
ATG	191 (17)	37 (42)	89 (79)	88
Cyclosporin	104 (11)	18 (25)	79 (74)	270
Diagnosis–BMT interval months: median (range)	2 (<1–258)	4 (<1–367)	12 (<1–245)	14
PreBMT transfusion				
Any transfusion	1130 (99)	90 (96)	132 (100)	97
>10 donor exposures	859 (78)	70 (82)	115 (93)	157
Median exposures (range)	25 (1–833)	45 (2–641)	56 (3–716)	77
Neutrophil count				
At diagnosis $\times 10^9$/l	0.42 (0–5.9)	0.52 (0–2.1)	0.47 (0–2.4)	729
Prior to conditioning $\times 10^9$/l	0.27 (0–7.2)	0.16 (0–3.5)	0.30 (0–4.6)	229

Notes:

[a] Entries as number (%) unless otherwise specified.

[b] For transfused patients.

* Patients in multiple registries were assigned to the most complete data source.

ALTFAM = other related donor BMT (ALTFAM-BMT); ID sibling = HLA-identical sibling donor BMT (ID-BMT); unrelated = unrelated donor BMT (UD-BMT).

Table 13.2. Donor variables in allogeneic bone marrow transplantation for severe aplastic anemia

Variable	ID sibling (n = 1155)	ALTFAM (n = 119)	Unrelated donor (n = 195)	Data missing
Median donor age: years (range)	20 (1–59)	28 (1–72)	35 (20–53)	141
HLA match				
HLA ID sib	1155 (100)	32 (28)	105 (75)	59
Matched related		84 (72)	34 (25)	
Mismatched related				
Matched unrelated				
Mismatched unrelated				
Gender match				
Male into male	385 (33)	30 (26)	55 (29)	13
Male into female	250 (22)	21 (18)	38 (20)	
Female into male	318 (28)	41 (36)	53 (28)	
Female into female	201 (17)	23 (20)	41 (22)	
Sensitized donor	139 (13)	26 (31)	30 (34)	218

the serological level and alternative donor-recipient pairs are described as either 'HLA-matched' or 'HLA-mismatched' based on these data. As expected, unrelated donors were significantly older than related donors ($P = 0.0001$). Gender matching of donor-recipient pairs was similar among the three groups. In the ALTFAM-BMT group 32 (28%) were HLA-phenotypically matched and in the UD-BMT group 105 (75%) were HLA-phenotypically matched.

Transplant data

The number of BMT per calendar year, BMT conditioning protocols, and acute GVHD prophylaxis are shown in Table 13.3. Most patients receiving ID-BMT (62%) were transplanted with nonirradiation protocols. In contrast, only 41 (37%) and 36 (20%) of ALTFAM-BMT and UD-BMT recipients respectively did not receive irradiation ($P = <0.001$). Total body irradiation was most frequently used in the unrelated donor BMT group, (108 cases, 59%), compared with 32 cases (29%) in the ALTFAM-BMT and 62 (5%) in the ID-BMT group. Limited field irradiation was used in 21–32% of cases in all groups (Table 13.3). Most patients received cyclosporin, with or without other agents, as GVHD prophylaxis. Only 39 (3%) of patients in the ID-BMT group received T-cell-depleted marrow as GVHD prophylaxis, whereas 21 (19%) of the ALTFAM-BMT group and 41 (28%) of the UD-BMT group received T-cell-depleted marrow ($P = <0.001$).

Table 13.3. Transplant variables for patients receiving allogeneic bone marrow transplantation for severe aplastic anemia

Variable	ID sibling ($n=1155$)	ALTFAM ($n=119$)	Unrelated donor ($n=195$)	Data missing
Year of BMT				
1986–87	273 (24)	32 (27)	9 (5)	0
1988–89	300 (26)	37 (31)	30 (15)	
1990–91	260 (23)	16 (13)	52 (27)	
1992–93	225 (20)	20 (17)	61 (31)	
1994–95	97 (8)	14 (12)	43 (22)	
Conditioning				
No irradiation	716 (62)	41 (37)	36 (20)	25
TBI	62 (5)	32 (29)	108 (59)	
LFR	372 (32)	38 (34)	39 (21)	
GVHD prophylaxis				
MTX ± other	36 (3)	1 (1)	0 (0)	54
CyA ± other	338 (29)	22 (20)	32 (22)	
MTX + CyA ± other	721 (63)	67 (60)	74 (50)	
T-depletion ± other	39 (3)	21 (19)	41 (28)	
Other/none	20 (2)	1 (1)	2 (1)	

Notes:
CyA = cyclosporin; LFR = limited filed irradiation; MTX = methotrexate; TBI = total body irradiation.

Outcomes analyzed

The primary study endpoint was probability of survival at 3 years. Nonengraftment was defined as failure to reach a postBMT peripheral-blood neutrophil count of $0.5 \times 10^9/l$. The probability of graft failure (defined as nonengraftment or late development of recurrent aplasia) was estimated for evaluable patients. Grade II–IV AGVHD was defined in patients with engraftment by published criteria (Glucksberg et al., 1974). Chronic GVHD was defined by published criteria (Atkinson et al., 1990) and was evaluated in patients surviving beyond 100 days with engraftment. Interstitial pneumonitis was defined as previously published (Weiner et al., 1986).

Statistical methods

Patients were grouped according to donor source and descriptive tables were prepared to examine differences in characteristics of the patient, disease, and trans-

Table 13.4. Outcomes after bone marrow transplantation for severe aplastic anemia: probability (95% confidence interval)

Variable	ID sibling ($n = 1155$)	ALTFAM ($n = 119$)	Unrelated donor ($n = 195$)	P value	Data missing
ANC $>0.5 \times 10^9$/l (at 28 days)	87 (85–89)%	71 (60–80)%	80 (72–85)%	<0.0001	88
Graft failure (3 years)	14 (12–16)%	27 (17–37)%	19 (13–27)%	<0.0001	84
Grade II–IV acute GVHD (day 100)	22 (19–24)%	36 (25–47)%	56 (47–64)%	<0.0001	112
Chronic GVHD (3 years)	34 (31–37)%	42 (26–57)%	56 (40–70)%	0.0045	114
Interstitial pneumonia	11 (9–13)%	21 (12–31)%	27 (18–38)%	<0.0001	115
Survival (3 years)	69 (66–71)%	45 (36–54)%	33 (26–40)%	<0.0001	3

Notes:
ANC = absolute neutrophil count; GVHD = graft versus host disease.

plant. Medians and ranges are listed for continuous variables, as is the percentage of the total for categorical variables. Groups were compared using the chi-square and Fisher exact tests for categorical variables, and the Mann–Whitney U-test for continuous variables. Univariate analyses of transplant outcomes were done using the Kaplan–Meier estimator, with the log-rank test utilized to compare outcomes by donor group. Multivariate analyses were not performed.

Results

The analysis of the main outcomes is shown in Table 13.4. The probability of survival at 3 years for the three groups of patients is also shown in Figure 13.1.

Survival

The probability of survival at 3 years was significantly lower in both the ALTFAM-BMT group (45%; 95% confidence interval 36–54%) and the UD-BMT group (33%; 26–40%) when compared with the ID-BMT group (69%; 66–71%) ($P<0.0001$; Figure 13.1, Table 13.4). Patients transplanted from phenotypically matched ALTFAM donors also had a lower survival at 3 years (52%; 32–69%) when compared to the ID-BMT group ($P=0.046$) (Table 13.5). The time between diagnosis and transplant inversely correlated with survival after ID-BMT ($P<0.0005$). Surprisingly our analyses did not show a similar relationship in the ALTFAM-BMT and UD-BMT cohorts (Table 13.6).

Engraftment

The probability of peripheral blood recovery to 0.5×10^9/l neutrophils by day 28 was 87% (85–89%) in the ID-BMT group, 71% (60–80%) in the ALTFAM-BMT

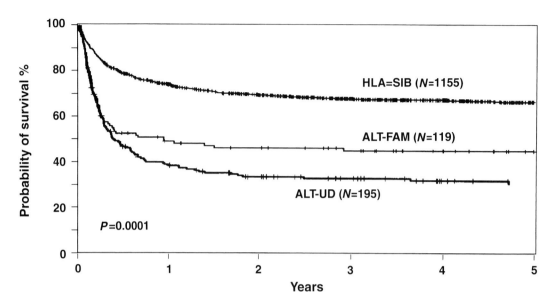

Figure 13.1. Kaplan–Meier plot of survival after bone marrow transplantation for severe aplastic anemia. 'HLA = SIB' = HLA-identical sibling donors; ALT-FAM = allogeneic family donors other than HLA-identical siblings; ALT-UD = unrelated donors.

group and 80% (72–85%) in the UD-BMT donor group ($P<0.0001$). The probability of graft failure at 3 years was 14% (12–16%) in the ID-BMT group, 27% (17–37%) in the ALTFAM-BMT group, and 19% (13–27%) in the UD-BMT group ($P<0.0001$). Univariate analysis showed no impact of HLA matching on the probability of graft failure after alternative donor BMT (Table 13.5).

The 3-year probability of graft failure after UD-BMT was higher in those patients who received conditioning protocols without irradiation (41%; 21–61%) compared to those who received limited field irradiation (10%; 3–24%) or TBI (15%; 7–24%). The use of total body irradiation appeared to reduce graft failure after ALTFAM-BMT to 15%, a level similar to that seen after ID-BMT without irradiation. Limited field irradiation did not appear to reduce graft failure in the ALTFAM-BMT group. The GVHD prophylaxis protocol had no apparent impact on the probability of graft failure after ALTFAM-BMT; however, using cyclosporin plus methotrexate was associated with a significantly lower probability of graft failure after UD-BMT.

Acute GVHD

The probability of grades II–IV AGVHD at 100 days postBMT was 22% (19–24%) for ID-BMT recipients. AGVHD was more frequent after ALTFAM-BMT (36%; 25–47%) and significantly higher after UD-BMT (56%; 47–64%) ($P<0.0001$) (Table 13.4). The probability of AGVHD was highest in all groups when cyclo-

Table 13.5. Effect of HLA matching on outcomes of alternative donor bone marrow transplants for severe aplastic anemia: probability (95 % confidence interval)

	ALTFAM		Unrelated	
	($n = 119$)	P value	($n = 195$)	P value
Probability of survival (3 years)				
0–mismatch	52 (32–69)%	0.27	34 (25–43)%	0.53
1,2–mismatch	44 (33–54)%		32 (17–48)%	
Probability of graft failure				
0–mismatch	35 (13–57)%	0.43	12 (6–20)%	0.22
1,2–mismatch	19 (10–30)%		22 (8–40)%	
Probability grade II–IV AGVHD (100 day)				
0–mismatch	21 (7–41)%	0.18	56 (44–67)%	0.99
1,2–mismatch	41 (27–54)%		53 (29–72)%	

Table 13.6. Effects of age and diagnosis–transplant interval on survival after bone marrow transplantation for severe aplastic anemia: probability (95% confidence interval)

	ID–BMT	ALTFAM–BMT	UD–BMT
Age <18 years			
Diagnosis–BMT: <12 months	78 (74–82)%	47 (34–60)%	41 (27–54)%
: ≥12 months	65 (50–76)%	33 (10–59)%	31 (18–44)%
Age ≥18 years			
Diagnosis–BMT: <12 months	64 (60–68)%	50 (32–66)%	30 (17–45)%
: ≤12 months	54 (43–63)%	29 (6–58)%	28 (16–41)%

sporin was given without methotrexate, intermediate in patients who received cyclosporin plus methotrexate, and lowest in patients who received T-cell-depleted marrow (data not shown).

Chronic GVHD

There was increased probability of chronic GVHD after alternative donor BMT compared to ID-BMT (Table 13.4). Univariate analyses did not reveal associations between recipient age or year of transplant and the probability of chronic GVHD.

Table 13.7. Causes of death after bone marrow transplantation for severe aplastic anemia

Cause of death	ID sibling ($n=368$)	ALTFAM ($n=64$)	Unrelated donor ($n=129$)
New malignancy	5 (1)	1 (2)	2 (2)
Acute GVHD	39 (11)	5 (8)	11 (9)
Chronic GVHD	21 (6)	0 (0)	2 (2)
GVHD and IP	21 (6)	6 (9)	6 (5)
IP	19 (5)	4 (6)	7 (5)
Infection	67 (18)	20 (31)	20 (16)
ARDS	11 (3)	0 (0)	2 (2)
Aplasia	108 (29)	21 (33)	15 (12)
Organ failure	27 (7)	2 (3)	6 (5)
Hemorrhage	22 (6)	3 (5)	6 (5)
Drug induced	2 (1)	1 (2)	0 (0)
Other	17 (5)	0 (0)	8 (6)
Unknown	9 (2)	1 (2)	44 (34)

Notes:

ARDS = acute respiratory distress syndrome; GVHD = graft-versus-host disease; IP = interstitial pneumonitis.

Cause of death

The causes of death after HLA-identical sibling BMT and after alternative donor BMT are shown in Table 13.7.

Discussion

This is the largest analysis of alternative donor BMT for SAA so far reported. The transplant era 1986–95 was chosen to include cases which were recent enough to reflect current protocols and supportive care but with long enough follow-up to allow meaningful analysis. The ID-BMT cohort was included to provide a 'gold standard' to compare with the results of alternative donor transplants. Figure 13.1 and Table 13.4 show that survival after alternative donor BMT is inferior to that after ID-BMT ($P<0.0001$), graft failure is increased ($P<0.0001$), AGVHD is more probable ($P<0.0001$), and interstitial pneumonitis is more frequent ($P<0.0001$).

From Table 13.1 it can be seen that before the transplant the ID-BMT, ALTFAM-BMT, and UD-BMT patient populations were similar in gender, etiology, and Karnofsky scores at the time of BMT. In contrast, the UD-BMT and ALTFAM-BMT groups had significantly longer diagnosis-to-transplant intervals than the ID-BMT group. This delay of BMT was presumably the result of time needed for the unrelated donor search as well as a greater likelihood of receiving one or more trials of immunosuppressive therapy prior to referral for BMT. The UD-BMT and ALTFAM-BMT cohorts also received more transfusions than the ID-BMT patients. These factors are associated with poorer survival after ID-BMT (Champlin et al., 1989; Storb et al., 1980) and may be responsible in part for the inferior survival and increased graft failure after alternative donor BMT observed in this study.

There was surprisingly little evidence for an impact of recipient age on survival after alternative donor BMT in this analysis. This contrasts with IBMTR and single-center results, in which older patient age was a strong, independent predictor of poor survival (Passweg et al., 1997). The multiple data sources and missing data points prohibited multivariate analyses. Such analyses are needed to probe accurately for correlations between outcomes and variables related to the patient, donor, and transplant. For these reasons we only present univariate analyses of limited factors in this chapter. Even these univariate analyses should be treated with caution.

A higher proportion of alternative donor BMT recipients compared with ID-BMT recipients received intensive conditioning protocols including irradiation. Irradiation reduced graft failure but was not associated with improved survival.

Although T-cell depletion was associated with some reduction in grade II–IV AGVHD in the unrelated donor group, this was not associated with a survival advantage. Again, the promising results of the Milwaukee team using T-cell depletion (Margolis et al., 1996) require confirmation by other centers studying a broader age range of patients.

The survival of the 32 patients with phenotypically matched family donors was significantly worse than that of the ID-BMT group and marginally better ($P=$ns) than that of the 84 patients transplanted from partially HLA-matched family donors. These data are somewhat at variance with the conclusions of previously published reports (Bacigalupo et al., 1988*a*; Wagner et al., 1996). The interval between diagnosis and BMT in both subgroups was similar to and statistically greater than that of the ID-BMT group. More experience with phenotypically identical family donors is needed before firm recommendations can be made.

There is no evidence that HLA matching in the unrelated donor group affects survival. Matching was based on serological typing in this study which is insensitive and, even when donor-recipient pairs were apparently matched, it is probable that HLA mismatches occurred. Occult HLA mismatch is readily detected by current high-resolution deoxyribonucleic acid (DNA) typing techniques based on the polymerase chain reaction (Bidwell, 1994). It has recently been shown that the HLA match defined by high-resolution DNA typing is associated with significantly better survival after unrelated donor BMT for leukemia than in cases where occult mismatch is detected (Speiser et al., 1996). It is likely that the results of unrelated donor BMT for SAA could be improved by better donor selection based on DNA-based, high-resolution HLA typing.

The probability of 5-year survival after immunosuppressive treatment has improved in the past decade (Bacigalupo et al., 1988*b*, 1995; Frickhoven et al., 1991). In a recent study, patients who were treated with a combination of ATG, cyclosporin and granulocyte colony-stimulating factor (G-CSF) had an 85% probability of 3-year survival (Bacigalupo et al., 1995). However, 20–50% of patients with an initial response to immunosuppression have a relapse of their marrow aplasia. In addition, studies from the EBMT group indicate a 35% probability of clonal disease at 8 years after immunosuppressive treatment (Tichelli et al., 1988). In cases that clonally evolve, about 15% develop myelodysplastic syndrome or acute myeloblastic leukemia, and 20% paroxysmal hemoglobinuria (PNH). At least 50% of the patients with a PNH clone do not have clinically significant disease. Despite the long-term risks of relapse or clonal evolution, immunosuppressive treatment remains first-line therapy for all patients with SAA who lack a HLA-identical sibling donor.

The optimal protocol for alternative donor BMT for SAA cannot be established from this analysis. The inclusion of irradiation in pretransplant preparation reduces graft failure in unrelated donor BMT. It is not certain whether limited field irradiation or total body irradiation is preferable. The Milwaukee experience suggests that patients younger than 25 years old may tolerate the toxicity of full-dose total body irradiation combined with ATG and high-dose chemotherapy to reduce graft failure, with T-cell depletion to ameliorate AGVHD (Camitta et al., 1989; Margolis et al., 1996). The Milwaukee team is currently investigating whether shielding the head during total body irradiation decreases neurological and endocrine complications while preserving their excellent overall results. In association with the National Marrow Donor Program the Seattle group is investigating the effect on survival after UD-BMT of nonablative doses of total body irradiation given with cyclophosphamide (50mg/kg×4) and ATG (30mg/kg×3) as a less toxic approach which may benefit older adults. The dose of total body irradiation given to the first cohort of patients was 200cGy×3, de-escalating to 200cGy×2 and then 200cGy×1 in subsequent cohorts. The GVHD prophylaxis regimen is cyclosporin plus methotrexate without T-cell depletion. Preliminary results are encouraging with 14 of 26 (54%) of patients surviving at 2–36 months postBMT (Deeg et al., 1997).

At this time alternative donor BMT is not recommended as first-line treatment for patients with SAA who lack an HLA-identical sibling. Patients who lack an HLA-identical sibling should receive some form of immunosuppression as initial therapy. When possible, patients should be entered into prospective studies designed to improve the outcome of immunosuppressive therapy. At the time the patient commences treatment, family HLA typing should be reviewed and either an extended family donor search or a preliminary unrelated donor search initiated. This action will save valuable time if there has been no response by 3–6 months after immunosuppressive therapy and alternative donor BMT is considered. The current guideline from the EBMT SAA working party is that two courses of immunosuppression should be given before considering alternative donor BMT, as approximately 35% of nonresponders after one course will respond to a second course of immunosuppression (Schrezenmeier et al., 1995).

Future directions

Transfusion policy in patients with SAA

The dual problems of HLA mismatch and sensitization to HLA antigens at the B-cell and T-cell level through multiple transfusions are a major barrier to progress in alternative donor transplantation. Use of leukocyte-poor blood products reduces sensitization effectively in patients who have not been previously immunized through prior transfusion earlier in life or through pregnancy, and in some presensitized patients as well (Slichter, for the trial to reduce alloimmunization to platelets study group, 1997).

Despite careful transfusion practice sensitization may still occur, as patients with SAA generally retain good cellular and humoral alloimmunity despite immunosuppressive therapy for their disease. A novel approach to overcome the problem of sensitization is by identification, analysis, and avoidance of response-inducing epitopes in the HLA molecules of potential donors (Laundy and Bradley 1995).

HLA molecular epitope analysis

Parham and others have suggested that amino acid sequences within the HLA molecule that define antigenic epitopes reactive with cytotoxic antibodies may be partly or completely different from the epitopes that stimulate T-cells (Parham, 1992). Short sequences of amino acids have been shown to define molecular epitopes, which, when mismatched in the transplant situation, can trigger alloreactive responses. In contrast, other epitopes have been identified that, when mismatched, are associated with nonreactivity after mismatched transplants (Laundy and Bradley, 1995). The first step towards 'intelligent mismatching' in alternative donor BMT for SAA is to perform high-resolution DNA typing and HLA sequencing on donor-recipient pairs (Bidwell, 1994). Secondly, pilot studies to correlate alloreactivity with transplant outcome have to be undertaken for the same donor-recipient pairs. Computer programs exist that can then be used to identify T-cell-response-inducing and nonresponse-inducing mismatches. A database of information could then be compiled of response-inducing (unsafe) and nonresponse-inducing epitopes which can be safely mismatched even when the potential recipient is sensitized through pregnancy and/or blood transfusion. Such a database would be valuable for selecting alternative donors for patients with SAA.

Conclusion

The decision to proceed with alternative donor BMT is complex. Hematologists are encouraged to discuss cases with centers specializing in the management of SAA. The correct timing of alternative donor BMT, the upper age limit for recipients and the level of acceptable mismatch have not been defined. The authors recommend that alternative donor BMT be considered within 6 months of the diagnosis of SAA in patients who are less than 30 years of age and have not responded to immunosuppressive therapy.

References

Atkinson, K., Horowitz, M. M., Gale, R. P. et al. (1990) Risk factors for chronic graft versus host disease after HLA identical sibling bone marrow transplantation. *Blood*, **73**, 2459–67.

Bacigalupo, A., Hows, J., Gordon–Smith, E. C. et al. (1988*a*) Bone marrow transplantation for severe aplastic anemia from donors other than HLA identical siblings: a report of the BMT Working Party. *Bone Marrow Transplantation*, **3**, 531–5.

Bacigalupo, A., Hows, J., Gluckman, E. et al. (1988*b*) Bone marrow transplantation (BMT) versus immunosuppression for the treatment of severe aplastic anaemia (SAA): a report of the EBMT SAA Working Party. *British Journal of Haematology*, **70**, 177–82.

Bacigalupo, A., Broccia, G., Corda, G. et al. (1995) Antilymphocyte globulin, cyclosporin and granulocyte colony-stimulating factor in patients with acquired severe aplastic anemia (SAA): a pilot study of the EBMT SAA Working Party. *Blood*, **85**, 1348–53.

Beatty, P. G., Dahlberg, S., Michelson, E. M. et al. (1988) Probability of finding HLA matched unrelated donors. *Transplantation*, **45**, 714–21.

Bidwell, J. L. (1994) Advances in DNA-based HLA typing methods. *Immunology Today*, **15**, 303–7.

Camitta, B. M., Thomas, E. D., Nathan, D. G. et al. (1976) Severe aplastic anemia: a prospective study of the effect of early marrow transplantation on acute mortality. *Blood*, **48**, 63–70.

Camitta, B. M., Ash, R., Menitove, J. et al. (1989) Bone marrow transplantation for children with severe aplastic anemia: use of donors other than HLA-identical siblings. *Blood*, **74**, 1852–7.

Champlin, R. E., Horowitz, M. M., van Bekkum, D. W. et al. (1989) Graft failure following bone marrow transplantation for severe aplastic anemia: risk factors and treatment results. *Blood*, **73**, 606–13.

Deeg, H. J., Schloch, G., Ramsay, N. et al. (1997) Marrow transplantation from unrelated donors for patients with aplastic anemia (AA) who fail immunosuppressive therapy. *Blood*, **90** [Suppl. 1], A1763.

Flowers, M. E. D., Pepe, M. S., Longton, G. et al. (1990) Previous donor pregnancy as a risk factor for acute graft-versus-host disease in patients with aplastic anaemia treated by allogeneic marrow transplantation. *British Journal of Haematology*, **74**, 492–6.

Frickhoven, N., Kaltwasser, J. P., Schrezenmeier, H. et al. for the German Aplastic Anemia Study Group(1991). Treatment of aplastic anemia with antilymphocyte globulin and methylprednisolone with or without cyclosporine. *New England Journal of Medicine*, **324**, 1297–303.

Gluckman, E., Socié, G., Devergie, A. et al. (1991) Bone marrow transplantation in 107 patients with severe aplastic anemia using cyclophosphamide and thoraco-abdominal irradiation for conditioning: long-term follow-up. *Blood*, **78**, 2451–5.

Gluckman, E., Horowitz, M. M., Champlin, R. E. et al. (1992) Bone marrow transplantation for severe aplastic anemia: influence of conditioning and graft-versus-disease prophylaxis regimens on outcome. *Blood*, **79**, 269–75.

Glucksberg, H., Storb, R., Fefer, A. et al. (1974) Clinical manifestations of graft versus host disease in human recipients of bone marrow transplantation. *Transplantation*, **18**, 295–302.

Hows, J., Downie, T., Nunn, A. et al. (1996) Fate of patients undergoing unrelated donor searches in the UK. *Bone Marrow Transplantation*, **17**, A579.

Hows, J. M., Yin, J. L., Marsh, J. et al. (1986) Histocompatible unrelated volunteer donors compared with HLA non-identical family donors in marrow transplantation for aplastic anemia and leukemia. *Blood*, **68**, 1322–8.

Kernan, N. A., Bartsch, G., Ash, R. et al. (1993) Analysis of 462 transplantations from unrelated donors facilitated by the National Marrow Donor Program. *New England Journal of Medicine*, **328**, 593–602.

Laundy, G. J. and Bradley, B. A. (1995) The predictive value of epitope analysis in highly sensitized patients awaiting renal transplantation. (1995) *Transplantation*, **59**, 1207–13.

Margolis, D., Camitta, B., Pietryga, D. et al. (1996) Unrelated donor bone marrow transplantation to treat severe aplastic anaemia in children and young adults. *British Journal of Haematology*, **94**, 65–72.

McGlave, P. B., Haake, R., Miller, W. et al. (1987) Therapy of severe aplastic anemia in young adults and children with allogeneic bone marrow transplantation. *Blood*, **70**, 1325–30.

Parham, P. (1992) Typing for class I HLA polymorphism: past, present and future. *European Journal of Immunogenetics*, **19**, 347–59.

Passeweg, J. R., Socié, G., Hinterberger, W. et al. (1997) Bone marrow transplantation for severe aplastic anemia: has outcome improved ? *Blood*, **90**, 858–64.

Schipper, R. F., D'Amaro, J. and Oudshoorn, M. (1996) The probability of finding a suitable related donor for bone marrow transplantation in extended families. *Blood*, **87**, 800–4.

Schrezenmeier, H., Hinterberger, W., Hows, J. M. et al. (1995) Second immunosuppressive treatment for patients with aplastic anaemia not responding to the first course of immunosuppression (IS): a report for the Working Party on Severe Aplastic Anaemia of the EBMT. *Bone Marrow Transplantation*, **15** [Suppl. 2], A65.

Slichter, S. J. for the trial to reduce alloimmunization to platelets study group. (1997) Leukocyte reduction and ultra violet B irradiation of platelets to prevent alloimmunization and refractoriness to platelet transfusions. *New England Journal of Medicine*, **337**, 1861–9.

Speiser, D. E., Tiercy, J. M., Rufer, N. et al. (1996) High resolution HLA matching associated with decreased mortality after unrelated bone marrow donor transplantation. *Blood*, **87**, 4455–63.

Storb, R., Thomas, E. D., Buchner, C. D. et al. (1980) Marrow transplantation in 30 'untransfused' patients with severe aplastic anemia. *Annals of Internal Medicine*, **92**, 30–8.

Storb, R., Prentice, R. L., Thomas, E. D. et al. (1983*a*) Factors associated with graft rejection after HLA-identical marrow transplantation for aplastic anaemia. *British Journal of Haematology*, **55**, 573–85.

Storb, R., Prentice, R. L., Buckner, C. D. et al. (1983*b*) Graft-versus-host disease and survival in patients with aplastic anemia treated by marrow grafts from HLA-identical siblings. Beneficial effect of a protective environment. *New England Journal of Medicine*, **308**, 302–7.

Storb, R., Etzioni, R., Anasetti, C. et al. (1994) Cyclophosphamide combined with antithymocyte globulin in preparation for allogeneic marrow transplants in patients with aplastic anemia. *Blood*, **84**, 941–9.

Tichelli, A., Gratwohl, A., Wursch, A. et al. (1988) Late haematological complications in severe aplastic anaemia. *British Journal of Haematology*, **69**, 413–18.

Wagner, J. L., Deeg, H. J., Seidel, K. et al. (1996) Bone marrow transplantation for severe aplastic anemia from genotypically HLA-nonidentical relatives. *Transplantation*, **61**, 54–61.

Weiner, R. S., Bortin, M. M., Gale, R. P. et al. (1986) Interstitial pneumonia after bone marrow transplantation. Assessment of risk factors. *Annals of Internal Medicine*, **104**, 168–75.

14

Treatment of children with acquired aplastic anemia

Anna Locasciulli

Ospedale San Gerardo, Monza

Introduction

Bone marrow transplantation (BMT), when HLA-identical siblings are available, and immunosuppressive therapy are the main therapeutic modalities currently used to treat pediatric patients with acquired aplastic anemia. Children who fail to respond can be treated with alternative therapies, including transplantation of bone marrow from unrelated or mismatched family donors and, more recently, hemopoietic growth factors. Reports on the outcome of immunosuppressive therapy in children are often controversial. Some authors have illustrated good response rates in adults and children older than 5 years, while others have shown the opposite (Doney et al., 1997; Matloub et al., 1994). When choosing which therapy to use to treat children with severe aplastic anemia (SAA), one should consider the possible late effects that are peculiar to pediatric patients, such as growth failure and other endocrine problems, as well as the risk of malignancies, which may occur if the conditioning regimen before BMT involves irradiation.

This chapter will cover the results and possible consequences of these treatments in childhood acquired aplastic anemia.

BMT from HLA-identical siblings

Allogeneic BMT from an HLA-identical sibling is thought to be the main treatment choice for young patients with acquired SAA. We analyzed the results of this therapeutic procedure in a large series of pediatric patients (less than 16 years of age) treated in Europe between 1970 and 1996. The SAA Registry of the European Blood and Marrow Transplantation Group (EBMT) contains data on 935 such patients, of whom 497 have received transplants from an HLA-identical sibling. Their clinical characteristics and treatment protocols are shown in Table 14.1. Briefly, patients were grouped according to age (younger than 5,

Table 14.1. Clinical characteristics of 497 children with acquired severe aplastic anemia (SAA) treated with allogeneic bone marrow transplant (BMT) from HLA-identical sibling donors in Europe

		No. of patients	(%)
Age (years)	≤5	87	(18)
	6–10	180	(36)
	>10	230	(46)
Gender	Male	273	(54)
	Female	215	(44)
	Not specified	9	(2)
Severity (PMN $\times 10^9$/l)	≤0.2	153	(31)
	0.2–0.5	52	(10)
	>0.5	55	(11)
	Not specified	237	(48)
Treatment protocols			
Conditioning regimen	Cyclophosphamide	298	(60)
	+ ALG	33	(7)
	+ ALG + others	2	(0.5)
	+ Others	15	(3)
	+ Irradiation	165	(33)
	Not specified	49	(9.5)
GVHD prophylaxis	MTX	113	(23)
	CSA	140	(28)
	CSA + MTX	85	(17)
	CSA + others	25	(5)
	Not specified	134	(27)

Notes:
ALG = antilymphocye globulin; CSA = cyclosporin;
MTX = methotrexate; PMN = peripheral blood neutrophils $\times 10^9$/l.

6–10 and older than 10 years) and classified according to the degree of granu-locytopenia (less than 0.2, 0.2–0.5, $>0.5 \times 10^9$/l neutrophils for very severe, severe and moderately severe aplastic anemia, respectively). Most condition-ing regimens included cyclophosphamide, while 165 of the children also received irradiation treatment (total lymphoid, total body, thoracoabdominal). Prophylaxis against graft-versus-host disease (GVHD) was carried out using methotrexate alone ($n = 113$), or cyclosporin either alone ($n = 140$) or in

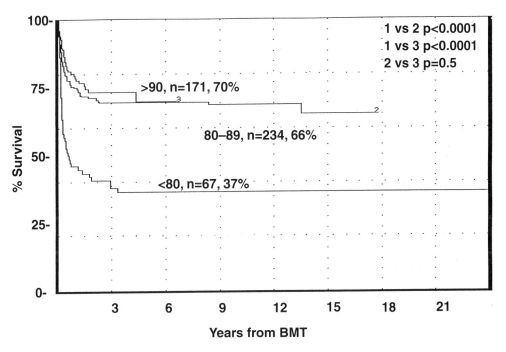

Figure 14.1. Overall survival of 472 children with acquired aplastic anemia treated with bone marrow transplantation (BMT) from HLA-identical siblings, according to year of BMT.

combination with methotrexate ($n=85$) or other drugs ($n=25$). Figure 14.1 outlines the overall survival of 472 of 497 children for whom there were sufficient data, stratified according to the year when BMT took place. Transplant results have improved considerably over time, from 37% obtained for patients treated between 1970 and 1980, compared with 66% in 1980–89 and 70% from then on. This reflects the changes in transplant protocols instigated over the years and, above all, the use of cyclosporin for GVHD prophylaxis, introduced in 1980. Indeed, major improvements began in 1980 ($P<0.0001$), whilst results during the 1990s were not significantly better than those observed between 1980 and 1989 ($P=0.5$, Figure 14.1). The sharp fall in transplant-related mortality, from more than 60% to 21 %, has not only come about through use of cyclosporin. Other factors are optimization of conditioning regimens, better supportive care, more appropriate treatment of infectious complications, and giving the BMT sooner after diagnosis than was done previously. Furthermore, these observations are also supported by the recent finding that decreasing the risks of other complications, such as rejection, interstitial pneumonia and other infections, as well as GVHD, has reduced mortality (Figure 14.2). Recent analysis reveals that the age does not influence survival, in line with previous observations (Locasciulli et al., 1990).

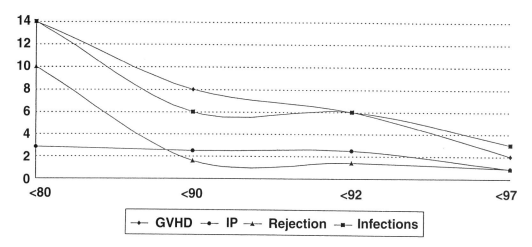

Figure 14.2. Leading causes of death of children undergoing BMT from HLA-identical siblings; changes over time. GVHD = graft-versus-host disease; IP = interstitial pneumonia.

BMT from alternative donors

Allogeneic BMT from a phenotypically identical family member or a matched unrelated donor has been proposed as a method for treating those children with SAA who do not have an HLA-identical sibling and who do not respond to immunosuppression. The SAA Registry of the EBMT contains data on 91 such patients, under 16 years of age, who underwent this procedure between 1970 and 1997. Their clinical characteristics and treatment protocols are summarized in Table 14.2. Of these 91 patients, the majority were male and the age distribution was similar in the three groups. The severity of the disease, classified according to the absolute neutrophil count at diagnosis, was not indicated in most cases. This is understandable, considering that these patients are to undergo the very high-risk procedure because the first-line therapy has failed, and they have very severe disease irrespective of the number of peripheral blood neutrophils (PMN) at diagnosis. It is interesting to note that the same data were missing for most patients receiving transplants from an HLA-identical sibling; however, here the data were not included because allogeneic BMT is indicated as the first treatment of choice for children who have an HLA-identical sibling regardless of the severity of disease: (Locasciulli et al., 1990). Furthermore, the number of PMN at diagnosis has been demonstrated not to affect outcome significantly for patients treated with BMT (Doney et al 1997; Locasciulli et al., 1990). Figure 14.3 outlines the overall survival for 86 of 91 children for whom sufficient data were available, stratified in two groups, according to the year of BMT (before or after 1990). These results are very poor, with an overall survival of 24%, which did not change over time. The rather discouraging finding that, unlike BMT from an HLA-identical sibling donor, alter-

Table 14.2. Clinical characteristics in 91 children with acquired SAA treated with BMT from alternative donors in Europe

		No. of patients	(%)
Age (years)	≤5	25	(28)
	6–10	35	(38)
	>10	31	(34)
Gender	Male	56	(62)
	Female	35	(38)
Severity (PMN ×10^9/l)	≤0.2	22	(24)
	0.2–0.5	10	(11)
	>0.5	8	(9)
	Not specified	51	(56)
Treatment protocols			
Conditioning regimen	Cyclophosphamide	3	(33)
	+ ALG	5	(6)
	+ ALG + others	2	(2)
	+ Others	15	(16)
	+ Irradiation	40	(44)
	Not specified	39	(43)
GVHD prophylaxis	MTX	—	—
	CSA	16	(18)
	CSA + MTX	17	(19)
	CSA + others	15	(16)
	Not specified	43	(47)

Notes:
ALG = antilymphocyte globulin; CSA = cyclosporin; MTX = methotrexate;
PMN = peripheral blood neutrophils ×10^9/l.

native donor BMT did not improve with time may be explained in part by the fact that this treatment is still considered as a rescue therapy, performed when other therapeutic protocols have failed. For this reason, patients undergoing this treatment are in a serious clinical condition, heavily transfused, and often infected.

Immunosuppressive treatment

Antilymphocyte (ALG) and antithymocyte (ATG) globulins, given as single agents or, more appropriately, in combination with cyclosporin and/or methylprednisolone, are the most important and definitive therapies for treating children with

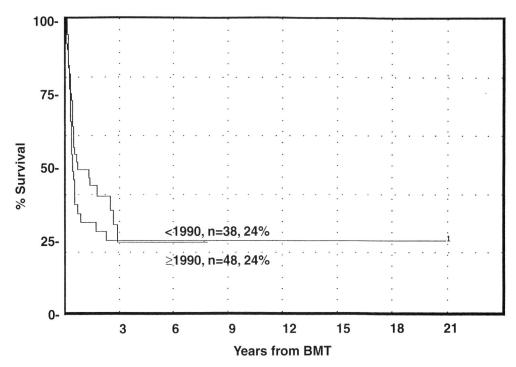

Figure 14.3. Overall survival of 86 children with acquired aplastic anemia treated with BMT from alternative donors, according to year of BMT.

acquired aplastic anemia who do not have an HLA-identical sibling. The SAA Registry of the EBMT contains data on 347 such patients who received immunosuppressive therapy between 1970 and 1997. Their clinical characteristics and treatment protocols are shown in Table 14.3. The age distribution was not homogeneous in this cohort, as about half of the cases are children older than 10 years. Interestingly the majority of patients presented with severe disease: in fact only 17% of children had granulocyte counts greater than 0.5×10^9 /l; this finding is significant when considering that data on the degree of severity were available in most cases (83%) for the whole therapy group. More than 90% of the patients (316 out of 347) were immunosuppressed with ALG, either alone or combined with cyclosporin, methylpredisolone or androgens. Growth factors, mostly granulocyte colony-stimulating factor (G-CSF), were included in 84 such cases treated more recently, but in this series no-one received any growth factor as a unique treatment. Figure 14.4 illustrates the overall survival of the 347 children, according to the years of treatment (before 1980, curve 1; 1980–89, curve 2; and after 1990, curve 3). Survival significantly improved over time, from 29% for cases treated before 1980 to 43% in children undergoing immunosuppression between 1980 and 1989 and 59% after 1990: $P = 0.009$ (1 versus 2), $P = 0.0001$ (1 versus 3), $P = 0.04$ (2 versus 3). Results were even better when the analysis was restricted to

Table 14.3. Clinical characteristics in 347 children with acquired SAA treated with immunosuppression in Europe

		No. of patients	(%)
Age (years)	≤5	84	(24)
	6–10	100	(29)
	>10	163	(47)
Gender	Male	194	(56)
	Female	153	(44)
Severity (PMN $\times 10^9$/l)	≤0.2	166	(48)
	0.2–0.5	77	(22)
	>0.5	60	(17)
	Not specified	44	(13)
Treatment protocols	ALG ± CSA ± MP ± androgens	232	(67)
	ALG ± CSA ± MP + growth factors	84	(24)
	CSA + MP	3	(1)
	Others	22	(6)
	Not specified	6	(2)

Notes:

ALG = antilymphocyte globulin; CSA = cyclosporin;

MP = methylprednisolone; PMN = peripheral blood neutrophils $\times 10^9$/l.

the 283 children with severe disease (PMN counts $<0.5 \times 10^9$/l): from 33% survivors at 5 years in cases treated before 1980, to 60% in patients undergoing immunosuppression between 1980 and 1989, and 70% for those treated more recently (Figure 14.5). These findings contradict previous conclusions based on the analysis of the SAA Registry of the EBMT, which included children treated up to 1988. In fact, in that study survival did not change over the time span considered and it depended greatly on disease severity; as children with PMN counts $<0.2 \times 10^9$/l, especially those younger than 5 years, responded so poorly to immunosuppression (11%), we suggested an early search for matched unrelated donors for children in that category (Locasciulli et al., 1990). In the present analysis, changes were more consistent, as treatment protocols were notably modified after 1988: one or more drugs, such as cyclosporin, androgens and G-CSF, have been added to ALG. Results have improved accordingly; the effect of age and the impact of severity of disease have become insignificant and the outcome for severe cases is even better than that of the whole population. The median time to transfusion independence is 80 days from immunosuppression for children treated more

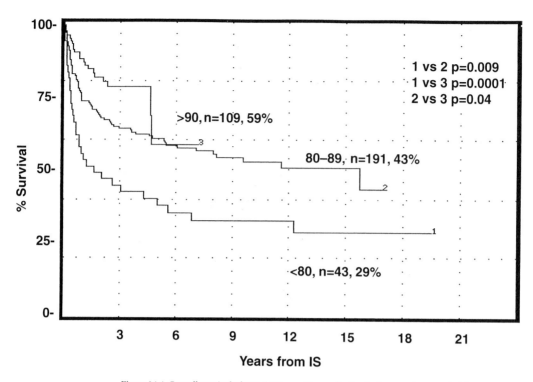

Figure 14.4. Overall survival of 347 children with acquired aplastic anemia treated with immunosuppression, according to year of treatment.

recently with ALG, cyclosporin and G-CSF, with a range of from 7 to 409 days (Figure 14.6). This variability implies that the response should never be evaluated before the third month after treatment, as recovery can still occur several months later in about half of these children.

Hemopoietic growth factors

Recently, administering recombinant hemopoietic growth factors, including G-CSF, granulocyte/macrophage colony-stimulating factor, interleukins 3, 1, and 6, and erythropoietin, has been proposed for treating SAA, either as adjuvant therapy for severe infections or combined with immunosuppression. The use of growth factors alone has produced only transient, if any, hematological responses, and is thought to be inappropriate because it delays the start of more established therapies, possibly compromising the prognosis of patients with SAA (Marsh et al., 1994). However, including G-CSF in immunosuppressive therapy has led to remarkable results both in adults and children (Bacigalupo et al., 1995), and this approach of combined immunosuppressive and cytokine therapy may

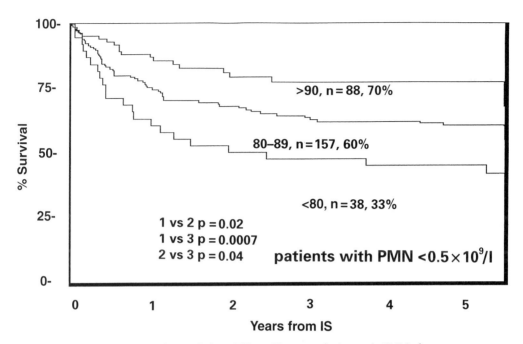

Figure 14.5. Percentage year actuarial survival of 283 children with severe aplastic anemia (SAA) [polymorphonuclear cell (PMN) $<0.5 \times 10^9/l$] treated with immunosuppression (IS), according to year of treatment.

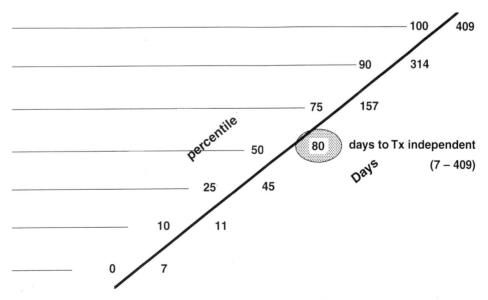

Figure 14.6. Time to transfusion independence from immunosuppression with antilymphocyte globulin (ALG), cyclosporin and granulocyte colony-stimulating factor in children with SAA.

Table 14.4. Occurrence of malignant or nonmalignant diseases in children with acquired aplastic anemia treated with immunosuppression or BMT from matched sibling donors

	Immunosuppression		BMT	
	With G-CSF	Without G-CSF	With IRR	Without IRR
Total number (%)	84	263	165	332
Leukemia	0	5 (2)	1 (0.6)	0
MDS	0	6 (2.3)	1 (0.6)	0
Solid tumor	0	1 (0.4)	4 (2.4)	0
NHL	0	1 (0.4)	0	0
AIDS	0	0	7 (4.2)	0
PNH	0	7 (2.7)	0	0

Notes:
AIDS = acquired immunodeficiency syndrome; IRR = irradiation; MDS = myelodysplastic syndrome; NHL = nonHodgkin lymphoma; PNH = paroxysmal nocturnal hemoglobinuria.

currently offer the best chances of a cure for a large proportion of patients with SAA. On the other hand, there is some concern about using these agents, especially in children, because of the possible impact on the later development of clonal disorders, as recently reported by Japanese investigators (Ohara et al., 1997). Our EBMT data on 84 children receiving immunosuppression and G-CSF did not support these findings, as no patient developed either cytogenetic alterations or clinical clonal disease after a median follow-up of 4 years from the administration of G-CSF (Table 14.4).

Late effects on children

The occurrence of long-term sequelae in children cured of SAA remains a matter of concern, given that, besides survival, their quality of life (including normal growth and development, endocrine function and fertility) is of high priority. As regards to BMT therapy, children who receive cyclophosphamide alone grow and develop normally (Sanders et al., 1994). However, irradiation has been shown to provoke significant long-term complications, such as growth failure, thyroid dysfunction, sterility and development of secondary malignancies, as well as a higher prevalence of chronic GVHD. To overcome these problems, major changes in conditioning regimens have been made over the years. In fact, before 1980, irradiation was used for 16% of children undergoing BMT; this figure rose to approximately 40% until 1992, as it was shown that its inclusion in the conditioning regimen decreased the prevalence of graft failure and rejection. After that time, reports derived from large series of patients strongly suggested that irradiation was a major risk factor for posttransplant malignancies in patients with aplastic anemia (Socié et al., 1993), and consequently its inclusion in treatment protocols has been decreased to less than 15%. Our data, derived from the analysis of 497 children given a transplant from a sibling donor in European BMT Units, confirm these observations (Table 14.4): of the 332 children transplanted without irradiation, none developed late malignancies, compared to six out of 165 irradiated cases. Seven additional patients in the latter group developed acquired immunodeficiency syndrome (AIDS), but this event was caused by an outbreak of human immunodeficiency virus (HIV) infection, transmitted by blood transfusion, occurring in centers that first introduced irradiation for conditioning regimen for SAA patients.

Besides recurrent aplasia, the long-term complications of immunosuppressive therapy include evolution to myelodysplastic syndrome, acute leukemia and the development of paroxysmal nocturnal hemoglobinuria (PNH) (Tichelli et al., 1989), a likely consequence of stressing hemopoiesis for a long time. It has been suggested that administering growth factors might promote the development of these clonal diseases (Ohara et al., 1997). The analysis we carried out on 347 children treated with immunosuppression alone ($n=263$) or in combination with G-CSF ($n=84$) showed that these events occurred only in the group that did not receive growth factors (Table 14.4): secondary malignancies, including leukemia, myelodysplastic syndrome, solid tumors and nonHodgkin lymphoma, were diagnosed in 13 out of 263 (5%) children and PNH in 7 cases (2.7%). It should be noted that the group receiving G-CSF has already reached a median observation period of 4 years. We therefore consider this combined therapy safe enough to be recommended to treat childhood SAA, although long-term studies are certainly required to clarify this point.

Treatment results obtained in the last 5 years in Europe

Treatment protocols employed in prospective clinical trials by the EBMT-SAA Working Party over the last 5 years have been modified as follows. For patients undergoing BMT from HLA-identical siblings, irradiation is not given. The ongoing EBMT-SAA Working Party protocol for such patients includes cyclophosphamide for conditioning and cyclosporin with or without methotrexate, for GVHD prophylaxis. Bone marrow transplants from an alternative donor do not have unified treatment regimens, as the pros and cons of the different protocols are still a matter of debate and concern, probably because of the poor results so far obtained with this procedure. With regard to immunosuppression, two prospective trials designed for patients with moderate or severe aplasia, which investigated the merits of ALG plus cyclosporin versus cyclosporin alone, and ALG plus

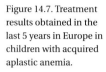

Figure 14.7. Treatment results obtained in the last 5 years in Europe in children with acquired aplastic anemia.

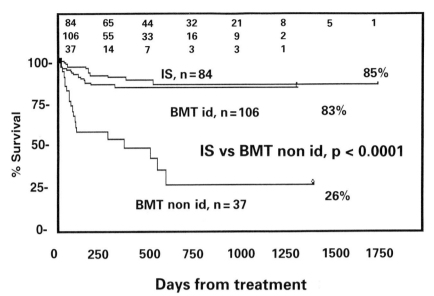

cyclosporin versus ALG plus cyclosporin plus G-CSF, have recently closed. During the trials, 227 children with SAA were treated in Europe, according to the guidelines described above. One hundred and six children received a bone marrow transplant from an HLA-identical sibling, 84 were immunosuppressed and 37 received an alternative donor BMT. Overall survival (Figure 14.7) did not differ significantly between the first two treatment arms (85% and 83%, respectively), while it remained very poor (26%) and significantly worse when compared to immunosuppression ($P<0.0001$) of children receiving an alternative donor BMT, unlike other experiences (Margolis et al., 1996).

Conclusion

Based on these results, we still recommend allogeneic BMT as a first-line therapy for children with an HLA-identical sibling and immunosuppression combined with G-CSF in cases without. BMT from alternative donor should be considered only for selected cases who did not respond to repeated immunosuppression.

References

Bacigalupo, A., Broccia, G., Corda, G., Arcese, W., Carotenuto, M., Gallamini, A., Locatelli, F., Mori, P. G., Saracco, P., Todeschini, G., Coser, P., Iacopino, P., Van Lint, M. T., Gluckman, E. for the European Group for Blood and Marrow Transplantation (EBMT) Working Party on

SAA. (1995) Antilymphocyte globulin, cyclosporin, and granulocyte colony-stimulating factor in patients with acquires severe aplastic anemia (SAA): a pilot study of the EBMT SAA Working Party. *Blood*, **85**, 1348–53.

Doney, K., Leisenring, W., Storb, R. and Appelbaum, F. R. (1997) Primary treatment of acquired aplastic anemia: outcomes with bone marrow transplantation and immuno-suppressive therapy. *Annals of Internal Medicine*, **126**, 107–15.

Locasciulli, A., van't Veer, L., Bacigalupo, A., Hows, J., Van Lint, M. T., Gluckman, E., Nissen, C., Vossen, J., Schrezenmeier, H., Hinteberger, W. and Marin, P. (1990) Treatment with marrow transplantation or immunosuppression of childhood acquired severe aplastic anemia: a report from the EBMT SAA Working Party. *Bone Marrow Transplantation*, **6**, 211–17.

Margolis, D., Camitta, B. and Pietryga, D. (1996) Unrelated donor bone marrow transplantation to treat severe aplastic anaemia in children and young adults. *British Journal of Haematology*, **94**, 65–72.

Marsh, J. C. W., Socié, G., Schrezenmeier, H., Tichelli, A., Gluckman, E., Ljungman, P., McCann, S. R., Raghavachar, A., Marin, P., Hows, J. M., Bacigalupo, A. for the European Bone Marrow Transplant Working Party for Severe Aplastic Anaemia. (1994) Haematopoietic growth factors in aplastic anaemia: a cautionary note. *Lancet*, **344**, 172–3.

Matloub, Y. H., Bostrom, B., Golembe, B., Priest, J. and Ramsay, N. K. C. (1994) Antithymocyce globulin, cyclosporin, and prednisone for the treatment of severe aplastic anemia in children. *American Journal of Pediatric Hematology Oncology*, **16**, 104–6.

Ohara, A., Kojima, S., Hamajima, N., Tsuchida, M., Imashuku, S., Ohta, S., Sasaki, H., Okamura, J., Sugita, K., Kigasawa, H., Kiriyama, Y., Akatsuka, J. and Tsukimoto, I. (1997) Myelodysplastic syndrome and acute myelogenous leukemia as a late clonal complication in children with acquired aplastic anemia. *Blood*, **90**, 1009–13.

Sanders, J. E., Storb, R., Anasetti, C., Deeg, H. J., Doney, K., Sullivan, K. M., Witherspoon, R. P. and Hansen, J. (1994) Marrow transplant experience for children with severe aplastic anemia. *American Journal of Pediatric Hematology Oncology*, **16**, 43–9.

Socié, G., Henry–Amar, M., Bacigalupo, A., Hows, J., Tichelli, A., Ljungman, P., McCann, S. R., Frickhofen, N., van't Veer K. E. and Gluckman, E. (1993) Malignant tumors occurring after treatment of aplastic anaemia. European Bone Marrow Transplantation – Severe Aplastic Anaemia Working Party. *New England Journal of Medicine*, **329**, 1152–7.

Tichelli, A., Gratwohl, A., Würsch, A., Nissen, C. and Speck, B. (1989) Late haematological complications in severe aplastic anaemia. *British Journal of Haematology*, **73**, 121–6.

15

Long-term follow-up of patients with aplastic anemia: clonal malignant and nonmalignant complications

André Tichelli

University Hospitals, Basel

and

Gérard Socié

Hôpital Saint-Louis, Paris

Introduction

Recent progress in the treatment of aplastic anemia has dramatically changed the previously grim prognosis for these patients, so that today the 2-year survival is 60–90% (Bacigalupo et al., 1988, 1995; Camitta and Doney, 1990; Doney et al., 1997; Gluckman et al., 1992*a,b*; Paquette et al., 1995; Passweg et al., 1997; Young, 1994). Improved results following bone marrow transplantation or immunosuppression increase the number of long-term survivors so that immediate survival is no longer the sole concern. Indeed, quality of life and late complications are becoming increasingly important (Deeg, 1990*a,b*; Duell et al., 1997; Kolb and Bender–Gotze, 1990). However, there are basic differences between both treatment modalities, resulting in their having specific effects on late morbidity and long-term survival.

Patients are likely to be cured of aplastic anemia by successful marrow transplantation. Late effects are caused by the treatment used to prepare the patient for transplantation, and the extent of chronic graft-versus-host disease and its treatment rather than the underlying disease. In contrast, after immunosuppression recovery often takes several months and stigmata of the disease persist despite clinical remission (Marsh et al., 1990, 1991; Nissen et al., 1980, 1993; Rudivic et al., 1985). Although immunosuppression allows autologous reconstitution of hemopoiesis, it leaves the patient with a fragile bone marrow prone to the development of a clonal disorder, such as myelodysplastic syndrome (MDS) or paroxysmal nocturnal hemoglobinuria (PNH). Late effects caused by the treatment itself may occur after immunosuppressive treatment; however, their consequences are usually much more harmless than those observed after transplantation.

In this chapter, clinical studies of the long-term evolution of patients treated with bone marrow transplantation or immunosuppression are discussed. Among late effects, new secondary malignancies such as MDS or leukemia and solid cancers, as well as clonal nonmalignant diseases such as PNH are of particular clinical concern. Long-term morbidity and mortality due to nonclonal complications are discussed in Chapters 10,12 and 13; therefore, they are not reviewed here.

Historical background

A relationship between aplastic anemia, leukemia, MDS and PNH has been suspected for a long time. For instance, leukemia and aplastic anemia share etiological risk factors such as irradiation, chemicals, and chromosomal abnormalities. The occurrence of leukemia as a complication of aplastic anemia has been reported on several occasions (Manoharan et al., 1981; Mir and Geary, 1980; Mufti et al., 1983; Orlandi et al., 1988; Tichelli et al., 1988a). Furthermore, those with PNH may develop aplastic anemia and vice versa: they are clearly clinically related syndromes. A number of patients with pancytopenia and hypoplastic marrow test positive for either the sucrose hemolysis test or the Ham's test (Conrad and Barton, 1979; Lewis and Dacie, 1967). More than 30 years ago, the distinguished hematologist and first editor of the journal *Blood*, William Dameshek, tackled the problem with a rather provocative question (Dameshek, 1967), 'What do aplastic anaemia, paroxysmal nocturnal haemoglobinuria and hypoplastic leukaemia have in common?'. He came to the conclusion that a single insult to the marrow might result in different morphological abnormalities, sometimes occurring together, sometimes sequentially. Nevertheless, before effective treatment for aplastic anemia was available, clonal evolution only rarely occurred after aplastic anemia.

Secondary MDS or leukemia

In 1988 two single-center studies described the evolution of acquired aplastic anemia into MDS or leukemia in patients treated with immunosuppression. In the Leiden study, five of 35 aplastic anemia patients surviving for two or more years developed a MDS (De Planque et al., 1988). All five patients had a normal karyotype at the time of first diagnosis: three of them were treated with antilymphocyte globulin (ALG), corticosteroids and androgens, and two received corticosteroids and androgens and were splenectomized. A pattern of evolution could be identified in patients with secondary hematological malignancy. The aplastic marrow first showed an improvement in hemopoiesis and subsequently developed dysplastic features in one or more cell lines, predominantly dyserythropoiesis. Refractory anemia evolved into chronic myelomonocytic leukemia in two patients, and refractory anemia with an excess of blasts in one patient. Three patients presented an abnormal karyotype with monosomy 7 at the time of the secondary MDS. Overall 10% of all patients surviving for 2 years eventually developed a leukemic disorder.

Similarly, the Basel group reviewed late hematological disorders in 137 patients with aplastic anemia (Tichelli et al., 1988b). One hundred and three patients were treated with ALG, and 34 with bone marrow transplantation. Twenty of the 103 patients treated with immunosuppression presented a clonal evolution (8 MDS; 12 PNH; 1 MDS together with PNH), but this did not occur in any of the patients treated with bone marrow transplantation. The risk of developing a hematological complication after immunosuppressive treatment was 57% at 8 years. In a subsequent follow-up study, it was found that cytogenetic analysis at diagnosis was normal in 13 patients who developed MDS/leukemia. At the time of transformation into a leukemic disease, five of the patients presented a clonal abnormality on karyotype analysis: monosomy 6 was found in two patients, and three others presented monosomy 7, deletion 7, deletion 14, or translocation t(8;21) respectively (Tichelli et al., 1994).

Long-term follow-up was evaluated in a large retrospective multicenter European Blood and Bone Marrow Transplantation (EBMT) group study including 468 aplastic anemia patients treated with ALG (De Planque et al., 1989). After immunosuppressive treatment of both severe and moderate aplastic anemia, the survival curve followed a biphasic pattern. The death rate was high in the first 2 years after treatment, but after that mortality gradually declined. Of the 245 patients who survived for 2 years, 21 died later. Thirteen patients died from a hemorrhage or infection due to persistent pancytopenia, four from the consequences of PNH and four from leukemia. Between the second and third years, pancytopenia due to aplastic anemia was still the major cause of death of the long-term survivors; after the third year posttreatment, leukemia and MDS became the primary cause of death. Twelve patients developed MDS/leukemia at a median of 4.6 years after immunosuppression. The actuarial mortality of long-term survivors was 22% at 8 years, but so far no plateau has occurred. The 5-year actuarial probability of developing MDS was between 15% and 20%. In comparison to single-center studies, the incidence of a clonal disease may have been underestimated, since these diagnoses are easily missed in the absence of symptoms without the appropriate and systematic blood and marrow tests.

These clinical observations indicate that there is a relationship between aplastic anemia and leukemic disorders, and all centers who routinely tested patients at regular intervals reported an actuarial risk of MDS and leukemia of between 10% and 20% at 10 years (Orlandi et al., 1988; Paquette et al., 1995). Furthermore, no age-related difference could be demonstrated; in particular the risk of secondary leukemia was similar for children and adults (Führer et al., 1998). The higher frequency of clonal complications observed since the mid-1980s can be accounted for by two factors: first, the improved survival of patients treated with immunosuppression, who otherwise would have died from pancytopenia, and, secondly, by the systematic search for MDS in long-term patients. Indeed, studies that observed patients for only a short follow-up period failed to demonstrate an increased risk of leukemia (Crump et al., 1992; Doney et al., 1992; Frickhofen et al., 1991; Gluckman et al., 1992*b*; Rosenfeld et al., 1995).

Hematological clonal complications are not usually observed after successful bone marrow transplantation, in contrast to immunosuppression (Paquette et al., 1995; Speck et al., 1990). In a Seattle Group study, none of 168 transplanted patients developed a leukemic disorder. Meanwhile 20 of 227 patients who received immunosuppressive treatment presented with a secondary MDS or leukemia ($P = 0.001$) (Doney et al., 1997). In fact, leukemia secondary to successful bone marrow transplantation is extremely rare. A previous study from Seattle showed that only one of over 400 patients transplanted for aplastic anemia whose conditioning regimen included cyclophosphamide developed acute leukemia of host cells 7 months after the transplant (Klingemann et al., 1986). A second case was reported by the Royal Postgraduate Medical School in London, where a patient with aplastic anemia developed an acute myeloid leukemia 5 years after bone marrow transplantation. Unfortunately it was not possible to obtain their cytogenetic analysis, and therefore it is not known whether the leukemia was in a donor or recipient cell line (Hughes et al., 1988). Finally and fascinatingly, cytogenetics and polymerase chain reaction of microsatellites sequences proved that, in two instances, donor cell leukemia developed after transplantation (Browne et al., 1991) (M. Lawler, personal communication).

To examine the incidence of hematological cancers and solid tumors in a large cohort of long-term survivors after treatment of aplastic anemia, the EBMT Severe Aplastic Anemia (SAA) Working Party studied the cases reported to the registry (Socié et al., 1993). The results on solid tumors will be discussed in the section entitled '*New solid cancers*'. The study population consisted of 860 patients treated with immunosuppression and 748 patients who had received bone marrow transplants. The risk of malignancy was analyzed overall and according to treatment relative to the risk in the general population. Thirty-four of the 860 patients who received immunosuppressive treatment developed MDS or leukemia (19 MDS, 15 leukemia), as did two of the 748 patients who received bone marrow transplants. The risk factors for MDS or acute leukemia after immunosuppressive treatment included being older (relative risk or RR = 1.03), being treated in or after 1982, as compared with in or before 1981 (RR = 3.01), having a splenectomy (RR=3.65), and receiving multiple courses of immunosuppression (RR=2.26). The addition of androgens to the immunosuppressive treatment was associated with a lower risk (RR=0.28). This study definitively proved the increased risk of developing MDS and leukemia after immunosuppressive treatment. Furthermore, based on a large number of patients, it could also demonstrate, for the first time, that even those who have had a bone marrow transplant are at greater risk of developing MDS/leukemia than the general population.

It is not clear whether aplastic anemia is a preleukemic disorder (Marsh and Geary, 1991; Socié, 1996). Clinical and biological evidence currently support the existence of a clear link between aplastic anemia and leukemia. Therefore, the high frequency of secondary leukemia is because of the disease rather than the immunosuppressive treatment. A number of historical publications describe secondary leukemia in patients with untreated aplastic anemia. It is difficult to distinguish between aplastic anemia and hypoplastic MDS. Therefore, some of the patients diagnosed as having aplastic anemia and secondary leukemia may in fact have hypoplastic MDS. The presence in bone marrow trephine biopsy samples of dysplastic micromegakaryocytes, focal increases of megakaryocyte numbers, and increased levels of reticulin is associated with a high risk of transformation to leukemia. Such cases might better be classified as hypoplastic MDS (Fohlmeister et al., 1985). However, MDS and aplastic anemia may share similar dysplastic features, including macrocytosis, dyserythropoiesis, ringed sideroblasts, atypical monocytes, and abnormal megakaryocytes in particular (Frisch et al., 1975; Kansu and Erslev, 1976; Lewis, 1979; Tichelli et al., 1992).

Distinguishing between hypoplastic MDS and aplastic anemia is helped by the detection of a leukemic clone. Cytogenetic analysis can demonstrate clonal changes before overt MDS or leukemia develops. An abnormal karyotype was detected in seven of 183 (4%) patients with otherwise morphologically typical aplastic anemia. Three of the seven patients were treated with immunosuppression and two developed late MDS or leukemia. Among the 169 patients with typical aplastic anemia and no cytogenetic anomalies, five (3%) subsequently presented a leukemic transformation (Appelbaum et al., 1987). In an Italian study, bone marrow cells from 69 patients with acquired aplastic anemia were analyzed cytogenetically at diagnosis and after immunosuppressive treatment (Mikhailova et al., 1996). Fifty-one patients (74%) were normal and remained normal, and 18 patients (26%) had at least one abnormal karyotype. Remarkably, three patterns of evolution were observed. In seven patients the anomaly was acquired after treatment, in three patients it was present at diagnosis and persisted during evolution, and in eight patients there was a transient posttreatment abnormality. The most frequent abnormality was trisomy 8 ($n=8$), followed by monosomy 7 ($n=2$). The three patients with the persistent cytogenetic abnormality all developed leukemia.

The EBMT SAA Working Party retrospectively evaluated cytogenetic anomalies in aplastic anemia patients treated with immunosuppression between 1974 and 1994 (Tichelli et al., 1996). One hundred and seventy evaluable karyotypes from six European centers were reported for analyses [Basel ($n=36$), Dublin ($n=13$), Genoa ($n=35$), London ($n=37$) and Paris ($n=49$)]. The median number of metaphases evaluated per karyoptype was 12 (range 6–100). One hundred and forty-six patients had a normal karyotype and one patient had a somatic chromosomal defect [46,XY,t(4;12)(q34;21)], confirmed by family karyotyping. In 23 (11.7%) cases a chromosomal aberration on hemopoietic cells could be demonstrated. This anomaly was clonal in 19 of the 23 (11.1%) cases. The chromosomal defect concerned all metaphases in six cases; a mosaic of normal and abnormal chromosomes was found in the 17 remaining cases. The defect was simple in 18 patients and complex in the remaining one. Trisomy 8 was observed in five cases and is therefore the most frequent single anomaly. Trisomy 6 was found in two patients, 5q– in another two patients and an anomaly on chromosome 7 in three others (monosomy 7; deletion 7; isochromosome 7). All other anomalies were seen in single cases. Follow-up of the karyotype for a selected group of patients was reported. At diagnosis, four of 31 cases presented a clonal anomaly (one case with monosomy 8); at the first analysis after therapy eight of 23 patients had a clonal anomaly (three cases with monosomy 8), as did 12 of 78 cases at the last analysis (four cases with monosomy 8). In Japan, monosomy 7 was the main chromosomal anomaly reported to occur in children treated with G-CSF and cyclosporin (Ohsaka et al., 1995; Tsuzuki et al., 1997; Yamazaki et al., 1997). Out of 11 children who developed MDS/leukemia, eight had a monosomy 7, two a monosomy 7 together with a monosomy 21 and one a monosomy 21.

All these reports show that a single clonal chromosomal defect in hemopoietic cells is not infrequent in aplastic anemia at presentation. Trisomy 8 and monosomy 7 are the most usual aberrations. However, cytogenetic analysis of empty marrow may be technically difficult. Classic karyotyping upon diagnosis of severe aplastic anemia is often not possible because of a lack of metaphases. The interphase fluorescent in situ hybridization (FISH) technique may detect anomalies such as trisomies and monosomies, even in marrow from patients in which no metaphases are found.

It is reasonable to conclude that an acquired clonal cytogenetic anomaly in a patient with otherwise typical aplastic anemia indicates that they are at a high risk of leukemic transformation, and therefore they should be considered as being in a preleukemic state. However, it is not clear how these fluctuating anomalies should be interpreted. The spontaneous disappearance of a clonal cytogenetic marker, such as monosomy 7 or trisomy 8, has been reported to occur in patients with MDS (Benaim et al., 1995; Matsuda et al., 1998; Renneboog et al., 1996. In patients with monosomy 7, the hematological improvement relates closely with the disappearance of the cytogenetic anomaly. This is not the case for patients with trisomy 8, whose hematology does not improve after the trisomy 8 disappears, as shown by conventional cytogenetics and FISH analysis (Iwabuchi et al., 1992; Matsuda et al., 1998). Therefore, trisomy 8 might not be related directly to the pathogenesis of MDS, but may represent a second step transformation, as in chronic myeloid leukemia. Similarly, the disappearance of trisomy 8 in aplastic anemia does not necessarily indicate that the malignant clone has gone.

Could the treatment of aplastic anemia favor the development of a clonal evolution? Before ALG and cyclosporin were available to treat aplastic anemia, few patients developed a secondary leukemia after successful treatment with oxymetholone (Delamore and Geary, 1971; King and Burns, 1972). However, because of the rarity of the disease and its complications, a causal relationship between treatment and the onset of leukemia could not be established. As already discussed, androgens were ruled out as initiating leukemia by the retrospective EBMT study of malignant tumor development after treatment of aplastic anemia. However, Socié et al. (1993) showed that treatment with multiple courses of immunosuppression and splenectomy is associated with an increased risk of hematological cancers.

Some recent findings suggest that administering G-CSF is associated with the development of MDS/leukemia (Imashuku et al., 1995; Kojima et al., 1992; Ohsaka et al., 1995; Tsuzuki et al., 1997, Yamazaki et al., 1997). Arguments supporting the theory of G-CSF's involvement in the occurrence of clonal disorders come mainly from Japan (Ohara et al., 1997). In a study of 167 children with aplastic anemia, 11 of 50 patients treated with G-CSF and cyclosporin developed MDS/leukemia. Of the group of children treated with G-CSF or cyclosporin alone, none presented this complication. The 7-year probability of developing MDS/leukemia was $47 \pm 17\%$ for patients treated with growth factors as compared to $15.9 \pm 6.2\%$ for the whole cohort. Furthermore, patients treated for longer periods or with a higher cumulative dose seemed to be at an increased risk. Finally, eight of the 11 late clonal disorders developed within 36 months, much earlier than is usually reported. However, these results do not corroborate with those of the prospective pilot study from Europe that includes 40 patients treated with G-CSF, ALG and cyclosporin (Bacigalupo et al., 1995). In a recent up-date, the frequency of MDS/leukemia in the 100 patients treated with this combination had not increased (personal communication, A. Bacigalupo). So, the debate continues as to whether G-CSF is involved in leukemic transformations in immunosuppressive-treated patients. Perhaps ethnic predisposition is significant for a subgroup of patients. Indeed, most publications supporting G-CSF as a risk factor for secondary leukemia come from pediatrics institutions in Japan. Further studies are needed to identify risk factors for developing MDS/leukemia in patients with aplastic anemia given new combinations of immunosuppressive treatment.

New solid cancers

Among late effects occurring after allogeneic bone marrow transplantation, solid cancers cause particular clinical concern, and need to be determined in a large population at risk. A retrospective EBMT study evaluated the incidence of new malignancies in 1211 patients, of whom 195 with aplastic anemia received transplants in 45 European centers and were alive 5 years after treatment (Kolb et al., 1995, 1996). New malignancies were observed in 47 patients, including glioblastoma ($n=4$), lymphoma ($n=3$), and neoplasms of the skin ($n=13$), oral cavity ($n=8$), uterine cervix ($n=5$), breast ($n=5$), oesophagus ($n=2$), and other tissues ($n=9$). Compared to an age- and sex-matched European population, the rate was significantly increased for neoplasms of the skin, oral cavity, oesophagus, uterine cervix, and brain.

The risk of developing a new solid cancer was also evaluated in a large retrospective multicenter IBMTR study, including 19,229 patients, 2159 with aplastic anemia who received bone marrow transplantation between 1964 and 1992 (Curtis et al., 1997). The transplant recipients were at a significantly higher risk of developing new solid cancers than the general population ($P<0.001$). The risk was 8.3 times higher than expected among those who survived 10 years after transplantation. The cumulative incidence rate was 2.2% at 10 years and 6.7% at 15 years. The risk was significantly elevated ($P<0.05$) for malignant melanoma and cancers of the buccal cavity, liver, brain or other parts of the central nervous system, thyroid, bone, and connective tissue. In multivariate analyses, higher doses of total-body irradiation were associated with a higher risk of solid cancers. Chronic graft-versus-host disease and being male were strongly linked with an increased risk of squamous-cell cancers of the buccal cavity and skin. These results show that patients undergoing bone marrow transplantation have an increased risk of developing new solid cancers later in life.

Since the conditioning regimen for patients with aplastic anemia is basically different from that for other patients requiring allogeneic bone marrow transplants, the risk of developing solid tumors had to be determined specifically for this cohort. In a study from the Hospital St. Louis, Paris, 147 patients with aplastic anemia (107 with acquired aplastic anemia; 40 with Fanconi's anemia) transplanted between 1980 and 1989 were evaluated for new cancers. The conditioning regimen included cyclophosphamide and thoracoabdominal irradiation (Socié et al., 1991). Four of the 147 patients developed a solid malignant tumor, all within the radiation field. The 8-year cumulative incidence rate was 22%. Meanwhile, in Seattle five of 330 transplanted patients with aplastic anemia developed secondary cancers: 318 patients had acquired aplastic anemia, and 12 patients Fanconi's anemia. The cumulative incidence of secondary cancers was 1.4% at 10 years, and 4.2% at 15 years. This latter report illustrates a remarkably lower risk of secondary tumors, as compared to the results from Paris. This difference may be accounted for by the exclusion of irradiation from the conditioning regimen and the lower proportion of Fanconi's anemia patients in the Seattle group compared with the Paris study (4% as compared to 27% in the French cohort) (Socié et al., 1991; Witherspoon et al., 1992). The influence of graft-versus-host disease and its treatment could not be determined.

Socié et al. (1992) evaluated the clinical outcome of patients who developed malignant solid tumors after bone marrow transplantation for severe aplastic anemia at the Hospital Saint Louis (Paris) between 1974 and 1991. Five cases of solid tumor occurred in 245 consecutive transplant patients. All five patients were treated with surgery and/or irradiation. The clinical course was unexpectedly difficult in four of these patients, whose secondary cancer relapsed early. Socié et al. (1992) focus on the unusually poor clinical outcome for patients who develop malignant tumors after bone marrow transplantation for severe aplastic anemia.

As previously presented for hematological cancers, the EBMT SAA Working Party examined the incidence of solid tumors in long-term survivors after treatment of aplastic anemia (Socié et al., 1993). The risk of cancer was analyzed overall, and according to treatment, relative to the risk in the general population. Eight solid tumors developed in the 860 patients who received immunosuppressive treatment (one nonHodgkin's lymphoma, seven solid tumors), and seven tumors in the 748 patients who received bone marrow transplants. The overall relative risk of cancer, including MDS and leukemia, was 5.50 ($P<0.001$) as compared with that in the general European population; the risk was 5.15 ($P<0.001$) after immunosuppressive treatment and 6.67 ($P<0.001$) after transplantation. The 10-year cumulative incidence rate of cancer was 18.8% after immunosuppressive treatment and 3.1% after transplantation. Risk factors for solid cancers after bone marrow transplantation were found to be age (RR = 1.11 per year) and the use of irradiation as a conditioning regimen before transplantation (RR = 9.56); such tumors occurred only in male patients. Despite the similar incidences of solid tumor after immunosuppression and bone marrow transplantation, transplanted patients have a greater overall risk of developing a malignant solid tumor compared with the general population.

As the risk factors for developing new malignancies after marrow transplantation had not been fully defined, a retrospective joint Seattle and Paris analysis was performed on data from 700 patients treated with allogeneic bone marrow transplantation (Deeg et al., 1996). Twenty-three patients developed a malignancy 1.4–221 months after transplantation, with an actuarial probability at 20 years of 14%. Five cases were lymphoid malignancies occurring at a median time of 3 months posttransplant, and 18 were solid tumors presenting at a median time of 99 months. Risk factors for solid tumors identified in multivariate analysis were chronic graft-versus-host disease treated with azathioprine, and the diagnosis of Fanconi's anemia. Azathioprine and irradiation were found to be significant risk factors for those with acquired aplastic anemia. The highest risk of developing a solid tumor was associated with the diagnosis of Fanconi's anemia.

Animal studies suggest that solid tumors occur after transplantation, but after a considerable delay. By extrapolation, secondary cancers in humans are expected to develop one or more decades after transplantation. In particular, squamous cell carcinoma of the skin and cancer of the oropharyngeal mucosa were observed. Irradiation is the major risk factor, but chronic graft-versus-host disease and its treatment are also associated with an increased incidence of secondary tumors. Therefore avoiding irradiation and preventing chronic graft-versus-host disease should reduce the risk of posttransplant tumors in aplastic anemia patients (Deeg and Socié, 1998).

Paroxysmal nocturnal hemoglobinuria

Paroxysmal nocturnal hemoglobinuria (PNH) is an acquired clonal disorder of hemopoietic stem cells caused by somatic mutation in the X-linked *PIG-A* gene, which encodes a protein involved in the synthesis of the glycosylphosphatidyl-inositol (GPI) anchor, by which many proteins are attached to the membrane. Aplastic anemia and PNH are clearly clinically related syndromes, sometimes called the aplastic anemia–PNH syndrome. Two pattern of evolution have been described. First, cases of PNH that present as a progressive pancytopenia with marrow failure, and, second, patients with primary aplastic anemia, in whom signs of PNH become manifest later (Conrad and Barton, 1979; Gardner, 1978; Lewis and Dacie, 1967; Thollot et al. 1984). This chapter presents data from clinical studies of PNH in aplastic anemia patients; further discussions of PNH in aplastic anemia are provided in Chapter 5.

In a study of late hematological disorders, including 137 patients with aplastic anemia, 12 of the 103 patients treated with ALG developed PNH, and one patient MDS together with PNH (Tichelli et al., 1988*b*). Four of the 13 patients with PNH only had biological anomalies, i.e., a positive sucrose test and/or Ham's test, and nine patients presented clinical symptoms of the disease. The cumulative risk of developing PNH at 15 years was 25% (Tichelli et al., 1994). To start with, the disease was usually limited to biological anomalies; however, most patients became symptomatic with time. The clinical evidence of PNH in aplastic anemia patients was hemolytic anemia with hemoglobinuria, abdominal or thoracic pain crisis, iron deficiency without any evidence of bleeding in multitransfused patients, and recurrent thromboses. Budd–Chirari syndrome, a particularly frequent complication in de novo PNH, was observed in three of six patients with recurrent thrombosis.

The development of PNH has also been evaluated in the large retrospective multicenter EBMT study on the long-term follow-up of 468 aplastic anemia patients treated with ALG (De Planque et al., 1989). PNH developed in 19 patients, and was diagnosed earlier in the course of the disease, at a median of 3 years after immunosuppression, compared with MDS (at a median of 4.6 years). The 5-year actuarial probability of developing PNH was between 15% and 20%.

The French Cooperative Group for the Study of Aplastic and Refractory Anemias reported data on the long-term evolution of a cohort of 156 nongrafted patients receiving androgen therapy (Najean and Haguenauer, 1990). Twenty-one of the 156 patients died 5 years or later after diagnosis. The cause of death was infection or hemorrhage secondary to pancytopenia in 12 patients, leukaemia in five, late side-effects following transfusion in two, and nonHodgkin's lymphoma or myocardial infarction in one each. Overall, 13 patients developed PNH, three of them exhibiting only biological anomalies. The probability of developing PNH at 12 years was about 10%. This unique recent study on the late effects in aplastic anemia patients not treated with bone marrow transplantation or immunosuppressants demonstrates that the aplastic anemia itself brings about the PNH, rather than the immunosuppressive treatment.

A large retrospective multicenter study (Socié et al., 1996) investigated factors that influence survival and the risk of complications in 220 patients with PNH diagnosed over a 46-year period (1950–1995) at participating French centers. An unequivocally positive Ham's test at least was required for disease diagnosis. Sixty-five of the 220 (30%) patients had a previous history of aplastic anemia. The 10-year survival estimate after diagnosis was 65%, and the cumulative probability of developing pancytopenia at 8 years was 15%, thrombosis 28%, and MDS 5%. Multivariate analysis revealed that survival was better for patients who developed aplastic anemia before PNH [RR = 0.32 (0.14–0.72), $P<0.02$]. Further factors associated with survival are the occurrence of thrombosis (RR = 10.2), evolution to pancytopenia (RR = 5.5), development of secondary MDS or acute leukemia (RR = 19.1), being older than 55 at diagnosis (RR = 4), needing additional treatment (RR = 2.1), and being thrombocytopenic at diagnosis (RR = 2.2). Factors associated with an increased risk of thrombosis during the disease course are thrombosis at diagnosis (RR = 5.1), being older than 54 years (RR = 2.6), and having an infection at diagnosis (RR = 2.6). The risk factors for progression to pancytopenia are not being anemic (RR = 4.03) or neutropenic (RR = 2.45) at diagnosis. The risk factors for developing MDS or acute leukemia are presenting with an abdominal pain crisis (RR = 10.5) and being diagnosed after 1983 (RR = 8.45). The better prognosis among patients with aplastic anemia before diagnosis of PNH is surprising. The only difference between these two groups of patients is that all those who had had aplastic anemia had been treated for it before they developed PNH. It is not yet clear whether the difference in outcome is because aplastic anemia–PNH syndrome and de novo PNH are separate diseases, or because the aplastic anemia patients had previously received immunosuppressive treatment.

In contrast to secondary MDS/leukemia or new solid cancers, PNH may present as an asymptomatic disease in those with aplastic anemia, with patients having only a positive Ham's test, or unspecific complaints. Therefore, centers who do not routinely perform regular PNH tests might miss the diagnosis. Today, flow cytometry analysis of peripheral blood cells is a simple and reliable method for establishing the diagnosis of PNH. Furthermore, the analysis of GPI-linked proteins is more sensitive than classic PNH tests and can be interpreted even in multitransfused patients (Kwong et al., 1994; Navenot et al., 1996). Granulocytes and monocytes appear to be the first cells affected, at a time when the erythrocytes are normal and the Ham's test negative (Schubert et al., 1991). During follow-up, the GPI-linked protein deficiency may appear in all types of peripheral blood cells (Fujioka and Yamada, 1993). The PNH clone may be detected in bone marrow cells before affected cells become evident in peripheral blood (Nakakuma et al., 1995). Using flow cytometry, GPI-deficient cells were observed in the bone marrow of four of ten patients with aplastic anemia, but not in their blood cells. More recently, Vu et al. (1996) demonstrated a deficiency of GPI-linked proteins in the platelets of eight out of nine patients with de novo PNH, and in five of 26 aplastic anemia patients.

According to immunophenotype analysis, the number of aplastic anemia patients with a clonal PNH defect is much higher than previously suspected (Schubert et al., 1994). A GPI-linked protein deficiency was identified in 27 out of 52 (52%) patients with aplastic anemia, affecting at least one cell population (Schrezenmeier et al., 1995). Granulocytes were involved in 25, monocytes in 18, lymphocytes in seven, and erythrocytes in seven of the 27 patients with a PNH clone. Normal cells and abnormal cells with a GPI-linked protein deficiency usually coexist, with a mean of 33% cells being affected (Griscelli–Bennaceur et al., 1995). Meanwhile, it has become evident that a PNH clone can be present when aplastic anemia is diagnosed; however, these patients do not usually present with a clinical hemolysis, because of the lack of cells during aplasia. However, flow cytometric analysis of granulocytes and monocytes allows the GPI-linked protein deficiency to be detected.

The behavior of a PNH clone may vary, presenting as an increase or a decrease. Spontaneous clinical long-term remissions have been observed in 12 of 80 (15%) patients with PNH (Hillmen et al., 1995). The Ham's test became negative for all nine patients who were tested, with flow cytometry revealing remission for erythrocytes in all five patients and for neutrophils in four. Furthermore, treatment with immunosuppression or growth factors might affect the behavior of this clone. Two of four patients with typical PNH responded to cyclosporin treatment, one presenting a hematological improvement, the other becoming transfusion independent (van Kamp et al., 1995). The correction of aplastic anemia complicating PNH was further observed in two of three patients treated with cyclosporin. However, the abnormal PNH clone persisted, despite the hematological improvement (Stoppa et al., 1996). Finally, one PNH patient with severe pancytopenia was treated with G-CSF and cyclosporin. Within 8 weeks, a trilineage response of hemopoiesis was observed. In this case, the proportion of normal to GPI-deficient granulocytes and monocytes increased significantly (Schubert et al., 1995). These observations suggest that some patients with aplastic anemia–PNH syndrome may benefit from being treated with immunosuppression or growth factors.

As retrospective studies show, aplastic anemia patients with deficient GPI-linked protein expression do not respond uniformly to standard immunosuppressive treatment. Schrezenmeier et al. (1995) described how GPI-deficient patients had a significantly lower response rate compared with nondeficient patients. The response rates were 30.4% and 85.7%, respectively ($P<0.0003$). It was postulated that a stem cell defect in patients with an abnormal PNH clone renders them resistant to immunosuppression. Similar data were observed by another German group (Schubert and Schmidt, 1993). Remission of the aplastic anemia after immunosuppression was observed in 13 of 17 patients who did not have a GPI-anchored protein defect, and in only three of 11 patients who did (Schubert and Schmidt, 1993). However, De Lord et al. (1998), studying patients from St. George's Hospital Medical School, London, did not find that those with a GPI-anchored protein defect had a similarly poor prognosis. A GPI-anchored protein defect was identified in 17 of 111 (15%) patients with aplastic anemia who had a negative Ham's test. Twelve patients received bone marrow transplantation, 94 patients were treated with immunosuppression, and 12 patients had neither transplantation nor immunosuppression. GPI-anchored protein expression status prior to immunosuppression did not appear to influence the response rate to treatment (50% response rate in those with GPI-anchored protein deficiency versus 75% in those without). The survival at 12 years after diagnosis was similar in both groups, at 90%.

Conclusion

After immunosuppressive treatment, there is an increased risk of developing a MDS/leukemia, with a 5-year actuarial probability between 15% and 20%. The risk factors for such a clonal complication include being older, having a splenectomy, or receiving multiple courses of immunosuppression. In 13–26% of the patients with secondary MDS or leukemia, chromosomal defects are observed. Trisomy 8 and monosomy 7 are the most frequent single anomaly. Secondary MDS/leukemia after aplastic anemia are also observed in untreated patients. Therefore, this clonal evolution seems to be related to the disease itself rather than the consequence of the immunosuppressive treatment. So far it is uncertain whether the administration of G-CSF favors the development of a secondary

MDS/leukemia. After successful bone marrow transplantation, MDS/leukemia is not usually observed, suggesting that transplanted patients might be cured from their disease.

After allogeneic bone marrow transplantation, there is a significantly higher risk of developing new solid cancers than in a general population. The cumulative incidence rate is between 1.4% and 22%, depending mostly on the type of conditioning regimen used for transplantation and on the number of Fanconi's anemia patients evaluated. New solid tumors occur after a considerable delay, and therefore their definite incidence still might be underestimated. The risk factors for solid cancers are found to be the age of the patient and the use of irradiation as a conditioning regimen. For this reason irradiation is no longer used as a standard regimen in treatments for aplastic anemia. After immunosuppression the risk of a new solid cancer is similar to that observed in a general population.

PNH is closely related to aplastic anemia. In the same patient, it can precede the onset of aplastic anemia, or in contrast appear during the course of the disease. After immunosuppressive treatment the cumulative risk of developing PNH at 10 years is between 15% and 25%. The clinical manifestations of PNH in patients with aplastic anemia may vary widely. PNH may present as an asymptomatic disease, with patients having only a positive Ham's test. In contrast, other patients develop severe thrombotic complications or pancytopenia leading to bleeding and infection. As for MDS or leukemia, PNH does not usually appear after successful bone marrow transplantation.

References

Appelbaum, F., Barrall, J., Storb, R., Ramberg, R., Doney, K., Sale, G. and Thomas, E. D. (1987) Clonal cytogenetic abnormalities in patients with otherwise typical aplastic anemia. *Experimental Hematology*, **15**, 1134–9.

Bacigalupo, A., Broccia, G., Corda, G., Arcese, W., Carotenuto, M., Gallamini, A., Locatelli, F., Mori, P. G., Saracco, P. and Todeschini, G. (1995) Antilymphocyte globulin, cyclosporin, and granulocyte colony-stimulating factor in patients with acquired severe aplastic anemia (SAA): a pilot study of the EBMT SAA Working Party. *Blood*, **85**, 1348–53.

Bacigalupo, A., Hows, J., Gluckman, E., Nissen, C., Marsh, J. C. W., Van Lint, M. T., Congiu, M., De Planque, M. M., Ernst, P., McCann, S., Ragavachar, A., Frickhofen, N., Würsch, A., Marmont, A. M. and Gordon–Smith, E. C. (1988) Bone marrow transplantation (BMT) versus immunosuppression for the treatment of severe aplastic anaemia: a report of the EBMT SAA Working Party. *British Journal of Haematology*, **70**, 177–82.

Benaim, E., Hvizdala, E. V., Papenhausen, P. and Moscinski, L. C. (1995) Spontaneous remission in monosomy 7 myelodysplastic syndrome. *British Journal of Haematology*, **89**, 947–8.

Browne, P. V., Lawler, M., Humphries, P. and McCann, S. R. (1991) Donor–cell leukemia after bone marrow transplantation for severe aplastic anemia. *New England Journal of Medicine*, **325**, 710–13.

Camitta, B. M. and Doney, K. (1990) Immunosuppressive therapy for aplastic anemia: indi-
    cations, agents, mechanisms, and results. *American Journal of Pediatric Hematology/
    Oncology*, **12**, 411–24.

Conrad, M. E. and Barton, J. C. (1979) The aplastic anemia–paroxysmal nocturnal hemo-
    globinuria syndrome. *American Journal of Hematology*, **7**, 61–7.

Crump, M., Larratt, L. M., Maki, E., Curtis, J. E., Minden, M. D., Meharchand, J. M., Lipton,
    J. H. and Messner, H. A. (1992) Treatment of adults with severe aplastic anemia: primary
    therapy with antithymocyte globulin (ATG) and rescue of ATG failures with bone marrow
    transplantation. *American Journal of Medicine*, **92**, 596–602.

Curtis, R. E., Rowlings, P. A., Deeg, H. J., Shriner, D. A., Socié, G., Travis, L. B., Horowitz, M.
    M., Witherspoon, R. P., Hoover, R. N., Sobocinski, K. A., Fraumeni, J. F. J. and Boice, J. D. J.
    (1997) Solid cancers after bone marrow transplantation [see comments]. *New England
    Journal of Medicine*, **336**, 897–904.

Dameshek, W. (1967) Riddle: what do aplastic anemia, paroxysmal nocturnal hemoglobi-
    nuria and hypoplastic leukemia have in common? *Blood*, **30**, 251–4.

De Lord, C., Tooze, J. A., Saso, R., Marsh, J. C. and Gordon–Smith, E. (1998) Deficiency of gly-
    cosylphosphatidyl inositol-anchored proteins in patients with aplastic anaemia does not
    affect response to immunosuppressive therapy. *British Journal of Haematology*, **101**, 90–3.

De Planque, M. M., Bacigalupo, A., Würsch, A., Hows, J., Devergie, A., Frickhofen, N., Brand,
    A. and Nissen, C. (1989) Long-term follow-up of severe aplastic anaemia patients treated
    with antilymphocyte globulin. *British Journal of Haematology*, **73**, 121–6.

De Planque, M. M., Kluin–Nelemans, H. C., Van Krieken, H. J. M., Kluin, P. M., Brand, A.,
    Beverstock, G. C., Willemze, R. and Van Rood, J. J. (1988) Evolution of acquired severe
    aplastic anaemia to myelodysplastic and subsequent leukaemia in adults. *British Journal
    of Haematology*, **70**, 55.

Deeg, H. J. (1990*a*) Delayed complications and long-term effects after bone marrow trans-
    plantation. *Hematology and Oncology Clinics of North America*, **4**, 641–57.

Deeg, H. J. (1990*b*) Early and late complications of bone marrow transplantation. *Current
    Opinions in Oncology*, **2**, 297–307.

Deeg, H. J. and Socié, G. (1998) Malignancies after hemopoietic stem cell transplantation:
    many questions, some answers. *Blood*, **91**, 1833–44.

Deeg, H. J., Socié, G., Schoch, G., Henry–Amar, M., Witherspoon, R. P., Devergie, A., Sullivan,
    K. M., Gluckman, E. and Storb, R. (1996) Malignancies after marrow transplantation for
    aplastic anemia and Fanconi anemia: a joint Seattle and Paris analysis of results in 700
    patients. *Blood*, **87**, 386–92.

Delamore, I. W. and Geary, C. G. (1971) Aplastic anaemia, acute myeloblastic leukaemia,
    and oxymetholone. *British Medical Journal*, **2**, 743–5.

Doney, K., Leisenring, W., Storb, R. and Appelbaum, F. R. (1997) Primary treatment of
    acquired aplastic anemia: outcomes with bone marrow transplantation and immuno-
    suppressive therapy. *Annals of Internal Medicine*, **126**, 107–15.

Doney, K., Pepe, M., Storb, R., Bryant, E., Anasetti, C., Appelbaum, F. R., Buckner, C. D.,
    Sanders, J., Singer, J., Sullivan, K. M., Weiden, P. and Hansen, J. (1992) Immunosuppressive
    treatment of aplastic anemia: results of a prospective randomized trial of antilymphocyte
    globulin (ATG), methylprednisolone, and oxymetholone to ATG, very high-dose methyl-
    prednisolone, and oxymetholone. *Blood*, **79**, 2566–71.

Duell, T., Van Lint, M. T., Ljungman, P., Tichelli, A., Socié, G., Apperley, J. F., Weiss, M., Cohen, A., Nekolla, E. and Kolb, H. J. (1997) Health and functional status of long-term survivors of bone marrow transplantation. *Annals of Internal Medicine*, **126**, 184–92.

Fohlmeister, J., Fischer, R., Modder, B., Rister, M. and Schaefer, M. E. (1985) Aplastic anaemia and the hypocellular myelodysplastic syndrome: histomorphological, diagnostic and prognostic features. *Journal of Clinical Pathology*, **38**, 1218–24.

Frickhofen, N., Kaltwasser, J. P., Schrezenmeier, H., Ragavachar, A., Vogt, H. G., Herrmann, F., Freund, M., Meusers, P., Salama, A. and Heimpel, H. (1991) Treatment of aplastic anemia with antilymphocyte globulin and methylprednisolone with or without cyclosporine. *New England Journal of Medicine*, **324**, 1297–304.

Frisch, B., Lewis, S. M. and Sherman, D. (1975) The ultrastructure of dyserythropoiesis in aplastic anaemia. *British Journal of Haematology*, **29**, 245–51.

Fujioka, S. and Yamada, T. (1993) Decay-accelerating factor and CD59 expression in peripheral blood cells in aplastic anaemia and report of a case of paroxysmal nocturnal haemoglobinuria secondary to aplastic anaemia. *British Journal of Haematology*, **83**, 660–2.

Führer, M., Rampf, U., Ebell, W., Friedrich, W., Gadner, H., Haas, R., Janka, G., Niemeywer, C., Zeidler, C. and Bender–Götze, C. (1998) Immunosuppressive therapy and bone marrow transplantation for aplastic anemia in children: results of the German/Austrian SAA 94 Study. *Bone Marrow Transplantation*, **21** [Suppl 1], S45.

Gardner, F. (1978) Aplastic anemia syndrome in paroxysmal nocturnal hemoglobinuria (PNH). In *Aplastic anemia*, ed. S. Hibano, F. Takaku, N. T. Shahidi, pp. 273–82. Baltimore, MD: University Park Press.

Gluckman, E., Horowitz, M. M., Champlin, R. E., Hows, J., Bacigalupo, A., Biggs, J. C., Camitta, B., Gale, R. P., Gordon–Smith, E., Marmont, A. M., Masaoka, T., Ramsay, N. K., Rimm, A. A., Rozman, C., Sobocinski, K. A., Speck, B. and Bortin, M. M. (1992*a*) Bone marrow transplantation for severe aplastic anemia: influence of conditioning and graft-versus-host disease prophylaxis regimens on outcome. *Blood*, **79**, 269–75.

Gluckman, E., Esperou–Bourdeau, H., Baruchel, A., Boogaerts, M., Briere, J., Donadio, D., Leverger, G., Leporrier, M., Reiffers, J. and Janvier, M. (1992*b*) Multicenter randomized study comparing cyclosporin-A alone and antithymocyte globulin with prednisone for treatment of severe aplastic anemia. *Blood*, **79**, 2540–6.

Griscelli–Bennaceur, A., Gluckman, E., Scrobohaci, M. L., Jonveaux, P., Vu, T., Bazarbachi, A., Carosella, E. D., Sigaux, F. and Socié, G. (1995) Aplastic anemia and paroxysmal nocturnal hemoglobinuria: search for a pathogenetic link. *Blood*, **85**, 1354–63.

Hillmen, P., Lewis, S. M., Bessler, M., Luzzatto, L. and Dacie, J. V. (1995) Natural history of paroxysmal nocturnal hemoglobinuria. *New England Journal of Medicine*, **333**, 1253–8.

Hughes, R. T., Milligan, D., Smith, G. M., Leyland, M. J. and Gordon–Smith, E. (1988) A second bone marrow transplant for acute myeloid leukaemia after transplantation for aplastic anaemia. *British Journal of Haematology*, **68**, 391.

Imashuku, S., Hibi, S., Kataoka–Morimoto, Y., Yoshihara, T., Ikushima, S., Morioka, Y. and Todo, S. (1995) Myelodysplasia and acute myeloid leukaemia in cases of aplastic anaemia and congenital neutropenia following G-CSF administration. *British Journal of Haematology*, **89**, 188–90.

Iwabuchi, A., Ohyashiki, K., Ohyashiki, J. H. et al., (1992) Trisomy of chromosome 8 in mye-lodysplastic syndrome. Significance of fluctuating trisomy 8 population. *Cancer Genetics and Cytogenetics*, **62**, 70–4.

Kansu, E. and Erslev, A. J. (1976) Aplastic anaemia with 'hot pockets'. *Scandinavian Journal of Haematology*, **17**, 326–34.

King, J. B. and Burns, D. G. (1972) Aplastic anaemia, oxymetholone and acute myeloid leu-kaemia. *South African Medical Journal*, **46**, 1622–3.

Klingemann, H. G., Storb, R., Sanders, J., Deeg, H. J., Appelbaum, F. and Thomas, E. D. (1986) Acute lymphoblastic leukaemia after bone marrow transplantation for aplastic anaemia. *British Journal of Haematology*, **63**, 47–50.

Kojima, S., Tsuchida, M. and Matsuyama, T. (1992) Myelodysplasia and leukemia after treat-ment of aplastic anemia with G–CSF. *New England Journal of Medicine*, **326**, 1294.

Kolb, H. J. and Bender–Gotze, C. (1990) Late complications after allogeneic bone marrow transplantation for leukaemia. *Bone Marrow Transplantation*, **6**, 61–72.

Kolb, H. J., Duell, T., Socié, G., Van Lint, E., Carreras, A., Tichelli, A., Ljungman, P., Jacobson, J. F., Apperley, B., Hertenstein, M., Weiss, M., Nekolla, E. and Goldstone, A. H. (1995) New malignancies in patients surviving more than 5 years after bone marrow transplantation. *Blood*, **86**, 460a.

Kolb, H. J., Socié, G., Duell, T., Van Lint, M. T., Tichelli, A., Weiss, M., Nekolla, E., Ljungman, P., Apperley, J. F., Jacobsen, N., Van Weel–Sipman, M., Carreras, E. and Goldstone, A. H. (1996) New malignancies in patients surviving more than 5 years after marrow transplan-tation. *Bone Marrow Transplantation*, **17** [Suppl. 1], S143.

Kwong, Y. L., Lee, C. P., Chan, T. K. and Chan, L. C. (1994) Flow cytometric measurement of glycosylphosphatidyl-inositol-linked surface proteins on blood cells of patients with par-oxysmal nocturnal hemoglobinuria. *American Journal of Clinical Pathology*, **102**, 30–5.

Lewis, S. M. (1979) Dyserythropoiesis in aplastic anaemia. In *Aplastic anemia*, ed. C. G. Geary, pp. 82–107. London: Ballière Tindall.

Lewis, S. M. and Dacie, J. V. (1967) The aplastic anaemia–paroxysmal nocturnal haemoglob-inuria syndrome. *British Journal of Haematology*, **13**, 236–51.

Manoharan, A., Horsley, R. and Pitney, W. R. (1981) Myelomatosis in aplastic anaemia – a true association of fortuitous occurrence. *Pathology*, **13**, 771–3.

Marsh, J. C. and Geary, C. G. (1991) Is aplastic anaemia a pre-leukaemic disorder? [edito-rial]. *British Journal of Haematology*, **77**, 447–52.

Marsh, J. C., Chang, J., Testa, N. G., Hows, J. and Dexter, T. M. (1990) The hemopoietic defect in aplastic anemia assessed by long-term marrow culture. *Blood*, **76**, 1–10.

Marsh, J. C., Chang, J., Testa, N. G., Hows, J. and Dexter, T. M. (1991) In vitro assessment of marrow 'stem cell' and stromal cell function in aplastic anaemia. *British Journal of Haematology*, **78**, 258–67.

Matsuda, A., Yagasaki, F., Jinnai, I., Kusumoto, S., Murohashi, I., Bessho, M. and Hirashima, K. (1998) Trisomy 8 may not be related to the pathogenesis of myelodysplastic syn-dromes: disappearance of trisomy 8 with refractory anaemia without haematological improvement. *European Journal of Haematology*, **60**, 260–1.

Mikhailova, N., Sessarego, M., Fugazza, G., Caimo, A., De Filippi, S., Van Lint, M. T., Bregante, S., Valeriani, A., Mordini, N., Lamparelli, T., Gualandi, F., Occhini, D. and Bacigalupo, A. (1996) Cytogenetic abnormalities in patients with severe aplastic anemia. *Haematologica*, **81**, 418–22.

Mir, M. A. and Geary, C. G. (1980) Aplastic anaemia: an analysis of 174 patients. *Postgraduate Medical Journal*, **56**, 322–9.

Mufti, G. J., Hamblin, T. J. and Lee–Potter, J. P. (1983) The aplasia–leukaemia syndrome: aplastic anaemia followed by dyserythropoiesis, myeloproliferative syndrome and acute leukaemia. *Acta Haematologica*, **69**, 349–52.

Najean, Y. and Haguenauer, O. (1990) Long-term (5 to 20 years) Evolution of nongrafted aplastic anemias. The Cooperative Group for the Study of Aplastic and Refractory Anemias. *Blood*, **76**, 2222–8.

Nakakuma, H., Nagakura, S., Iwamoto, N., Kawaguchi, T., Hidaka, M., Horikawa, K., Kagimoto, T., Shido, T. and Takatsuki, K. (1995) Paroxysmal nocturnal hemoglobinuria clone in bone marrow of patients with pancytopenia. *Blood*, **85**, 1371–6.

Navenot, J. M., Bernard, D., Harousseau, J. L., Muller, J. Y. and Blanchard, D. (1996) Expression of glycosyl-phosphatidylinositol-linked glycoproteins in blood cells from paroxysmal nocturnal haemoglobinuria patients: a flow cytometry study using CD55, CD58 and CD59 monoclonal antibodies. *Leukemia and Lymphoma*, **21**, 143–51.

Nissen, C., Cornu, P., Gratwohl, A. and Speck, B. (1980) Peripheral blood cells from patients with aplastic anaemia in partial remission suppress growth of their own bone marrow precursors in culture. *British Journal of Haematology*, **45**, 233–43.

Nissen, C., Gratwohl, A., Tichelli, A., Stebler, C., Wursch, A., Moser, Y., dalle Carbonare, V., Signer, E., Buser, M. and Ritz, R. (1993) Gender and response to antilymphocyte globulin (ALG) for severe aplastic anaemia. *British Journal of Haematology*, **83**, 319–25.

Ohara, A., Kojima, S., Hamajima, N., Tsuchida, M., Imashuku, S., Ohta, S., Sasaki, H., Okamura, J., Sugita, K., Kigasawa, H., Kiriyama, Y., Akatsuka, J. and Tsukimoto, I. (1997) Myelodysplastic syndrome and acute myelogenous leukemia as a late clonal complication in children with acquired aplastic anemia. *Blood*, **90**, 1009–13.

Ohsaka, A., Sugahara, Y., Imai, Y. and Kikuchi, M. (1995) Evolution of severe aplastic anemia to myelodysplasia with monosomy 7 following granulocyte colony-stimulating factor, erythropoietin and high-dose methylprednisolone combination therapy [see comments]. *Internal Medicine*, **34**, 892–5.

Orlandi, E., Alessandrino, E. P., Caldera, D. and Bernasconi, C. (1988) Adult leukemia developing after aplastic anemia: report of 8 cases. *Acta Haematologica*, **79**, 174–7.

Paquette, R. L., Tebyani, N., Frane, M., Ireland, P., Ho, W. G., Champlin, R. E. and Nimer, S. D. (1995) Long-term outcome of aplastic anemia in adults treated with antithymocyte globulin: comparison with bone marrow transplantation. *Blood*, **85**, 283–90.

Passweg, J. R., Socié, G., Hinterberger, W., Bacigalupo, A., Biggs, J. C., Camitta, B. M., Champlin, R. E., Gale, R. P., Gluckman, E., Gordon–Smith, E. C., Hows, J. M., Klein, J. P., Nugent, M. L., Pasquini, R., Rowlings, P. A., Speck, B., Tichelli, A., Zhang, M. J., Horowitz, M. M. and Bortin, M. M. (1997) Bone marrow transplantation for severe aplastic anemia: has outcome improved? *Blood*, **90**, 858–64.

Renneboog, B., Hansen, P., Heimann, A., Mulder, D., Janssen, F. and Ferster, A. (1996) Spontaneous remission in a patient with therapy-related myelodysplastic syndrome (t-MDS) with monosomy 7. *British Journal of Haematology*, **92**, 696–8.

Rosenfeld, S. J., Kimball, J., Vining, D. and Young, N. S. (1995) Intensive immunosuppression with antithymocyte globulin and cyclosporin as treatment for severe acquired aplastic anemia. *Blood*, **85**, 3058–65.

Rudivic, R., Jovcic, G., Bilijanovic–Paunovic, L., Stojanovic, N., Mijoric, A. and Partivic Kentera, V. (1985) Myelopoiesis and erythropoiesis of bone marrow cells cultured in vitro in patients recovered from aplastic anaemia. *British Journal of Haematology*, **70**, 55–62.

Schrezenmeier, H., Hertenstein, B., Wagner, B., Raghavachar, A. and Heimpel, H. (1995) A pathogenetic link between aplastic anemia and paroxysmal nocturnal hemoglobinuria is suggested by a high frequency of aplastic anemia patients with a deficiency of phosphatidylinositol glycan anchored proteins. [Published erratum appears in *Experimental Hematology*, 1995, **23**, 181.] *Experimental Hematology*, **23**, 81–7.

Schubert, J., Alvarado, M., Uciechowski, P., Zielinska–Skowronek, M., Freund, M., Vogt, H. and Schmidt, R. E. (1991) Diagnosis of paroxysmal nocturnal haemoglobinuria using immunophenotyping of peripheral blood cells. *British Journal of Haematology*, **79**, 487–92.

Schubert, J. and Schmidt, R. E. (1993) The GPI-anchoring defect characteristic for paroxysmal nocturnal hemoglobinuria in patients with aplastic anemia. In *Aplastic anemia: current perspectives on the pathogenesis and treatment*, ed. A. Raghavchar, H. Schrezenmeier and N. Frickhoven, pp. 49–57. Vienna: Blackwell MZV.

Schubert, J., Scholz, C. and Schmidt, R. E. (1995) Experimental therapy of hypoplastic paroxysmal nocturnal hemoglobinuria. *Immun. Infekt.*, **23**, 65–6.

Schubert, J., Vogt, H. G., Zielinska–Skowronek, M., Freund, M., Kaltwasser, J. P., Hoelzer, D. and Schmidt, R. E. (1994) Development of the glycosylphosphatitylinositol-anchoring defect characteristic for paroxysmal nocturnal hemoglobinuria in patients with aplastic anemia. *Blood*, **83**, 2323–8.

Socié, G. (1996) Could aplastic anaemia be considered a pre-pre-leukaemic disorder? *European Journal of Haematology Supplement*, **60**, 60–3.

Socié, G., Henry–Amar, M., Bacigalupo, A., Hows, J., Tichelli, A., Ljungman, P., McCann, S. R., Frickhofen, N., Van't Veer–Korthof, E. and Gluckman, E. (1993) Malignant tumors occurring after treatment of aplastic anemia. European Bone Marrow Transplantation – Severe Aplastic Anaemia Working Party. *New England Journal of Medicine*, **329**, 1152–7.

Socié, G., Henry–Amar, M., Cosset, J. M., Devergie, A., Girinsky, T. and Gluckman, E. (1991) Increased incidence of solid malignant tumors after bone marrow transplantation for severe aplastic anemia [see comments]. *Blood*, **78**, 277–9.

Socié, G., Henry–Amar, M., Devergie, A., Wibault, P., Neiger, M., Cosset, J. M. and Gluckman, E. (1992) Poor clinical outcome of patients developing malignant solid tumors after bone marrow transplantation for severe aplastic anemia. *Leukemia and Lymphoma*, **7**, 419–23.

Socié, G., Mary, J. Y., de Gramont, A., Rio, B., Leporrier, M., Rose, C., Heudier, P., Rochant, H., Cahn, J. Y. and Gluckman, E. (1996) Paroxysmal nocturnal haemoglobinuria: long-term follow-up and prognostic factors. French Society of Haematology [see comments]. *Lancet*, **348**, 573–7.

Speck, B., Tichelli, A., Gratwohl, A. and Nissen, C. (1990) Treatment of severe aplastic anemia: a 12-year follow-up of patients after bone marrow transplantation or after therapy with antilymphocyte globulin. In *Aplastic anemia and other bone marrow failure syndromes*, ed. N. T. Shahidi, pp. 96–103. New York: Springer–Verlag.

Stoppa, A. M., Vey, N., Sainty, D., Arnoulet, C., Camerlo, J., Cappiello, M. A., Gastaut, J. A. and Maraninchi, D. (1996) Correction of aplastic anaemia complicating paroxysmal nocturnal haemoglobinuria: absence of eradication of the PNH clone and dependence of response on cyclosporin A administration. *British Journal of Haematology*, **93**, 42–4.

Thollot, F., Bordigoni, P. and Olive, D. (1984) Hémoglobinurie paroxystique nocturne et aplasie médullaire. *Archives Francaise de Pediatrie*, **41**, 197–200.

Tichelli, A., Gratwohl, A., Nissen, C., Signer, E., Stebler Gysi, C. and Speck, B. (1992) Morphology in patients with severe aplastic anemia treated with antilymphocyte globulin. *Blood*, **80**, 337–45.

Tichelli, A., Gratwohl, A., Nissen, C. and Speck, B. (1994) Late clonal complications in severe aplastic anemia. *Leukemia and Lymphoma*, **12**, 167–75.

Tichelli, A., Gratwohl, A., Wursch, A., Nissen, C. and Speck, B. (1988*a*) Secondary leukemia after severe aplastic anemia. *Blut*, **56**, 79–81.

Tichelli, A., Gratwohl, A., Würsch, A., Nissen, C. and Speck, B. (1988*b*) Late haematological complications in severe aplastic anaemia. *British Journal of Haematology*, **69**, 413–18.

Tichelli, A., Socié, G., Marsh, J. C., McCann, S., Hows, J., Schrezenmeier, H., Marín, P., Hinterberger, W., Ljungman, P., Ragavachar, A., Van't Veer–Korthof, E., Gratwohl, A. and Bacigalupo, A. (1996) Cytogenetic abnormalities in aplastic anaemia. *Bone Marrow Transplantation*, **17** [Suppl. 1], S56.

Tsuzuki, M., Okamoto, M., Yamaguchi, T., Ino, T., Ezaki, K. and Hirano, M. (1997) [Myelodysplastic syndrome with monosomy 7 following combination therapy with granulocyte colony–stimulating factor, cyclosporin A and danazole in an adult patient with severe aplastic anemia.] *Rinsho Ketsueki*, **38**, 745–51.

van Kamp, H., van Imhoff, G. W., de Wolf, J. T., Smit, J. W., Halie, M. R. and Vellenga, E. (1995) The effect of cyclosporin on haematological parameters in patients with paroxysmal nocturnal haemoglobinuria. *British Journal of Haematology*, **89**, 79–82.

Vu, T., Griscelli–Bennaceur, A., Gluckman, E., Sigaux, F., Carosella, E. D., Menier, C., Scrobohaci, M. L. and Socié, G. (1996) Aplastic anaemia and paroxysmal nocturnal haemoglobinuria: a study of the GPI-anchored proteins on human platelets. *British Journal of Haematology*, **93**, 586–9.

Witherspoon, R. P., Storb, R., Pepe, M., Longton, G. and Sullivan, K. M. (1992) Cumulative incidence of secondary solid malignant tumors in aplastic anemia patients given marrow grafts after conditioning with chemotherapy alone [letter; comment]. *Blood*, **79**, 289–91.

Yamazaki, E., Kanamori, H., Taguchi, J., Harano, H., Mohri, H. and Okubo, T. (1997) The evidence of clonal evolution with monosomy 7 in aplastic anemia following granulocyte colony-stimulating factor using the polymerase chain reaction. *Blood Cells, Molecules, and Diseases*, **23**, 213–18.

Young, N. (1994) Definitive treatment of acquired aplastic anemia. In *Aplastic anemia: acquired and inherited*, ed. N. Young and B. P. Alter, pp. 159–200. Philadelphia: WB Saunders.

16

Guidelines for treating aplastic anemia

Consensus Document of a group of international experts*

Decision making: immunosuppressive treatment versus allogeneic bone marrow transplantation as first-line treatment of aplastic anemia

The choice of primary treatment should be based on the availability of an HLA-identical sibling, the age of the patient and the severity of the disease. Patients without a donor should be given immunosuppressive therapy (IS) as the first-line therapy. When there is an available matched donor, and for those under 50 years of age, bone marrow transplantation (BMT) is probably the treatment of choice. Some thought that a first course of IS could also be considered for those above the age of 40 with high neutrophil counts.

Bone marrow transplantation

HLA-matched sibling transplantation

Five- to 10-year survivals of about 90% have been reported following BMT (see Chapter 12). There are at least two reasons for the recent improvement in survival of transplant patients. These include decreased incidences of marrow graft rejection, and of acute graft-versus-host disease (GVHD), the latter through better GVHD prevention regimens, e.g., methotrexate and cyclosporin. Rejection has decreased, in turn, because of several changes in the management of patients with aplastic anemia who are candidates for BMT. One change has been the more judicious use of transfusions before transplant, which are known to sensitize patients to minor histocompatibility antigens on donor cells. Also, removing sensitizing white blood cells from transfusion products has contributed to a reduced

---

* The speakers and discussion leaders of the Consensus Conference were:

H. Schrezenmeier, A. Bacigalupo, M. Aglietta, B. Camitta, N. Frickhofen, M. Führer, E. Gluckman, A. Gratwohl, H. Heimpel, J. Hows, S. Kojima, A. Locasciulli, A. Marmont, P. Marín, J. Marsh, S. McCann, J. Passweg, R. Pasquini, M. Podesta, G. Socié, R. Storb, A. Tichelli, B. Torok-Storb, A. Wodnar-Filipovicz, N. Young.

Bone marrow transplantation

Preparative regimen and posttransplant immunosuppression in HLA-matched sibling transplantation of aplastic anemia:

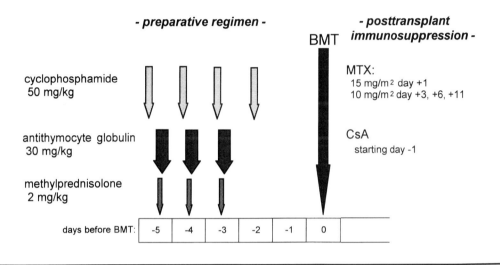

Figure 16.1. Schematic representation of the recommended conditioning regimen for allotransplantation of patients with aplastic anemia who are not entered in a clinical trial.

risk of sensitization and subsequent marrow graft rejection. Finally, the immunosuppressive qualities of the conditioning programs used to prepare patients for transplant have improved. While irradiation-based programs have been effective in reducing rejection, they have accomplished their goal at the price of increasing the incidence of transplant-related complications. A combination of cyclophosphamide and antithymocyte globulin was found to be as effective as irradiation at preventing rejection, and has a better long-term outcome. As for conditioning regimens, irridiation-based regimens should be avoided because of the higher associated likelihood of inducing secondary cancer, the deleterious effects on fertility, and the potential detrimental effects on growth and development, a policy that would be particularly important for pediatric patients.

Participation in the ongoing clinical trials by the European Blood and Bone Marrow Transplantation (EBMT) group and the International Bone Marrow Transplantation Registry (IBMTR) is encouraged. For patients not entered into a clinical trial, a preparative regimen with cyclophosphamide and ATG and posttransplant immunosuppression with methotrexate and cyclosporin A is recommended (see schema in Figure 16.1).

As for transfusing before marrow transplant, animal experiments suggest that in vitro irradiation of all blood products further reduces the risk of sensitization to minor histocompatibility antigens. Blood product irradiation is simple and should, therefore, become an integral part of managing aplastic anemia patients.

In addition, until a given patient's cytomegalovirus antibody status is known, all transfusions should be either from cytomegalovirus-antigen-negative individuals or infused through leukocyte filters, to reduce the risk of inadvertent transmission of this potentially pathogenic virus (see also Chapter 9).

For patients older than 50 years a number of participants favored front-line therapy with ATG, and cyclosporin, with or without hemopoietic growth factors. Then BMT should only be considered if that failed to accomplish a remission. Other participants pointed out that, while this approach is theoretically attractive, it may be difficult to accomplish practically. Difficulties may arise from the fact that patients who fail to respond to immunosuppressive therapy often have become infected, and refractory to random donor platelet transfusions, and these complications may jeopardize the success of subsequent marrow transplants.

Recent animal data were presented that emphasized the role of postgrafting immunosuppression not only for controlling GVHD, but also for minimizing host-versus-graft reactions, and thereby diminishing the risk of graft failure. In this regard, the combination of methotrexate and cyclosporin was found to be more effective then cyclosporin alone. Given these differences, future studies aimed at evaluating novel conditioning programs for transplantation must consider the effect of postgrafting immunosuppression on engraftment.

Finally, pretreatment work-up of any patient diagnosed with 'aplastic anemia' must rule out myelodysplastic syndrome. Patients with myelodysplastic syndrome should all be considered as marrow transplant candidates, given that transplant is the only current therapy that cures a high proportion of these patients.

The use of peripheral mobilized stem cells (PBSC) for primary allogeneic BMT in aplastic anemia should be considered experimental: the risk of chronic GVHD seems greater with PBSC and results with bone marrow are extremely good.

Unrelated and family-mismatched donor transplants

Alternative donor transplants are not indicated as first-line therapy for patients with severe aplastic anemia (SAA) of any age. The exception is a patient with an HLA-phenotypically matched family donor (see below).

Recent registry data (1989–94) from the IBMTR and the EBMT SAA Working Party, prospectively collected data from the International Marrow Unrelated Search and Transplant (IMUST) Study and single-center data from Seattle all indicate a 2-year posttransplant actuarial survival of 35–45%. Overall, patients were young, with a median age of 17–18 years in the different datasets. Unifactorial analysis of age and survival did not show a significant difference between patients older and younger than the median age. The EBMT data indicated significantly worse survival for patients transplanted more than 2 years from diagnosis (for details see Chapter 13).

Alternative donor transplants should be considered as salvage therapy for patients failing to respond to one or more courses of immunosuppressive therapy. A prospective study of patients failing one course of immunosuppressive therapy was proposed to compare survival of patients with a well-matched alternative donor with that of patients who lacked such a donor who would be treated with a second course of immunosuppressive therapy.

As to the choice between one HLA-A, -B, -DR-antigen-mismatched family donor and a phenotypically matched unrelated donor, comparative data are limited and neither IBMTR nor EBMT analyses favored unrelated compared with alternative family donors.

Recently, the results of unrelated donor transplants for leukemia have improved, because of using donors matched by high-resolution DNA typing for HLA. Application of high-resolution typing is now critically important for matching donors to patients with SAA. Seattle data indicate that a serological cross-match (patient serum with donor peripheral-blood mononuclear cells) should be performed in all cases where the recipient and donor are HLA mismatched. A positive crossmatch precludes the use of the potential donor.

Data presented from the IBMTR and from the IMUST studies showed that the probability of graft failure was in excess of 35% in alternative donor transplants using protocols without irradiation. Data from Seattle and the IMUST Study indicate that although engraftment was improved survival of patients treated with ablative doses of total-body irradiation (TBI) was reduced. In a series of alternative donor transplants in children receiving ablative TBI combined with partial T-cell depletion in the Milwaukee program, survival is excellent. However, innovative regimens using less intense TBI [either nonablative TBI (2×200 to 3×200 cGY) or limited field irradiation] should be developed in order to decrease both acute and chronic regimen-related toxicities. There are insufficient data to reach a consensus on the use of in vivo or in vitro T-cell depletion.

Data from Seattle indicate that the results of HLA phenotypically matched family donor transplants are close to the results obtained using HLA-identical sibling donors when combining ATG with cyclophosphamide in the pretransplant protocol and with cyclosporin and methotrexate as postgraft immunosuppression. Including irradiation in the protocol is not necessary. HLA phenotypically matched transplants should be carried out in the same way as HLA-identical sibling transplants.

Immunosuppression

Primary immunosuppressive treatment of patients with <u>vSAA / SAA</u>:

ATG (Lymphoglobulin Merieux): 0.75 ml/kg b.w. per day *
ATG (ATGAM): 40 mg/kg b.w. per day **

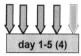

day 1-5 (4)

Methylprednisolone: 1mg/kg b.w. per day

| day 1-14 | tapering off until day 28 |

Cyclosporin: 5 mg/kg b.w. per day; blood level adjusted

| day 1 until day 112 (at least; further treatment depending on response) |

*   Lymphoglobulin is recommended for 5 consecutive days
** ATGAM is recommended for 4 consecutive days

Figure 16.2. Schematic representation of the recommended treatment schedule for patients with aplastic anemia not entered in a clinical trial.

Immunosuppressive treatment

Patients who do fulfill the eligibility criteria for primary allogeneic BMT should receive immunosuppressive treatment.

Many aspects of treatment for aplastic anemia warrant randomized prospective clinical trials. Since aplastic anemia is a rare disease, patients should be enrolled in ongoing multicentric trials. To guarantee the comparability of future clinical trials, we strongly recommend using uniform definitions of response criteria for forthcoming trials. The criteria proposed by the Consensus Conference are listed in Table 16.1.

As the first-line treatment of severe or very severe aplastic anemia an ATG-based regimen combined with cyclosporin A (CSA) is recommended (see Figure 16.2). Clinical trials with cyclosporin alone or cyclosporin plus granulocyte colony-stimulating factor (G-CSF) produced low response rates. The best response rates and survival were reported following ATG + CSA or ATG + CSA + G-CSF. The conventional schedule of ATG is 15–40 mg/kg per day (depending on the ATG brand) on each of four or five consecutive days. A randomized clinical trial and meta-analyses of clinical trials that used different doses or duration of treatment failed to suggest that intensifying the treatment by extending the ATG treatment period improves response rate or survival. Figure 16.2 summarizes immunosuppressive treatment regimens currently considered as standard treatment (see also Chapter 10).

The optimal source of ATG (horse versus rabbit) is still unclear and deserves to be studied.

Regimens based on ATG + CSA should be given as the first-line treatment of nonsevere aplastic anemia. The response rate to CSA alone is inferior to that to ALG + CSA. It is currently not clear whether patients with nonsevere aplastic anemia require a combined treatment with ATG + CSA up front.

Using growth factors (e.g., G-CSF and also early acting factors like stem factor or flt-3 ligand) to treat aplastic anemia should be evaluated in pilot studies. In particular, growth factors should not be used *alone* without immunosuppression. There are encouraging data on the use of G-CSF from a pilot study of the EBMT Working Party on Severe Aplastic Anemia. However, the final analysis of this EBMT trial as well as the analysis of the trial of the German Aplastic Anemia Study Group (comparing ALG + CSA with G-CSF + CSA) would be awaited before defining the role of G-CSF as an adjunct to immunosuppression in first-line treatment of aplastic anemia (for more details see Chapter 11).

The concern about an increased risk of secondary malignancies after long-term administration of G-CSF (in particular to children) is not supported by available data; neither is there convincing evidence that G-CSF increases the risk of cytogenetic abnormalities. The reported high incidence of secondary clonal disorders in reports from Japan may be caused partially by a failure to obtain cytogenetic data from patients before treatment. Baseline cytogenetic examination is recommended in aplastic anemia (see below), in particular for patients starting cytokine-containing treatment regimens (see Chapter 6).

Failures to respond to first-line treatment/relapse

Supportive treatment alone is not recommended for those patients who fail to respond to the first course of immunosuppression. Patients younger than 50 years who have an HLA-identical sibling donor should receive a bone marrow transplant; older patients or patients without a matched sibling donor should receive a second course of immunosuppression (including at least ATG + CSA). The role of matched unrelated donor transplants in this group of patients remains to be determined. An ongoing IBMTR/EBMT study will compare the outcome after matched unrelated donor BMT versus a second course of immunosuppression in patients failing to respond to a first course.

Repeated antilymphocyte globulin for relapsing patients or patients who fail to respond to the first course of immunosuppression is safe and feasible. Treatment can be repeated with the same ATG that was used in the first treatment protocol without increasing the risk of adverse events. A second course of immunosuppression for patients failing to respond to the first course is superior to supportive treatment, and 40% can be expected to respond (retrospective data of the EBMT Working Party on SAA). The majority of relapsing patients will respond when re-treated with the initial regimen. Repeated ATG treatment may be associated with an increased risk of clonal complications.

Relapse is relevant to the treatment of aplastic anemia. The actuarial risk of relapse is in excess of 30% in most of the studies with long-term follow-up. More than 70% of relapsing patients respond to re-treatment. Overall survival was not affected by relapse and re-treatment. This emphasizes the importance of careful follow-up and early re-treatment in cases of relapse.

Failures to respond to second-line treatment

There are currently no clear recommendations for how to treat patients who do not respond to salvage treatment. These patients might be enrolled in clinical trials evaluating the efficacy and toxicity of new immunosuppressive agents/regimens or new hemopoietic growth factors, or considered for matched unrelated donor transplantation if the patient is younger than 40 years of age.

Age limit for immunosuppressive treatment

There is no age limit for ATG treatment. The decision of whether to treat older patients with ATG should be based on their performance status. A retrospective analysis of the EBMT Working Party on SAA demonstrated that treating elderly patients (>60 years) with ATG is safe and feasible, and that the response rate of elderly patients is not different from that of younger patients (see Chapter 10).

Recent studies also indicate that the response rates to ATG ± CSA and to G-CSF do not differ between adults and children with aplastic anemia. There is currently no evidence that a different treatment strategy is required for children with aplastic anemia (see Chapter 14).

Myelodysplastic syndrome/leukemia after treatment

In order to improve our knowledge about the interrelationships between aplastic anemia and clonal disorders of hemopoiesis, we recommend cytogenetic examination at the start and during follow-up. Cytogenetic abnormalities indicate the presence of a clonal population. However, since cytogenetic abnormalities can be present in a subgroup of aplastic anemia patients, but appear only transiently, a cytogenetic abnormality does not always imply that there is a malignant population. Prospective trials (e.g., also including FISH analysis) are warranted to evaluate the prognostic implications of a clonal population in aplastic anemia. Storage of DNA for molecular analysis is recommended.

Conclusion

Aplastic anemia is a rare disease. Improvements of current treatment strategies can only be achieved by joint efforts. We encourage referral of patients early in the course of aplastic anemia to centers experienced in clinical trials of stem cell transplantation, where immunosuppressive treatment is ongoing (new conditioning regimens, hemopoietic growth factors, e.g. stem cell factor, and escalated immunosuppression with cyclophosphamide). These guidelines need to be updated when the final results of these trails are available.

Part IV

Fanconi's anemia

17

Clinical features and diagnosis of Fanconi's anemia

Blanche P. Alter

University of Texas Medical Branch, Galveston

Clinical suspicion of Fanconi's anemia

When Fanconi described a family with three children with birth defects and aplastic anemia (AA), he made the first clinical observation of what is now clearly a hematological syndrome (Fanconi, 1927). After a few more such families were recognized by others, Fanconi's name was assigned to this phenotype, which is now called Fanconi's anemia (abbreviated FA). In many ways, we have come a long way since then, with the knowledge that there may be at least eight genes responsible for this autosomal recessive condition (Joenje et al., 1997), the cloning of three and mapping of a fourth gene (de Winter et al., 1998; Lo Ten Foe et al., 1996; Strathdee et al., 1992*ab*; The Fanconi Anaemia/Breast Cancer Consortium, 1996; Whitney et al., 1995), and substantial insights into the evolution and treatment of many of the complications of this disorder (see Alter and Young, 1998; Young and Alter, 1994 for recent reviews). However, we still do not always know who to suspect of this condition, precisely how to definitively diagnose or exclude it, how to predict the course of a specific patient, and how to cure or even treat many patients. Given many caveats with regard to biased and possibly incorrect ascertainment, more than 1000 cases of FA have been reported in the literature, with a male:female ratio of 1.3:1. The average age at diagnosis is 7.8 years for males, and 8.8 years for females, with a range from birth to adults. Approximately 5% were diagnosed in the first year of life, and 10% were diagnosed at 16 years of age or more.

The first major problem in the diagnosis of FA is the selection of patients who should be tested. There is a high index of suspicion in children with AA who have physical abnormalities similar to those described in the early literature; this aspect has clearly skewed both the testing and the reporting of FA. Although the incidence of those anomalies is undoubtedly less than the >75% ascertained from literature reports (Alter and Young, 1998), the true figure will not be clear until all genes are cloned, and population screening can be performed. As a minimum, it is important that patients with characteristic birth defects be

Table 17.1. Physical abnormalities in Fanconi's anemia

Abnormality	All patients (%)	<1 year at diagnosis (%)	>16 years at diagnosis (%)
Skin	60	35	66
Short stature	57	50	59
Upper-limb anomalies	48	68	37
Hypogonads, male	37	42	47
Hypogonads, female	3	19	5
Head	27	38	16
Eyes	26	33	22
Renal	23	45	19
Birth weight <2500 g	12	50	7
Developmental delay	13	5	7
Lower limbs	8	15	4
Ears	10	25	10
Increased reflexes	7	3	3
Other skeletal anomalies	6	8	13
Cardiopulmonary	6	18	3
Gastrointestinal	4	30	0
Other anomalies	5	3	2
None, or not reported	20	15	20
Short stature only	1	0	0
Skin only	3	0	3
Short stature and skin only	4	3	5
Short stature and/or skin	8	3	9
Number of patients	955	40	91
Male:female	1.3:1	1.5:1	1.2:1

Notes:
Data represent percentage of patients with the abnormality. The proportions are underestimates, since some reports did not provide physical descriptions. Many patients had multiple anomalies. From Alter and Young, 1998.

identified as FA patients from the outset, for early treatment, and for genetic counseling with regard to subsequent pregnancies. Thus, any of the anomalies summarized in Table 17.1 should be triggers for consideration of the diagnosis of FA. As shown, there are age-related differences in the observation of some of the findings, such as stature and pigmentation. The most frequent abnormalities overall are short stature, hyperpigmented skin, café au lait spots or hypopigmented areas, thumb and radial deformities, microcephaly, microphthalmia, structural renal anomalies, and hypogonadism. Details of all the physical findings that have been reported are provided elsewhere (Alter and Young, 1998; Young and Alter, 1994). The incidence of FA in the absence of major anomalies may emerge from the International Fanconi Anemia Registry (IFAR, Butturini et al., 1994), but the IFAR is biased by the fact that many patients are only diagnosed after they develop AA or even leukemia, and thus the IFAR data may not indicate the true incidence of mild or asymptomatic homozygous FA. Studies of siblings suggest that 25% of patients lack major anomalies (Glanz and Fraser, 1982), while a review of IFAR patients found that 30% lacked congenital malformations, although minor malformations and particularly short stature, microsomy, skin pigmentation, and microphthalmia were almost as frequent in this group of patients as in those with significant birth defects (Giampietro et al., 1997).

The next group to be considered at risk of FA are all patients with AA, irrespective of their physical appearance. Most, although still not all (!), pediatric hematologists include testing for FA in the initial work-up of all children with newly diagnosed 'acquired' aplastic anemia. Were this to become a universal procedure for AA patients of all ages, the frequency of FA as the cause of AA could be ascertained. Reviews from two pediatric centers in the era before modern FA testing suggested that at least 25% of children with AA in fact had FA, but the diagnosis of FA was based on clinical phenotype, and thus those figures were clearly underestimates (Alter et al., 1978; Windass et al., 1987). The frequency of FA homozygotes has been estimated (without hard data) at one to three per million (Joenje et al., 1995). A 13-year study of childhood AA in the north of England suggested an annual incidence of acquired AA of 2 per million, and of AA due to FA of 1.4 per million; 42% of 24 children with AA had FA (Tweddle and Reid, 1996). There are no meaningful adult data, and adults with undiagnosed FA are usually considered to have acquired AA and are treated accordingly (and incorrectly). There are recent reports of adults diagnosed in their thirties to fifties (Kwee et al., 1997; Liu et al., 1991; Zatterale et al., 1995), and other cases known anecdotally to this author. Although the IFAR suggests a cumulative risk of AA of 98% in patients with FA (Butturini et al., 1994), the IFAR cannot provide the obverse figure, which is the frequency of FA as the cause of AA.

Diagnosis of FA

How can the diagnosis of FA be made at this time? The 'gold standard' for the diagnosis of FA was developed following the early observations of increased chromosomal fragility (Schroeder et al., 1964), which is enhanced in the presence of deoxyribonucleic acid (DNA) clastogenic agents such as mitomycin C (MMC) or diepoxybutane (DEB) (Auerbach et al., 1981; Cervenka et al., 1981). This method involves analysis of chromosome breakage in metaphase preparations of phytohemagglutinin-stimulated cultured peripheral blood lymphocytes to which the DNA crosslinker has been added for a specific time period. FA cells usually show a high frequency of breaks, gaps, rearrangements, exchanges, and endoreduplications. Cultured skin fibroblasts may also be used for this test. Diagnosis is fairly certain when chromosome breakage is positive with MMC or DEB, but a negative breakage test may not exclude FA.

Until recently, the chromosome breakage test was considered to be diagnostic, specific, and relatively sensitive. Approximately 10% of patients were classified as 'clonal', however, because of the presence of only a small proportion of cells with chromosome breaks, in a background of cells lacking breaks (Auerbach et al., 1989). Explanations for this phenomenon can now be evoked, and demonstrated at the molecular level. In compound heterozygotes for different mutations of the same gene, intragenic rearrangements or other molecular events, such as gene conversion in rapidly dividing hemopoietic cells, may lead to in vivo gene correction in clones of cells. This may result in a 'false-negative' test for chromosome breakage, such as was initially observed for one of two FA brothers (Dokal et al., 1996), and subsequently reported for seven additional mosaic patients (Lo Ten Foe et al., 1997). Since DNA studies (see below and Chapter 18) now permit definitive diagnosis in some cases, the 'gold standard' has been proven to be tarnished.

A different approach has been taken by several groups who examined cell cycle kinetics in FA. Progression through the cell cycle was delayed, and the proportion of lymphocytes arrested at G_2/M was increased in most FA patients after culture in nitrogen mustard (Berger et al., 1993); in that study the only negative results were in three FA patients with myelodysplasia or leukemia. Another group examined the cell cycle without adding a DNA crosslinker, and found nondiagnostic results only in three FA patients with leukemia (Seyschab et al., 1995). They also identified five cases in which the cell cycle delay was apparent, but classic chromosome breakage studies were normal, and suggested that those patients had atypical or mild FA disease which would have been missed by standard tests. Our own group has performed cell cycle studies using a nitrogen mustard dose/response curve, and found an abnormal result in a patient with normal DEB and MMC breakage studies, later found to be a mosaic, as discussed above (Arkin et al., 1993; S. Arkin, B. P. Alter and J. M. Lipton unpublished). All known FA patients had abnormal results in this test, and nonFA AA patients, such as those with acquired AA or dyskeratosis congenita, had normal results.

The molecular genetics of FA will be discussed in detail in Chapter 18, but a very brief summary cannot be omitted here, since this is the future of accurate diagnosis of FA. The genetic heterogeneity of FA was suggested by complementation analyses as early as 1980 (Yoshida, 1980). In those experiments, cells from various FA patients were fused and examined for correction of chromosome breakage. Cells which corrected came from patients who belonged to different complementation groups, while failure to correct indicated that they were from the same group. These studies were extensively expanded by Joenje and his colleagues, who have now found at least eight different groups (Joenje et al., 1997). The gene for FA group C, now called *FANCC*, was cloned in 1992, and mapped to 9q22.3 (Strathdee et al., 1992*a,b*). The FA group A gene, *FANCA*, cloned in 1996, maps to 16q24.3 (Lo Ten Foe et al., 1996; The Fanconi Anaemia/Breast Cancer Consortium, 1996). *FANCD* has been mapped to 3p22–26 (Whitney et al., 1995), but is not yet cloned. The third cloned gene, *FANCG*, was recently mapped to 9p13, and codes for XRCC9 (de Winter et al., 1998). The gene products, their cellular localization, and possible functions will be discussed elsewhere (Chapter 18).

Molecular methods are now widely and rapidly employed to identify the genetic defects in specific patients. Complementation analysis may be used to assign a patient to a specific group, and to determine population frequencies and founder effects (Joenje, 1996); for example, the high incidence of group A in Italy, Germany, Saudi Arabia, and in South African Afrikaans (The Fanconi Anaemia/Breast Cancer Consortium, 1996), the association of group C with Germany (Joenje, 1996), and a specific group C mutation at IVS4 A→T with Ashkenazi Jews (Whitney et al., 1994). Results in North America indicate 69% group A, 18% C, 4% D, and 9% B or E (Jakobs et al., 1997). Screening for specific mutations can be done with various molecular techniques, such as Southern blotting, oligonucleotide hybridization, restriction site assays, amplification refractory mutation, chemical cleavage mismatch analysis, and single-strand conformational polymorphism. Positive results from these tests, with exclusions of silent polymorphisms, serve to make a definite diagnosis of FA in a candidate patient. However, negative results do not exclude FA, since the mutation may not have been found by the technology that was employed. Nevertheless, when all of the genes and their mutations are elucidated, this approach should become the new 'gold standard'. In populations with a unique mutation, such as the IVS4 A→T in Ashkenazi Jews, the carrier frequency can be determined, and previously undiagnosed homozygotes identified. For example, carriers were shown to comprise 1% of Ashkenazi Jews in New York, and 0% of Israeli Iraqi Jews (Verlander et al., 1995). Molecular studies will also be invaluable for prenatal diagnosis in families in which the specific mutation is known, including those identified by population screening, rather than through a propositus.

Genotype/phenotype correlations are available so far only within the group C population studied in the IFAR (Gillio et al., 1997). Approximately 15% of the close to 400 patients screened belonged to group C. The largest number of major congenital malformations was found in those with the IVS4 A→T mutation, with the next in frequency in those with a mutation in exon 14, and the fewest malformations in those with a mutation in exon 1 (322delG). Those with mutations in exon 14 or IVS4 also had an earlier onset of hematological disease and a shorter median survival than the exon 1 patients. NonC patients, presumably mostly mutant in *FAA*, were similar to the exon 1 patients. Leukemia occurred earlier in the exon 14 and IVS4 patients than in the exon 1 group. Sensitivity to DEB-induced chromosome breakage had an unexplained negative correlation with genotype severity (e.g., the largest number of breaks per cell was seen in those with exon 1 mutations).

Prenatal diagnosis of FA can be done by analysis of clastogen-induced chromosome breakage in cultured fibroblasts, or in fetal lymphocytes obtained by percutaneous umbilical blood sampling (Auerbach and Alter, 1989). DNA-based diagnoses can be used with the methods already outlined, in situations in which the mutation has been identified in a propositus, or in the carrier parents. These diagnoses will be more reliable, and more rapid than the cell-culture-dependent methods used formerly.

Hematological manifestations

Peripheral blood manifestations of FA encompass the entire spectrum from normal to macrocytosis and/or increased fetal hemoglobin (Hb F) levels, to thrombocytopenia, neutropenia, and/or anemia, to trilineage pancytopenia. The blood smear may have large red cells, anisocytosis, mild poikilocytosis, and cytopenias. Red cell mean cell volume (MCV) and Hb F levels may be higher in FA than in acquired AA, but this distinction cannot be relied upon for individual cases. However, increased MCV or Hb F levels may be an early indicator of FA in an asymptomatic sibling of a propositus. Conversely, the MCV may be inappropriately normal in the presence of concomitant iron deficiency or thalassemia trait (Alter, 1998). Bone marrow examination may reveal evolving aplasia, with progressively decreasing cellularity, loss of normal myeloid hemopoietic elements, and relatively increased numbers of lymphocytes, reticulum cells, mast cells, and plasma cells. We attempted to classify FA patients according to their hematological status before any genotype information was available, in order to correlate in vitro culture data with the in vivo condition (Table 17.2; Alter et al., 1991*b*). This classification scheme may be useful with regard to correlation of the timing of the decline in hematological class with genotype. The only genotype/phenotype correlations for hematological status are limited to those cited already from the IFAR.

It is fair to state that the major problem for FA patients who have been diagnosed to date is the risk of AA. The only available 'cure' at this time is bone marrow transplantation, preferably from an HLA-matched sibling. For those for whom transplant is not currently an option, treatment possibilities include androgens and steroids ('standard of care'), to which there is a 50–75% response rate (Alter and Young, 1998), with the most frequent responses including a rise in hemoglobin, followed by a possible increase in platelet count; neutrophil improvement occurs less often. An alternative that will improve the white cell count in essentially all patients is the use of granulocyte colony-stimulating factor (G-CSF), but platelet and hemoglobin responses to this agent are usually not dramatic (Rackoff et al., 1996). Treatment modalities are examined in detail

Table 17.2. Clinical classification of Fanconi's anemia

Group	Transfusions	Androgen or cytokine treatment	Status
1	Yes	No	Severe aplastic anemia, failed or never received androgens
2	Yes	Yes	Severe aplastic anemia, currently on but not responding to androgens
3	No	Yes	Previously severe or moderate aplasia, responding to androgens or cytokines
4	No	No	Severe or moderate aplastic anemia, needs treatment
5	No	No	Stable, with some sign of marrow failure (e.g., mild anemia, neutropenia, thrombocytopenia, high red cell mean cell volume, high fetal hemoglobin)
6	No	No	Normal hematology ± normal fetal hemoglobin

Note:

From Alter et al., 1991*b*.

in Chapter 19, and gene therapy in Chapter 20. It must be pointed out that there are potentially serious side-effects to most of the treatments, such as the risk of secondary malignancies following bone marrow transplant or gene therapy, of liver tumors from androgens, and risk of leukemia from G-CSF.

Leukemia

Leukemia is reported to occur in approximately 10% of FA patients in the literature (Alter, 1996) at a mean age of 14 years, with a male:female ratio of 1.3:1 (Table 17.3). Leukemia was the presenting problem for 20 of the 84 patients with FA and leukemia. The major type was acute myeloid leukemia (AML), with 30 myeloblastic, 20 myelomonocytic, nine monocytic, seven erythroleukemia, six unspecified, six 'nonlymphocytic', one megakaryoblastic, and two chronic myelomonocytic (which may be classified under myelodysplasia, see later). Only three were reported to be acute lymphoblastic, although this is the type usually seen in children without FA. Five patients had coincidental liver tumors (see below), one an astrocytoma, and one a retinoblastoma. Only three long-term remissions were reported, for 2, 8, and >10 years. Chemotherapy was problematic, since the therapeutic index between toxicity to leukemic cells and sensitivity of normal

Table 17.3. Complications in Fanconi's anemia

	Leukemia	MDS	Cancer	Liver disease
Number of patients	84	68	47	37
Percentage of total	9%	7%	5%	4%
Male:female	1.3:1	0.9:1	0.3:1	1.6:1
Age* at diagnosis of FA				
mean	10	12	13	9
median	9	9	10	6
range	0.1–28	1–31	0.1–34	1–48
percentage >16 years	20%	21%	30%	11%
Age at complication				
mean	14	16	23	16
median	14	16	26	13
range	0.1–29	2–43	0.3–38	3–48
Number without pancytopenia (%)	21 (25%)	19 (28%)	8 (17%)	1 (3%)
Number without androgens (%)	40 (48%)	40 (63%)	18 (38%)	1 (3%)
Number reported deceased (%)	66 (79%)	36 (53%)	28 (60%)	32 (86%)

Notes:

* Ages are in years. 148 patients had one or more malignancy (myelodysplastic syndrome or MDS was not counted as a malignancy); the number of malignancies was 155. MDS cases include nine who developed leukemia; the others are not included in the total. Patients with tumors after bone marrow transplantation are not included. Adapted from Alter, 1996.

hemopoietic cells is very small. Bone marrow transplant was also difficult, with <40% survival. This topic will be discussed more extensively in Chapter 19.

The IFAR has attempted to address the risk of leukemia in a prospective manner (Butturini et al., 1994). Unfortunately, their report did not always distinguish leukemia from myelodysplastic syndrome (MDS, see later). They suggested that the cumulative risk of development of MDS/AML was 50% by the age of 35. However, since MDS may not necessarily mean the inevitable development of leukemia in the context of FA (see later), the distinction may be important. They did report a 9% incidence of AML (35 of 388 patients), and one patient with acute lymphoblastic leukemia, data resembling our literature review.

Myelodysplastic syndrome

The definition of MDS is generally based on the French–American–British classification scheme (Bennett et al., 1982), and usually involves pancytopenia with a cellular marrow, although there are some hypocellular myelodysplasias, based on morphologic dysplasia or clonal cytogenetics. Peripheral blood in MDS has hypochromic red cells, pelgeroid and hypogranular neutrophils, hypersegmented neutrophils with long filaments, circulating blasts, and circulating micromegakaryocytes and fragments (Elghetany et al., 1996). Bone marrow criteria for MDS include bi- or trilineage dysplasia, high numbers and irregular distribution of megakaryocytes, ring sideroblasts, or aggregates of blasts and marrow fibrosis (Fohlmeister et al., 1985). The most specific objective diagnostic feature is clonal cytogenetics.

The incidence of MDS in FA is not clear. Cross-sectionally, in two separate studies, we found cytogenetic clones in 8 of 18 and 2 of 14 patients (Alter et al., 1993; Rackoff et al., 1996; and unpublished). The IFAR reported clones in 23 of 68 patients (Butturini et al., 1994), and the French group noted them in 4 of 35 patients (Schaison et al., 1983). A mini 'meta-analysis' totals 37 of 135 patients, or 27%. Whether FA patients who develop leukemia all have a preceding clone cannot be determined without serial studies of all patients. However, since MDS occurs on average in older patients than does leukemia, MDS may not be a harbinger of leukemic transformation (Table 17.3).

While it is theoretically possible that a clonal cytogenetic marker in a patient with FA may mean impending development of leukemia, as it does in adult MDS, there are in fact no data to support this hypothesis for FA. Close to 70 FA patients were reported in the literature with the diagnosis of MDS, although the features and the French–American–British group were not always provided (Alter, 1996; Maarek et al., 1996). Ten patients did develop leukemia within 1.5 years of documentation of a clone, and nine died. All those who developed leukemia did so within 4 years after the clone was seen. In contrast, 58 patients with FA did not develop leukemia at up to 13 years, and 25 of those died, 11 from infection, five from bone marrow transplant complications, two from hemorrhage, one each from renal cancer, renal failure, and MDS with Sweet's syndrome, and four from unspecified causes.

An analysis of the chromosomes involved in the marrow clones in FA patients with leukemia alone (42 patients), MDS followed by leukemia (ten patients), and MDS alone (58 patients) is shown in Figure 17.1 (Alter, 1996; Maarek et al., 1996). In leukemia alone, 47% had abnormalities of chromosome 7, either monosomy 7 or 7q–; 40% had abnormalities involving chromosome 1, with additions, duplications, or translocations; and 19% had an abnormal chromosome 6. In those in whom MDS preceded leukemia, 40% had involvement of chromosome 1, and 20% chromosome 7. Among those with MDS in whom leukemia was not observed, chromosome 1 was abnormal in 31%, and chromosome 7 in 26%. These data suggest that there is no specific cytogenetic clonal abnormality which clearly predicts evolution to leukemia.

It must be emphasized that clonal findings in FA bone marrows are not stable, but fluctuate, including disappearance and reappearance, and serial studies are

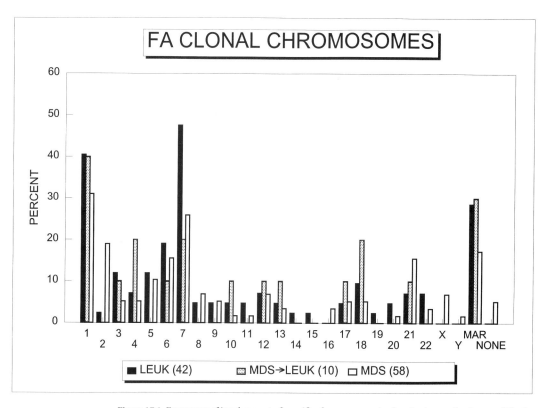

Figure 17.1. Frequency of involvement of specific chromosomes in clonal cytogenetic abnormalities in Fanconi's anemia (FA) patients with leukemia and/or myelodysplastic syndrome (MDS). Black bars, 42 patients with leukemia who had clonal abnormalities. Gray bars, 10 patients who had documented MDS prior to development of leukemia. Open bars, 58 patients who had MDS and had not developed leukemia. MAR, marker chromosome. None indicates that there were no abnormal chromosomes. Data show the proportions of patients in each category with involvement of the designated chromosomes. Many patients had more than one clonal pattern. From Alter, 1996.

very important. In addition to the ten literature cases with a clone on the first study who then developed leukemia, one patient with morphologic MDS developed a clone on a later study, and four with clones developed new independent clones on repeat studies. Among 22 patients with serial studies who did not develop leukemia, 13 had the appearance of new clones. Several patients had marrow examinations in which previously observed clones had disappeared, only to have the same or a different clone reappear later. Thus, detection of a clone may in part be coincidental, since a single patient might be termed 'clonal' or 'nonclonal', depending on the status of the fluctuation.

An International Scoring System was recently proposed in order to classify adult MDS according to cytogenetic findings (Greenberg et al., 1997). A good prognosis consisted of a normal pattern, or one of del(5q), del(20q), or –Y; intermediate was trisomy 8, single miscellaneous, or double abnormalities; while a poor prognosis was associated with complex anomalies (three or more), or anomalies of chromosome 7. Application of this system to the published FA MDS patient data led to an even division between intermediate and poor cytogenetics, both among those who did develop leukemia and those who did not. It appears that 'MDS' and/or clonal abnormalities in FA patients may not be comparable to adult primary MDS, and require their own interpretation. Hemopoiesis derives from a finite number of stem cells. At different time points, hemopoiesis may be derived from different stem cells. In FA, perhaps related to a defect in DNA repair, the stem cell clones may be identified by cytogenetic abnormalities. Clones may fluctuate, disappearing because of poor growth of mutant cells, or through overgrowth by normal or other mutant clones. Observation of a clone may represent a window in time, but the malignant implication of that clone remains to be demonstrated. The evidence that MDS is a prelude to leukemia is not convincing from the data available so far.

Cancer

Solid tumors are underemphasized in FA, perhaps because they usually occur in relatively older patients, and were not clinically important when patients were not surviving beyond their teens due to fatal AA. However, bone marrow transplant (and perhaps gene therapy) will result in a longer life expectancy. In addition, physicians are more sensitive to the diagnosis of FA, and patients are being diagnosed when older, as well as without characteristic physical anomalies. With all the caveats relative to the bias of literature reports, 55 tumors were reported in 45 patients, representing approximately 5% of the case reports (Alter, 1996). An unexpected observation is that the ratio of females to males was 3:1, even after exclusion of gynecologic malignancies. Most tumors were squamous cell carcinomas and occurred at a mean age of 23 years, which is much younger than when most of the same tumors are seen in the nonFA population. The major sites of the tumors were oropharyngeal, gastrointestinal, and gynecological, and the specific locations are summarized in Table 17.4. Eleven patients had two or more primaries, including two with liver cancer and two with leukemia.

These cancers were diagnosed when the FA patients were in their twenties, generally later than when most FA patients reported in the literature develop AA (mean age of 8 years), leukemia (14 years), liver tumors (16 years) and myelodysplasia (17 years) (Table 17.3). It thus appears that FA patients who do not succumb to AA remain at risk of other malignancies, with solid tumors coming last.

There are reports of at least six FA patients (equally males and females) whose hemopoietic disease was cured by bone marrow transplantation, but who developed solid tumors 2–12 years later (Bradford et al., 1990; Flowers et al., 1992;

Table 17.4. Types of cancer in Fanconi's anemia

Type	Number of tumors	Males	Females
Oropharyngeal	16	5	11
Cricoid	1	—	1
Gingiva	4	2	2
Gingiva, tongue	1	1	—
Jaw, benign	1	—	1
Mandible	1	—	1
Pharynx	1	1	—
Tongue	7	1	6
Gastrointestinal	15	4	11
Anus	3	—	3
Anus Bowen's	1	—	1
Colon, anus	1	—	1
Esophagus	8	2	6
Gastric adenoca	2	2	—
Gynecological	12	—	12
Breast	4	—	4
Cervix	1	—	1
Cervix, vulva	1	—	1
Vulva	6	—	6
Brain	4	1	3
Astrocytoma	2	—	2
Medulloblastoma	2	1	1
Other	9	1	8
Bone marrow lymphoma	1	—	1
Bronchopulmonary	1	1	—
Eyelid Bowen's	1	—	1
Renal	1	—	1
Skin	2	—	2
Bowen's	1	—	1
Wilms'	1	—	1
Retinoblastoma	1	—	1
Total	56	11	45

Notes:

Number of tumors (56) exceeds number of patients (47);
11 had > 2 primaries, including 2 with liver cancer and
2 with leukemia. Modified from Alter, 1996.

Millen et al., 1997; Murayama et al., 1990; Socié et al., 1991; Somers et al., 1994). Bone marrow transplantation preparation included irradiation (three) and cyclophosphamide (200 mg/kg in two, 20 mg/kg in the others), and four of the patients had chronic graft-versus-host disease (GVHD). One patient had independent cheek and tongue cancers 5 years apart, four had tongue cancer, and one had cheek cancer. The relative roles of the immunosuppressive preparation and GVHD are not clear; both may be blamed. In addition, since oropharyngeal cancers were the most common in the nontransplanted FA patients, these tumors may represent the natural history of FA, perhaps accelerated by bone marrow transplantation. The frequency of these tumors may already be as high as 5% of transplanted patients, with more to come.

Liver disease

Approximately 5% of reported FA patients had liver disease, usually a tumor (Alter, 1996). All but one had received androgens. Diagnoses were made at a mean of 16 years of age, and the male:female ratio was 1.6:1 (Table 17.3). The tumors were called 'hepatocellular carcinoma' or 'hepatoma' in 20 patients; two were called 'benign', two had adenomas, and only one had metastases and an increased level of alpha-fetoprotein. Six patients had adenomas, one of which had metastases, and two were unclassified. It is possible that these pathologic distinctions were not entirely clear-cut, but included dysplasia, similar to the apparent myelodysplasia seen in the bone marrows. Five patients also had leukemia, and one each tongue and esophageal cancer. Liver tumors were only found at autopsy following death from other causes in four patients. Six patients had peliosis hepatis with the tumors, while another seven had peliosis alone. Several patients stopped androgen therapy (including having bone marrow transplantation), and the tumors regressed. Eighty-five percent of those with liver tumors died, but not directly from their tumor; they died from the underlying hematological problems.

Reproduction

As discussed above, AA is not the only major problem for patients with FA, a condition which is considered to be premalignant. However, FA patients are living longer than before, and are being diagnosed with milder phenotypes. The complications summarized in Table 17.3 are not the only problems for the older patients.

Older females have nonmalignant gynecological problems, including delayed menarche, irregular menses, and early menopause, which can result in low estrogen levels and osteoporosis. Female fertility is probably reduced, but not absent. Twenty-nine pregnancies were reported in 19 women, with seven

Table 17.5. Median survival age in
Fanconi's anemia (FA)

Condition	Age (years)
All FA, 1927–94	19
All FA, 1991–94	30
Cancer	28
Liver disease	13
All leukemia	15
Leukemia with clone	19
MDS → leukemia	19
MDS no leukemia	25
MDS intermediate cytogenetics	21
MDS poor cytogenetics	35

miscarriages, 22 births, and 21 surviving children (Alter and Young, 1998; Alter et al., 1991d). Half of the mothers needed red blood cell and/or platelet transfusions during the pregnancies or at delivery. There were six Cesarean sections because of failure of labor to progress, and four cases with preeclampsia or eclampsia. No FA mother died intrapartum, but nine died later at ages 24–45 years, primarily from cancer.

In addition, males are small, with gonads that are underdeveloped, and abnormal spermatogenesis (Bargman et al., 1977). The number of FA males reported to have children is less than half a dozen (Alter and Young, 1998). Infertility is a frequent complaint among the older FA males, particularly for those diagnosed as adults. Indeed, documented infertility caused by azoospermia in a male with 'acquired' AA should lead to consideration of FA.

Prognosis

The survival of all patients with FA has improved with time (Table 17.5), with the median reaching more than 30 years of age recently. This reflects improvements in the management of AA (see Chapter 19), including better supportive care, but also the inclusion of patients whose phenotype is milder than that of the 'classic' patients of the early years. Figure 17.2 and Table 17.5 indicate median survivals for patients with various major complications, including leukemia, cancer, liver disease, and MDS. The older median survival age in patients with cancer, for example, does not necessarily imply that cancer has a good prognosis, but that the subset of patients who developed cancer may have had a milder phenotype, and did not succumb earlier to hematologic

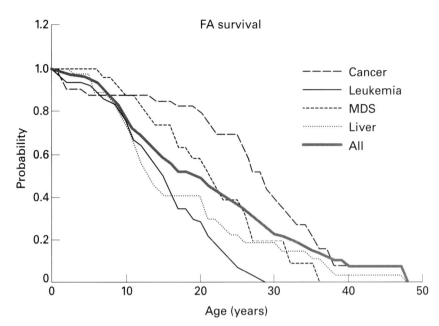

Figure 17.2.
Kaplan–Meier survival curves for all FA patients reported in the literature since 1927. The center line shows the curve for all patients. The marked lines are for patients with leukemia (Leuk), MDS, liver disease (mostly tumors), and solid tumors (Ca).

disease. The ability to offer prognoses in FA will improve as the diagnosis becomes more specific at the molecular level.

Conclusion

The diagnosis of FA is easily made in the 'textbook' patient who has AA and characteristic birth defects. This group may represent 75% of cases, but the actual number will remain unclear until all of the genes have been cloned, and all cases of AA at all ages are studied at the molecular level. The most important component of the diagnosis of FA is thinking of it, which leads to testing (currently done with chromosome breakage analysis), which will probably identify more than 90% of cases. The unusual presentations alluded to in this chapter include AA at an older age (i.e., cared for by adult not pediatric hematologists), or AML or solid tumor without antecedent AA, with or without the FA physical phenotype. The diagnosis of FA will be made by those who think of it in the atypical circumstances.

References

Alter, B. P. (1996) Fanconi's anemia and malignancies. *American Journal of Hematology*, **53**, 99–110.

Alter, B. P. (1998) Modulation of macrocytosis in aplastic anemia. *American Journal of Hematology*, **57**, 92.

Alter, B. P. and Young, N. S. (1998) The bone marrow failure syndromes. In *Hematology of infancy and childhood*, ed. D. G. Nathan, and S. H. Orkin, pp. 237–335. Philadelphia, PA: W. B. Saunders.

Alter, B. P., Potter, N. U. and Li, F. P. (1978) Classification and aetiology of the aplastic anaemias. *Clinical Haematology*, **7**, 431–65.

Alter, B. P., Frissora, C. L., Halpérin, D. S., Freedman, M. H., Chitkara, U., Alvarez, E., Lynch, L., Adler–Brecher, B. and Auerbach, A. D. (1991*a*) Fanconi's anemia and pregnancy. *British Journal of Haematology*, **77**, 410–18.

Alter, B. P., Knobloch, M. E. and Weinberg, R. S. (1991*b*) Erythropoiesis in Fanconi's anemia. *Blood*, **78**, 602–8.

Alter, B. P., Scalise, A., McCombs, J. and Najfeld, V. (1993) Clonal chromosomal abnormalities in Fanconi's anemia: what do they really mean? *British Journal of Haematology*, **85**, 627–30.

Arkin, S., Brodtman, D., Alter, B. P. and Lipton, J. M. (1993) A screening test for Fanconi anemia using flow cytometry. *Blood*, **82**, 176a.

Auerbach, A. D. and Alter, B. P. (1989) Prenatal and postnatal diagnosis of aplastic anemia. In *Methods in hematology: perinatal hematology*, ed. B. P. Alter, pp. 225–51. Edinburgh: Churchill Livingstone.

Auerbach, A. D., Adler, B. and Chaganti, R. S. K. (1981) Prenatal and postnatal diagnosis and carrier detection of Fanconi anemia by a cytogenetic method. *Pediatrics*, **67**, 128–35.

Auerbach, A. D., Rogatko, A. and Schroeder–Kurth, T. M. (1989) International Fanconi Anemia Registry: relation of clinical symptoms to diepoxybutane sensitivity. *Blood*, **73**, 391–6.

Bargman, G. J., Shahidi, N. T., Gilbert, E. F. and Opitz, J. M. (1977) Studies of malformation syndromes of man XLVII: disappearance of spermatogonia in the Fanconi anemia syndrome. *European Journal of Pediatrics*, **125**, 163–8.

Bennett, J. M., Catovsky, D., Daniel, M. T., Flandrin, G., Galton, D. A. G., Gralnick, H. R. and Sultan, C. (1982) Proposals for the classification of the myelodysplastic syndromes. *British Journal of Haematology*, **51**, 189–99.

Berger, R., Coniat, M. L. and Gendron, M. C. (1993) Fanconi anemia. Chromosome breakage and cell cycle studies. *Cancer Genetics and Cytogenetics*. **69**, 13–16.

Bradford, C. R., Hoffman, H. T., Wolf, G. T., Carey, T. E., Baker, S. R. and McClatchey, K. D. (1990) Squamous carcinoma of the head and neck in organ transplant recipients: Possible role of oncogenic viruses. *Laryngoscope*, **100**, 190–4.

Butturini, A., Gale, R. P., Verlander, P. C., Adler–Brecher, B., Gillio, A. P. and Auerbach, A. D. (1994) Hematologic abnormalities in Fanconi anemia: an International Fanconi Anemia Registry study. *Blood*, **84**, 1650–5.

Cervenka, J., Arthur, D. and Yasis, C. (1981) Mitomycin C test for diagnostic differentiation of idiopathic aplastic anemia and Fanconi anemia. *Pediatrics*, **67**, 119–27.

de Winter, J. P., Waisfisz, Q., Rooimans, M. A., van Berkel, C. G. M., Bosnoyan-Collins, L., Alon, N., Carreau, M., Bender, O., Demuth, I., Schindler, D., Pronk, J. C., Arwert, F., Hoehn, H., Digweed, M., Buchwald, M. and Joenje, H. (1998) The Fanconi anaemia group G gene *FANCG* is identical with *XRCC9*. *Nature Genetics*, **20**, 281–3.

Dokal, I., Chase, A., Morgan, N. V., Coulthard, S., Hall, G., Mathew, C. G. and Roberts, I. (1996) Positive diepoxybutane test in only one of two brothers found to be compound heterozygotes for Fanconi's anaemia complementation group C mutations. *British Journal of Haematology*, **93**, 813–16.

Elghetany, M. T., Hudnall, S. D. and Gardner, F. H. (1996) Peripheral blood picture in primary hypocellular refractory anemia and idiopathic acquired aplastic anemia: an additional tool for differential diagnosis. *Haematologica*, **82**, 21–4.

Fanconi, G. (1927) Familiäre infantile perniziosaartige Anämie (perniziöses Blutbild und Konstitution). *Jahrbuch Kinder*, **117**, 257–80.

Flowers, M. E. D., Doney, K. C., Storb, R., Deeg, H. J., Sanders, J. E., Sullivan, K. M., Bryant, E., Witherspoon, R. P., Appelbaum, F. R., Buckner, C. D., Hansen, J. A. and Thomas, E. D. (1992) Marrow transplantation for Fanconi anemia with or without leukemic transformation: an update of the Seattle experience. *Bone Marrow Transplantation*, **9**, 167–73.

Fohlmeister, I., Fischer, R., Modder, B., Rister, M. and Schaefer, H. E. (1985) Aplastic anaemia and the hypocellular myelodysplastic syndrome: histomorphological, diagnostic, and prognostic features. *Journal of Clinical Pathology*, **38**, 1218–24.

Giampietro, P. F., Verlander, P. C., Davis, J. G. and Auerbach, A. D. (1997) Diagnosis of Fanconi anemia in patients without congenital malformations: An International Fanconi Anemia Registry study. *American Journal of Medical Genetics*, **68**, 58–61.

Gillio, A. P., Verlander, P. C., Batish, S. D., Giampietro, P. F. and Auerbach, A. D. (1997) Phenotypic consequences of mutations in the Fanconi anemia FAC gene: an International Fanconi Anemia Registry study. *Blood*, **90**, 105–10.

Glanz, A. and Fraser, F. C. (1982) Spectrum of anomalies in Fanconi anaemia. *Journal of Medical Genetics*, **19**, 412–16.

Greenberg, P., Cox, C., LeBeau, M., Fenaux, P., Morel, P., Sanz, G., Sanz, M., Vallespi, T., Hamblin, T., Oscier, D., Ohyashiki, K., Toyama, K., Aul, C., Mufti, G. and Bennett, J. (1997) International scoring system for evaluating prognosis in myelodysplastic syndromes. *Blood*, **89**, 2079–88.

Jakobs, P. M., Fiddler–Odell, E., Reifsteck, C., Olson, S., Moses, R. E. and Grompe, M. (1997) Complementation group assignments in Fanconi anemia fibroblast cell lines from North America. *Somatic Cell and Molecular Genetics*, **23**, 1–7.

Joenje, H. (1996) Fanconi anaemia complementation groups in Germany and the Netherlands. *Human Genetics*, **97**, 280–2.

Joenje, H., Mathew, C. and Gluckman, E. (1995) Fanconi anaemia research: current status and prospects. *European Journal of Cancer*, **31A**, 268–72.

Joenje, H., Oostra, A. B., Wijker, M., di Summa, F. M., van Berkel, C. G. M., Rooimans, M. A., Ebell, W., van Weel, M., Pronk, J. C., Buchwald, M. and Arwert, F. (1997) Evidence for at least eight Fanconi anemia genes. *American Journal of Genetics*, **61**, 940–4.

Kwee, M. L., van der Kleij, J. M., van Essen, A. J., Begeer, J. H., Joenje, H., Arwert, F. and Ten Kate, L. P. (1997) An atypical case of Fanconi anemia in elderly sibs. *American Journal of Medical Genetics*, **68**, 362–6.

Liu, J. M., Auerbach, A. D. and Young, N. S. (1991) Fanconi anemia presenting unexpectedly in an adult kindred with no dysmorphic features. *American Journal of Medicine*, **91**, 555–7.

Lo Ten Foe, J. R., Rooimans, M. A., Bosnoyan–Collins, L., Alon, N., Wijker, M., Parker, L., Lightfoot, J., Carreau, M., Callen, D. E., Savoia, A., Cheng, N. C., van Berkel, C. G. M., Strunk, M. H. P., Gille, J. J. P., Pals, G., Kruyt, F. A. E., Pronk, J. C., Arwert, F., Buchwald, M. and Joenje, H. (1996) Expression cloning of a cDNA for the major Fanconi anaemia gene, FAA. *Nature Genetics*, **14**, 320–3.

Lo Ten Foe, J. R., Kwee, M. L., Rooimans, M. A., Oostra, A. B., Veerman, A. J. P., Van, W. M., Pauli, R. M., Shahidi, N. T., Dokal, I., Roberts, I., Altay, C., Gluckman, E., Gibson, R. A., Mathew, C. G., Arwert, F. and Joenje, H. (1997) Somatic mosaicism in Fanconi anemia: molecular basis and clinical significance. *European Journal of Human Genetics*, **5**, 137–48.

Maarek, O., Jonveaux, P., Le Coniat, M. and Berger, R. (1996) Faconi anemia and bone marrow clonal chromosome abnormalities. *Leukemia*, **10**, 1700–4.

Millen, F. J., Rainey, M. G., Hows, J. M., Burton, P. A., Irvine, G. H. and Swirsky, D. (1997) Oral squamous cell carcinoma after allogeneic bone marow transplantation for Faconi anaemia. *British Journal of Haematology*, **99**, 410–14.

Murayama, S., Manzo, R. P., Kirkpatrick, D. V. and Robinson, A. E. (1990) Squamous cell carcinoma of the tongue associated with Fanconi's anemia: MR characteristics. *Pediatric Radiology*, **20**, 347.

Rackoff, W. R., Orazi, A., Robinson, C. A., Cooper, R. J., Alter, B. P., Freedman, M. H., Harris, R. E. and Williams, D. A. (1996) Prolonged administration of granulocyte colony-stimulating factor (Filgrastim) to patients with Fanconi anemia: a pilot study. *Blood*, **88**, 1588–93.

Schaison, G., Leverger, G., Yildiz, C., Berger, R., Bernheim, A. and Gluckman, E. (1983) L'anémie de Fanconi. Fréquence de l'évolution vers la leucémie. *Presse Medicale*, **12**, 1269–74.

Schroeder, T. M., Anschütz, F. and Knopp, A. (1964) Spontane Chromosomenaberrationen bei familiärer Panmyelopathie. *Humangenetik*, **1**, 194–6.

Seyschab, H., Friedl, R., Sun, Y., Schindler, D., Hoehn, H., Hentze, S. and Schroeder–Kurth, T. (1995) Comparative evaluation of diepoxybutane sensitivity and cell cycle blockage in the diagnosis of Fanconi anemia. *Blood*, **85**, 2233–7.

Socié, G., Henry–Amar, M., Cosset, J. M., Devergie, A., Girinsky, T. and Gluckman, E. (1991) Increased incidence of solid malignant tumors after bone marrow transplantation for severe aplastic anemia. *Blood*, **78**, 277–9.

Somers, G. R., Tabrizi, S. N., Tiedemann, K., Chow, C. W., Garland, S. M. and Venter, D. J. (1994) Squamous cell carcinoma of the tongue in a child with Fanconi anemia: a case report and review of the literature. *Pediatric Pathology and Laboratory Medicine*, **15**, 597–607.

Strathdee, C. A., Duncan, A. M. V. and Buchwald, M. (1992*a*) Evidence for at least four Fanconi anaemia genes including FACC on chromosome 9. *Nature Genetics*, **1**, 196–8.

Strathdee, C. A., Gavish, H., Shannon, W. R. and Buchwald, M. (1992*b*) Cloning of cDNAs for Fanconi's anaemia by functional complementation. *Nature*, **356**, 763–7.

The Fanconi Anaemia/Breast Cancer Consortium (1996) Positional cloning of the Fanconi anaemia group A gene. *Nature Genetics*, **14**, 324–8.

Tweddle, D. A. and Reid, M. M. (1996) Aplastic anaemia in the northern region of England. *Acta Paediatrica*, **85**, 1388–9.

Verlander, P. C., Kaporis, A., Liu, Q., Zhang, Q., Selingsohn, U. and Auerbach, A. D. (1995) Carrier frequency of the IVS4 + 4 A→T mutation of the Fanconi anemia gene FAC in the Ashkenazi Jewish population. *Blood*, **86**, 4034–8.

Whitney, M. A., Jakobs, P., Kaback, M., Moses, R. E. and Grompe, M. (1994) The Ashkenazi Jewish Fanconi anemia mutation: incidence among patients and carrier frequency in the at-risk population. *Human Mutation*, **3**, 339–41.

Whitney, M., Thayer, M., Reifsteck, C., Olson, S., Smith, L., Jakobs, P. M., Leach, R., Naylor, S., Joenje, H. and Grompe, M. (1995) Microcell mediated chromosome transfer maps the Fanconi anaemia group D gene to chromosome 3p. *Nature Genetics*, **11**, 341–3.

Windass, B., Vowels, M. R., O'Gorman Hughes, D. and White, L. (1987) Aplastic anaemia in childhood: prognosis and approach to therapy. *Medical Journal of Australia*, **146**, 15–19.

Yoshida, M. C. (1980) Suppression of spontaneous and mitomycin C-induced chromosome aberrations in Fanconi's anemia by cell fusion with human fibroblasts. *Human Genetics*, **55**, 223–6.

Young, N. S. and Alter, B. P. (1994) *Aplastic anemia: acquired and inherited*, pp. 1–410. Philadelphia, PA: W. B. Saunders.

Zatterale, A., Calzone, R., Renda, S., Catalano, L., Selleri, C., Notaro, R. and Rotoli, B. (1995) Identification and treatment of late onset Fanconi's anemia. *Haematologica*, **80**, 535–8.

18

Genetic basis of Fanconi's anemia

Manuel Buchwald

University of Toronto

and

Madeleine Carreau

Centre Hospitalier Universitaire de Québec

Introduction

From its first description as an inherited disorder, progress in our understanding of Fanconi's anemia (FA) has depended heavily on exploitation of its genetic features. This chapter summarizes our knowledge of three aspects relating to the genetic basis of FA: cellular phenotypes, genetic heterogeneity, and the identification of defective genes.

Cellular phenotypes

The cellular features of chromosome instability and sensitivity to DNA crosslinking agents were the first to be systematically described in FA. Schroeder and coworkers (Schroeder et al., 1964, 1976) were the first to suggest that spontaneous chromosomal breakage is a cellular marker for FA. However, longitudinal studies have revealed variation in the frequency of baseline breakage within the same FA patient, ranging from no breakage to high levels, thus reducing the usefulness of this feature. Cellular phenotypes are much more specific to FA when DNA-damaging agents are used, especially those that lead to the formation of crosslinks. The sensitivity of FA cells to a variety of DNA crosslinking agents has been extensively studied (Auerbach and Wolman, 1976; Poll et al., 1982; Sasaki and Tonomura, 1973) and, as a result, the hypersensitivity of FA cells to the clastogenic effect of crosslinking agents is now considered to be a unique FA cellular marker.

Based on the work of Auerbach and colleagues on the sensitivity to diepoxybutane (DEB) (Auerbach, 1993), most investigators and clinicians consider that the diagnosis of FA requires an increased cellular sensitivity to one or more DNA crosslinking agents. The most commonly used are DEB and mitomycin C (MMC), but many studies have also used psoralen + UVA, *cis*-diaminedichloro-platinum

II (cis-DPP) and nitrogen mustard (NM). Clinical use of cyclophosphamide (also a crosslinking agent) as a conditioning agent for bone marrow transplantation revealed that FA patients also have an increased sensitivity to this compound (Gluckman et al., 1980).

As described below, somatic cell genetics have been used to classify FA patients into complementation groups; it is presumed that each group has a defect in a different gene. All patients whose cells have been classified into complementation groups have an increased sensitivity to crosslinking agents, since this feature is used in the complementation studies. The patients whose cell lines constitute the reference set for the eight published complementation groups also have been shown to have elevated spontaneous chromosomal instability and, in the case of FA-C, this feature is corrected by introduction of the cloned cDNA (Stavropoulos et al., 1996).

Because of the a priori assumption that the diagnosis of FA predicates an increased sensitivity to these agents, the relationship between the two features has not been extensively studied. For example, patients with clinical features of FA but with no increased sensitivity to DNA crosslinking agents have not been included in the International Fanconi Anemia Registry (IFAR) (Auerbach et al., 1989). However, the advent of molecular methods for identifying alterations in the FA genes now provides us with an independent assessment. Dokal et al. (1996) published the first example of discordant DEB sensitivity between two siblings who both have known deleterious mutations in *FANCC*. Such variability in phenotype is not surprising, since there are likely to be intermediate steps between the gene defect and the phenotype under study, and these steps can be modulated by other genetic or epigenetic events. However, given the extensive experience with FA (Auerbach et al., 1989), these are likely to be rare cases.

Genetic heterogeneity

Complementation of the hypersensitivity of FA cells to crosslinking agents has been studied in somatic cell hybrids. In this test, a positive result (complementation) is considered indicative of the existence of more than one gene causing FA. Successive analysis of cell lines that complement each other allows determination of the number of genes underlying the disease, as has been previously shown in the case of XP through the analysis of heterokaryons (Thompson, 1991).

Genetic heterogeneity in FA was first demonstrated in 1980 (Zakrzewski and Sperling, 1980), on the basis of complementation studies of hybrids between skin fibroblast strains derived from FA patients. A more developed set of complementation results were provided in the mid1980s on the basis of hybrids derived from lymphoblasts (Duckworth–Rysiecki et al., 1985). These latter cells had the advantage of being immortalized and easily distributed throughout the research community. Thus, this genetic classification has become standard in the field (Buchwald, 1995), strengthened recently by the cloning of three of the defective genes.

FA is characterized by extensive genetic heterogeneity. Lymphoblastoid cell lines from seven unrelated FA patients were investigated in the first systematic study (Duckworth–Rysiecki et al., 1986). A hprt⁻ouab^R derivative of one of these cell lines (HSC72) was used as a universal fusion partner in hybridizations with the other cell lines, allowing selective outgrowth of hybrids in culture medium containing hypoxanthine-aminopterin-thymidine (HAT) plus ouabain. MMC sensitivity versus resistance was used as a criterion for complementation in hybrids (Figure 18.1). Two groups of cell lines were distinguished: three that failed to complement the reference cell line HSC72 (termed 'A'), and three that fully complemented the defect (termed 'B' or 'nonA'). The correction of the drug sensitivity phenotype was confirmed by the analysis of both spontaneous and MMC-induced chromosomal breakage.

The latter three nonA cell lines were subsequently marked with dominant drug resistance markers, introduced by stable transfection with plasmids conferring hygromycin or neomycin resistance, and allowing the selection of fusion hybrids generated from combinations of these cell lines. Since all possible combinations yield crosslinker-resistant hybrids, each nonA cell line represents a separate complementation group, i.e., FA-B, FA-C and FA-D (Strathdee et al., 1992*a*). This analysis has been recently taken further: a cell line derived from a patient of Turkish ancestry complemented all four existing groups and therefore represents a fifth complementation group, FA-E (Joenje et al., 1997). Multiple patients were subsequently assigned to this group (Joenje, 1996) and a similar study then revealed even further heterogeneity. Analysis of four lines defined a minimum of three further groups, FA-F to FA-H, for a total of eight FA complementation groups (Joenje et al., 1997).

Complementation groups are considered to represent distinct disease genes. However, in the case of ataxia telangiectasia, also an autosomal recessive chromosomal instability disorder, this assumption has not been borne out, since mutations in the same gene (*ATM*) were found in patients previously assigned to four different complementation groups (Savitsky et al., 1995). In FA, however, at least four complementation groups (A, C, D and G) represent distinct genes on the basis of their separate positions in the human genetic map. *FANCC*, the first FA gene isolated by expression cloning methodology, was mapped to chromosome 9q22.3 by in situ hybridization (Strathdee et al., 1992*a*), while different map positions were subsequently established for *FANCA*, *FANCD* and *FANCG*.

FANCA was mapped by linkage studies with families classified as belonging to FA-A to markers positioned close to the telomere of chromosome 16 (16q24.3)

Complementation Assay

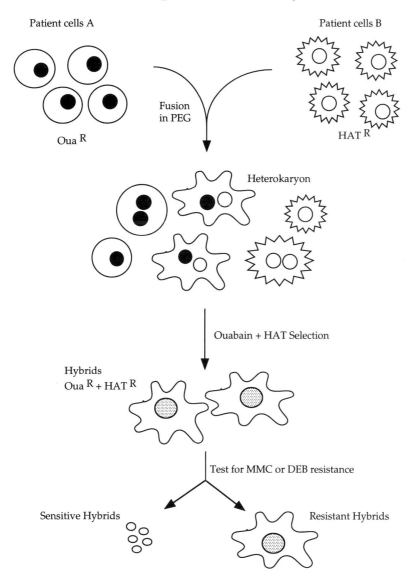

Figure 18.1. Schematic representation of a complementation test. Cells from two patients (A and B) are marked with dominant selectable markers (ouabain (Oua) and hypoxanthine-aminopterin-thymidine (HAT), in this case) and fused with polyethylene glycol (PEG). The resulting heterokaryons are selected in the presence of the two drugs; only viable hybrids containing the genetic constitution of both parental cell lines will survive (indicated by a gray nucleus). The hybrids are tested for their ability to grow in the presence of the drugs specific to Fanconi's anemia (mitomycin C (MMC) or diepoxybutane (DEB)). Cells that are resistant to these drugs have recovered the normal phenotype presumably due to the fact that the mutations in the two parental cells are in different genes. They are therefore placed in two different complementation groups. If the cells cannot grow in the presence of MMC or DEB, it is presumed that the mutations in the parental cells were in the same gene and thus the cells are classified in the same complementation group.

(Pronk et al., 1995). A genome-wide search using microsatellite markers led to the initial linkage to D16S520. More refined analysis, including other FA families, led to a LOD score of 8.01 at a theta value of 0.00 to marker D16S305. The *FANCD* locus was mapped to the short arm of chromosome (3p22–26) using microcell-mediated chromosome transfer (Whitney et al., 1995). These data suggest that for FA the 'one group = one gene' concept does seem to hold up (Buchwald, 1995). Results from the complementation studies thus strongly suggest that at least eight distinct genes, when defective, can cause FA. The recent identification of *XRCC9* as the equivalent of *FANCG* (de Winter et al., 1998) places the latter locus at 9p13.

Cell fusion studies are time-consuming and labor-intensive means of determining the genetic subtype of FA patients. Consequently, only a limited number of patients have been analyzed and the results may well be biased depending on their different ethnic backgrounds. The figures reported in a cumulative European/US/Canadian survey, based on 47 patients, indicate 66% to be group A, 4.3% as B, 12.7% as C, 4.3% as D and 12.7% as groups E–H. The results of a study of a racially and ethnically diverse mapping panel of 50 nonC IFAR families indicate that 73% are linked to marker D16S303, known be close to the location of *FANCA*, and are therefore likely to be in group A (The Fanconi Anaemia Breast Cancer Consortium, 1996). Since about 15% of IFAR patients are in group C, FA-A accounts for about 62% of patients in the IFAR, a figure similar to that obtained through complementation studies.

Identification of the FA genes

In view of the difficulties in defining the basic defect in FA through biochemical analysis of FA cells, various groups have attempted to clone the defective genes directly. The first approach used to identify the FA genes involved correcting the MMC sensitivity of FA cells by introducing genomic DNA from normal cells and then isolating the complementing DNA, a procedure successfully used to isolate the normal human version of several mutant genes in UV- and MMC-sensitive Chinese hamster ovary (CHO) cells (Thompson, 1991). Using mouse DNA, partial complementation of the MMC-sensitive phenotype of both FA-A and FA-D cells was reported (Diatloff–Zito et al., 1990; Moustacchi et al., 1990), but these initial studies did not lead to the identification of an FA gene (Buchwald and Clarke, 1991; Diatloff–Zito et al., 1994).

To circumvent the problems of using genomic DNA, which is incorporated at much lower levels in human cells in comparison to rodent cells, a cDNA expression cloning procedure was adapted and successfully used to initially clone the gene defective in FA-C cells (*FANCC*) and, subsequently, *FANCA* and *FANCG*.

Cloning of *FANCC*

The cDNA expression system uses an episomal shuttle vector (pREP4) to transfer DNA between bacterial and human cells. A set of cDNAs from a lymphoblast pREP4 cDNA library specifically complemented the MMC- and DEB-sensitivity of FA-C cells (Strathdee et al., 1992*b*). The cDNAs code for the same open reading frame (ORF); different forms of the cDNA contain three alternative 3'-untranslated regions (3'-UTRs), each terminated by a consensus polyadenylation signal, in combination with one of two 5'-UTRs. The 5'-UTRs reflect the presence of alternative transcriptional start sites spliced to a common downstream exon, since they all possess suitable splice donor sites only at their 3'-end (Savoia et al., 1995; Strathdee et al., 1992*b*). The murine, rat, and bovine cDNAs are also characterized by multiple 3'-UTRs (Wevrick et al., 1993; Wong and Buchwald, 1997); their significance is not yet known. The FA-C cells used in the selection of the *FANCC* cDNA carry a mutation that leads to an L554P substitution (Strathdee et al., 1992*b*) that inactivates the cDNA (Gavish et al., 1993). The second mutant allele of this cell line leads to a deletion of 327 base pairs (bp) that eliminates all putative ATG start codons, leading to a nonfunctional transcript (Parker et al., 1998). *FANCC* was localized to 9q22.3 by in situ hybridization (Strathdee et al., 1992*a*). The mapping of *FANCC* was confirmed by genetic analysis of known FA-C patients (Verlander et al., 1994; Whitney et al., 1993) which led to the identification of frame shift, splicing, amino acid substitutions, and chain termination mutations. In some cases (e.g., IVS4 $+4\,A\rightarrow T$), no protein is detected (Yamashita et al., 1994), while in others (e.g., L554P) a protein of normal size is seen (Youssoufian et al., 1996). Thus, a variety of protein modifications lead to the FA phenotype, suggesting that all alterations abrogate *FANCC* function. Table 18.1 summarizes known mutations and polymorphic sequence variations in *FANCC*.

The IVS4 $+4\,A\rightarrow T$ splice site mutation in *FANCC* is responsible for most of the cases of FA in the Ashkenazi Jewish population (Whitney et al., 1993; Yamashita et al., 1996). In a study of over 3000 Jewish individuals, primarily of Ashkenazi descent, the frequency of IVS4 carriers was shown to be 1 in 89 (Verlander et al., 1995). The high carrier frequency of the IVS4 mutation places FA-C in the group of so-called Jewish genetic diseases that include Tay–Sachs, Gaucher, and Canavan disease, among others. With a carrier frequency greater than 1% and simple testing available, the IVS4 mutation merits inclusion in the battery of tests routinely provided for the Jewish population. A recent abstract suggests that, in Japanese families, the IVS4 $+4A\rightarrow T$ mutation is not as severe, implying that other genetic factors, distributed differently among ethnic groups, can influence the effects of specific *FANCC* mutations. Group C is also relatively prevalent among Dutch patients, mainly exhibiting the exon 1 frameshift 322delG (Joenje, 1996), whereas group A is the prevalent complementation group represented in Italy (Savoia et al., 1996) as well as among the Afrikaans-speaking population of South

Table 18.1. FANCC mutations

Exons	Nucleotide changes	Amino acid changes	Mutation type
1	292C→T	Q13X	Stop codon
1	320G→A	W22X	Stop codon
1	322delG		Frameshift
4	IVS4+4A→T		RNA splicing
5	775C→T	R174X	AA substitution
6	808C→T	R185X	Stop codon
13	1742T→G	L496R	AA substitution
14	1806insA		Insertion
14	1897C→T	R548X	Stop codon
14	1916T→C	L554P	AA substitution

Note:
AA = amino acid.

Africa (Pronk et al., 1995). Once the genes for the different complementation groups have been identified, the relative prevalences of the groups in different parts of the world can begin to be estimated through mutation screening methods.

Function of FANCC

The predicted structure of FANCC (and Fancc) does not resemble that of any known protein or functional motifs that could serve as clues to its biological role (Strathdee et al., 1992b). Comparison of the primary sequences of the human, mouse, rat, and bovine proteins does not reveal, other than putative phosphorylation sites, any obvious regions of higher homology, precluding identification of more instructive functional domains (Wong and Buchwald, 1997).

The predicted *FANCC* ORF codes for a 63-kDa protein (558 amino acids) with a preponderance of hydrophobic amino acids but no predicted transmembrane domains (Strathdee et al., 1992b). In vitro transcription and translation of the cDNA produces a protein with an apparent molecular weight of 60 kDa and a protein of similar size is immunoprecipitated from lymphoblasts or transfected cells using antiFANC antibodies (Yamashita et al., 1994; Youssoufian, 1994). The protein is found in the cytoplasm (Yamashita et al., 1994; Youssoufian, 1994), arguing against a direct role in DNA repair, though a recent paper indicates that a proportion of FANCC may be located in the nucleus in association with FANCA (Kupfer et al., 1997a). If FANCC is directly targeted to the nucleus it is incapable of correcting the MMC sensitivity of FA-C cells (Youssoufian, 1996). This implies that FANCC may act as a sensor of crosslinking agents regulating DNA repair through binding of FANCA. The FA cellular phenotype of increased sensitivity to MMC can be recreated by introducing *FANCC* antisense oligonucleotides into wild-type cells (Segal et al., 1994), suggesting that FANCC plays a direct role in protecting cells against the cytotoxic and clastogenic action of this compound.

Immunoprecipitation of FANCC from cell extracts has identified a set of associated cytoplasmic proteins (Youssoufian et al., 1995) of approximately 70, 50 and 30 kDa. The existence of FANCC-binding proteins is also supported by the fact that overexpression of the L554P mutant FANCC protein leads to an FA-like phenotype, suggesting that the presence of elevated levels of an inactive mutant protein sequesters other functional proteins of the FA pathway (Youssoufian et al., 1996). FANCC has also been shown to interact with a cyclin-dependent kinase (cdc2), which regulates G2 progression of the cell cycle (Kupfer et al., 1997*b*). cdc2 specifically binds the carboxyl terminus portion of the FANCC protein but fails to bind the L554P mutant FANCC. This interaction may play an important role in cell cycle regulation after damage.

The cytoplasmic localization of FANCC has led to studies aimed at determining whether the protein has a function in apoptosis. Initial studies have focused on the possible role of FANCC in MMC-mediated apoptosis. Results suggest that FA-C cells may have a generalized defect in apoptosis, mediated by treatment with either MMC or gamma radiation and may involve a failure to induce p53, although conflicting results regarding p53 have been reported (Kruyt et al., 1996; Kupfer and D'Andrea, 1996; Rosselli et al., 1995). Human MO7e and mouse 32D hemopoietic cell lines overexpressing FANCC show a significant delay in cell death compared to the neomycin controls following interleukin-3 (IL-3) deprivation (Cumming et al., 1996). Thus, FANCC appears to play a role in the apoptotic pathway of hemopoietic cells, a role consistent with its cytoplasmic localization as well as its increased expression in hemopoietic precursors (Brady et al., 1995). A hypothesis that could explain these observations is that FANCC modulates the apoptosis that may occur during normal fluctuation of growth factor levels in the marrow microenvironment (Koury, 1992). More hemopoietic cells will die in FA-C patients than in normal individuals and, with time, will lead to hemopoietic failure. The high susceptibility of FA-C patients to AML still remains to be explained.

Patterns of *FANCC* and *fancc* expression

The analysis of gene expression can yield two types of useful information about gene function: the sites and levels where the gene functions and the mechanisms that mediate expression. In the case of FA-C, the pleiotropic phenotype of patients and the presence of multiple transcription start sites (Savoia et al., 1995;

Strathdee et al., 1992*b*) point to a complex regulation. Both human and mouse genes are ubiquitously expressed at low levels in adult tissues (Strathdee et al., 1992*b*; Wevrick et al., 1993). PCR-derived cDNA libraries from single hemopoietic cells have been used to show that higher levels of *Fancc* expression can be detected in less differentiated (multilineage progenitors) than in more differentiated (single lineage progenitors) cells (Brady et al., 1995). During mouse embryogenesis, *Fancc* expression is high in undifferentiated mesenchymal cells 8–10 days post conception. Starting at 13 days, expression becomes restricted to regions with rapidly replicating chondro- and osteoprogenitors (e.g., perichondrium), a pattern that persists to later stages (15–19.5 days), except in regions where differentiation has taken place (e.g., hypertrophic chondrocytes of the epiphyseal growth plate). As bone development proceeds, expression is seen in osteogenic and hemopoietic cells in the zone of calcification (Krasnoshtein and Buchwald, 1996).

Cloning of *FANCA*

FANCA has been cloned by two different approaches: functional complementation, as used to clone *FANCC*, and positional methods (Lo Ten Foe et al., 1996; The Fanconi Anaemia Breast Cancer Consortium, 1996). In the first approach, HSC72 (FA-A) cells were transfected and selected in hygromycin and MMC. A single cDNA that corrected the DNA crosslinking hypersensitivity of FA-A cells, but not of FA-C cells, was found in a surviving cell population that exhibited a wild-type level of resistance to MMC and was fully crossresistant to DEB and cis-DPP. Screening of a bacterial artificial chromosome library with the cDNA yielded a positive clone that was used to localize the gene by fluorescence in situ hybridization; a signal was observed at the telomere of chromosome 16q, which is the genetic map location established for *FANCA* (Pronk et al., 1995), thus strengthening the candidacy of this cDNA. To obtain further proof of identity of the candidate cDNA, cell lines from FA patients classified as FA-A by complementation analysis were screened for mutations in this gene. Sequence variations were seen in patients from different ancestral backgrounds; these were likely to be pathogenic on the basis of their severity and their segregation with the disease in three informative multiplex families. These data confirmed that the cDNA indeed represents the *FANCA* gene (Lo Ten Foe et al., 1996).

Positional cloning of *FANCA* was attempted subsequent to the mapping of the FA-A locus to 16q24.3 (Gschwend et al., 1996; Pronk et al., 1995). The candidate region was narrowed by further linkage studies and by allelic association analysis. A physical map of the critical region was developed by screening a chromosome 16 cosmid library with various tagged probes leading to an integrated cosmid contig of about 650 kb. The cosmids were used for exon trapping and direct selection of cDNAs; the products were used to probe high-density gridded cDNA clones, which resulted in the identification of a clone which contained a poly(A) tail and was located at the 3'-end of a candidate gene. An overlapping cDNA clone was then identified; together these two clones gave a combined sequence of 2.3 kb. Exon trapping identified potential additional exons, which were used to extend the sequence by RT-PCR and to screen cDNA libraries for larger clones. One of these was found to be partially deleted in an Italian FA-A patient, and was investigated in more detail as an *FANCA* candidate. Several additional mutations, all of which would be expected to disrupt the function of the protein, were observed in FA-A patients of various ethnic origins (The Fanconi Anaemia Breast Cancer Consortium, 1996). The sequence of this putative *FANCA* cDNA was found to be virtually identical to the cDNA isolated from the expression library described above. Table 18.2 lists reported mutations in *FANCA*.

The *FANCA* cDNA is composed of 43 exons ranging from 34 to 188 bp in length (Ianzano et al., 1997) and codes for a protein with a predicted molecular weight of 162 kDa (Lo Ten Foe et al., 1996). Although no homology was found between *FANCA* and known genes or proteins including FANCC, two functional domains were identified: a putative bipartite nuclear localization signal located in exon 1 and a putative leucine zipper domain in exon 32 (Lo Ten Foe et al., 1996). Furthermore, characterization of the 5'-region of the *FANCA* gene has revealed consensus sequences for binding of transcription factors (Ianzano et al., 1997). Initial localization analysis demonstrated cytoplasmic rather than an anticipated nuclear localization (Kruyt et al., 1997), although a more recent study suggests that FANCA and FANCC may colocalize to the nucleus (Kupfer et al., 1997a).

The basic defect of the various complementation groups

Our inability to understand the pathophysiology of FA could be due to each complementation group having a different basic defect. A review of the FA literature to establish whether specific complementation groups have clearly identifiable cellular or biochemical defects is essentially not possible because most of the cells used cannot be assigned to a complementation group. A similar situation arises when examining data from patient samples, usually lymphocytes. Given the relatively recent discovery of most complementation groups and the difficulty in classifying patients through complementation studies, it is not surprising to find no mention of genetic classification in the vast majority of papers. All of these published data mix individuals with different genetic defects and it is now impossible to review this literature appropriately. Knowledge about the fundamental defect(s) in FA should come from the use of cell lines from known complementation groups and, more specifically, using the available FA cDNAs.

Table 18.2. FANCA mutations

Exons	Nucleotide change	Amino acid change	Mutation type
1	24C→G	N8K	AA substitution
1	65C→G	W22X	Stop codon
4	401insC		Frameshift
6	542C→T	A181V	AA substitution
7	IVS7-1G→A		RNA splicing
7	IVS7-5G→T		RNA splicing
7	IVS7-5G→A		RNA splicing
8	732G→C	L244F	AA substitution
8	755A→G	D252G	AA substitution
10	938–1050del		Frameshift
11	987–990del		Frameshift
11	IVS11–1delG		RNA splicing
13	1115–1118del		Frameshift
14	1303 C→T	R435C	AA substitution
15	1391del1467		Frameshift
15	1459insC		Frameshift
16	1475A→G	H492G	AA substitution
16	1515del1670		Deletion
17	1615delG		Frameshift
18	1671–1944del		Frameshift
19	1771C→T	R591X	Stop codon
22	1944delG		Frameshift
23	1932del879		Deletion
24	2167–2169del		Deletion
26	2450T→C	L817P	AA substitution
27	2524delT		Frameshift
27	2534T→C	L845P	AA substitution
27	2535–2536del		Frameshift
28	2815–2816ins19		Frameshift
29	2840C→G	S947X	Stop codon
29	IVS29(–19)		RNA splicing
32	3091C→T	Q1031X	Stop codon
32	3164G→T	R1055L	AA substitution
32	3188G→A	W1063X	Stop codon
34	3349A→G	R1117G	AA substitution
34	3382C→G	Q1128E	AA substitution
34	3391A→G	T1131A	AA substitution
34	3396–3399del		Frameshift
36	3520–3522del		Deletion
37	3715–3729del		Deletion

Table 18.2 (*cont.*)

Exons	Nucleotide change	Amino acid change	Mutation type
37	3760–3761del		Frameshift
38	3788–3790del		Deletion
39	3884T→A	L1295X	AA substitution
39	3904T→C	W1302R	AA substitution
41	4069–4082del		Frameshift
42	4249C→G	H1417D	AA substitution

Animal models

Insight into the biological functions of genes whose absence leads to human genetic disorders can be obtained from the study of animal models, in particular mice, that are developed through disruption of the orthologous gene. Two mouse models have been developed for FA-C, through disruption of exons 8 or 9, respectively, and neither strain has Fancc present (Chen et al., 1996; Whitney et al., 1996). As with the human patients, the mice are characterized by an increased sensitivity to MMC and DEB, as tested in spleen lymphocytes and fibroblast strains developed from the mice. In addition, hemopoietic progenitor cells from Fancc−/− mice were found to be hypersensitive to interferon-γ, showing a reduced colony growth (Rathbun et al., 1997; Whitney et al., 1996). Neither mouse model shows evidence of congenital malformations, although this might represent the effects of null mutations. No specific models (e.g., L554P) have yet been established. Male and female mice both showed markedly reduced fertility, due to testicular atrophy in males and ovarian hypoplasia in females.

While no spontaneous bone marrow failure was detected up to 18 months of age, treatment of mice with low doses of MMC leads to progressive bone marrow failure (Carreau et al., 1998). Thus, under specific environmental conditions, the mice develop the same disease as human patients, suggesting that unknown environmental influences may also act on patients. This model may be especially useful for determining the efficacy of novel treatments for bone marrow failure, including gene therapy.

Conclusion

Significant progress in understanding the genetic basis of FA has occurred during the past decade. This includes a firm understanding of the degree of existing genetic heterogeneity and the identification of three novel genes that can cause this disease. Because patients with defects in these three genes account for about two-thirds to three-quarters of FA patients, the discovery of these genes has important diagnostic implications, which will be of benefit to families. What has proven to be more elusive is a better understanding of the biochemical and cellular basis of the disease, undoubtedly due to the fact that the three genes code for novel proteins, with no known homologs. Notwithstanding this, the next few years should see progress in defining the basic defect(s) of the disease, since work will be carried out using samples and cell lines with defined genetic constitutions. Comparisons of FA cells to those expressing the specific cDNA will eliminate effects of genetic background and will permit accurate comparisons of experiments performed in various laboratories. This new information will, hopefully, lead to improved diagnosis and treatment, for the benefit of patients and their families.

Acknowledgements

Work in our laboratory has been supported by grants from the Medical Research Council of Canada (MRC), National Institutes of Health (USA), National Cancer Institute of Canada, supported by the Canadian Cancer Society, the Fanconi Anemia Research Fund, Inc. and private donors.

References

Auerbach, A. D. (1993) Fanconi anemia diagnosis and the diepoxybutane (DEB) test. *Experimental Hematology*, **21**, 731–3.

Auerbach, A. D. and Wolman, S. R. (1976) Susceptibility of Fanconi's anaemia fibroblasts to chromosome damage by carcinogens. *Nature*, **261**, 494–6.

Auerbach, A. D., Rogatko, A. and Schroeder–Kurth, T. M. (1989) International Fanconi Anemia Registry: relation of clinical symptoms to diepoxybutane sensitivity. *Blood*, **73**, 391–6.

Brady, G., Billia, F., Knox, J., Hoang, T., Kirsch, I. R., Voura, E. B., Hawley, R. G., Cumming, R., Buchwald, M., Siminovitch, K. et al. (1995) Analysis of gene expression in a complex differentiation hierarchy by global amplification of cDNA from single cells. *Current Biology*, **5**, 909–22.

Buchwald, M. (1995) Complementation groups: one or more per gene? *Nature Genetics*, **11**, 228–30.

Buchwald, M. and Clarke, C. (1991) DNA-mediated transfer of a human gene that confers resistance to mitomycin C. *Journal of Cellular Physiology*, **148**, 472–8.

Carreau, M., Gan, O., Liu, L., Comming, R., Doedens, M., McKerlie, C., Dick, J. and Buchwald, M. (1998) Bone marrow failure in the Fanconi anemia group C mouse model following DNA damage. *Blood*, **91**, 2737–44.

Chen, M., Tomkins, D. J., Auerbach, W., McKerlie, C., Youssoufian, H., Liu, L., Gan, O., Carreau, M., Auerbach, A., Groves, T., Guidos, C. J., Freedman, M. H., Cross, J., Percy, D. H., Dick, J. E., Joyner, A. L. and Buchwald, M. (1996) Inactivation of Fac in mice produces inducible chromosomal instability and reduced fertility reminiscent of Fanconi anaemia. *Nature Genetics*, **12**, 448–51.

Cumming, R. C., Liu, J. M., Youssoufian, H. and Buchwald, M. (1996) Suppression of apoptosis in hemopoietic factor-dependent progenitor cell lines by expression of the *FAC* gene. *Blood*, **88**, 4558–67.

de Winter, J. P., Waisfisz, Q., Rooimans, M. A., van Berkel, C. G. M., Bosnoyan–Collins, L., Alon, N., Carreau, M., Bender, O., Schindler, D., Pronck, J. C., Arwert, F. R., Hoehn, H., Digweed, M., Buchwald, M. and Joenje, H. (1998) The Fanconi anemia group G gene is identical with human *XRCC9*. *Nature Genetics*, **20**, 281–3.

Diatloff–Zito, C., Rosselli, F., Heddle, J. and Moustacchi, E. (1990) Partial complementation of the Fanconi anemia defect upon transfection by heterologous DNA. Phenotypic dissociation of chromosomal and cellular hypersensitivity to DNA cross-linking agents. *Human Genetics*, **86**, 151–61.

Diatloff–Zito, C., Duchaud, E., Viegas–Pequignot, E., Fraser, D. and Moustacchi, E. (1994) Identification and chromosomal localization of a DNA fragment implicated in the partial correction of the Fanconi anemia group D cellular defect. *Mutation Research*, **307**, 33–42.

Dokal, I., Chase, A., Morgan, N. V., Coulthard, S., Hall, G., Mathew, C. G. and Roberts, I. (1996) Positive diepoxybutane test in only one of two brothers found to be compound heterozygotes for Fanconi's anaemia complementation group C mutations. *British Journal of Haematology*, **93**, 813–16.

Duckworth–Rysiecki, G., Cornish, K., Clarke, C. A. and Buchwald, M. (1985) Identification of two complementation groups in Fanconi anemia. *Somatic Cell and Molecular Genetics*, **11**, 35–41.

Duckworth–Rysiecki, G., Toji, L., Ng, J., Clarke, C. and Buchwald, M. (1986) Characterization of a simian virus 40-transformed Fanconi anemia fibroblast cell line. *Mutation Research*, **166**, 207–14.

Gavish, H., dos Santos, C. C. and Buchwald, M. (1993) A Leu554-to-Pro substitution completely abolishes the functional complementing activity of the Fanconi anemia (FACC) protein. *Human Molecular Genetics*, **2**, 123–6.

Gluckman, E., Devergie, A., Schaison, G., Bussel, A., Berger, R., Sohier, J. and Bernard, J. (1980) Bone marrow transplantation in Fanconi anaemia. *British Journal of Haematology*, **45**, 557–64.

Gschwend, M., Levran, O., Kruglyak, L., Ranade, K., Verlander, P. C., Shen, S., Faure, S., Weissenbach, J., Altay, C., Lander, E. S., Auerbach, A. D. and Botstein, D. (1996) A locus for Fanconi anemia on 16q determined by homozygosity mapping. *American Journal of Human Genetics*, **59**, 377–84.

Ianzano, L., D'Apolito, M., Centra, M., Savino, M., Levran, O., Auerbach, A., Cleton–Jansen, A., Doggett, N., Pronk, J., Tipping, A., Gibson, R., Mathew, C., Whitmore, S., Apostolou, S., Callen, D., Zelante, L. and Savoia, A. (1997) The genomic organization of the Fanconi anemia group A (FAA) gene. *Genomics*, **41**, 309–14.

Joenje, H. (1996) Fanconi anaemia complementation groups in Germany and the Netherlands. *Human Genetics*, **97**, 280–2.

Joenje, H., Oostra, A., Wijker, M., di Summa, F., van Berkel, C., Rooimans, M., Ebell, W., van Weel, M., Pronk, J., Buchwald, M. and Artwert, F. (1997) Evidence for at least eight Fanconi anemia genes. *American Journal of Human Genetics*, **61**, 940–4.

Koury, M. J. (1992) Programmed cell death (apoptosis) in hemopoiesis. *Experimental Hematology*, **20**, 391–4.

Krasnoshtein, F. and Buchwald, M. (1996) Developmental expression of the Fac gene correlates with congenital defects in Fanconi anemia patients. *Human Molecular Genetics*, **5**, 85–93.

Kruyt, F. A., Dijkmans, L. M., van den Berg, T. K. and Joenje, H. (1996) Fanconi anemia genes act to suppress a cross-linker-inducible p53-independent apoptosis pathway in lymphoblastoid cell lines. *Blood*, **87**, 938–48.

Kruyt, F. A., Waisfisz, Q., Dijkmans, L. M., Hermsen, M. A., Youssoufian, H. and Arwert, F. (1997) Cytoplasmic localization of a functionally active Fanconi anemia group A-green fluorescent protein chimera in human 293 cells. *Blood*, **90**, 3288–95.

Kupfer, G. M. and D'Andrea, A. D. (1996) The effect of the Fanconi anemia polypeptide, FAC, upon p53 induction and G2 checkpoint regulation. *Blood*, **88**, 1019–25.

Kupfer, G. M., Näf, D., Suliman, A., Pulsipher, M. and D'Andrea, A. D. (1997*a*) The Fanconi anaemia proteins, FAA and FAC, interact to form a nuclear complex. *Nature Genetics*, **17**, 487–90.

Kupfer, G. M., Yamashita, T., Näf, D., Suliman, A., Asano, S. and D'Andrea, A. D. (1997*b*) The Fanconi anemia polypeptide, FAC, binds to the cyclin–dependent kinase, cdc2. *Blood*, **90**, 1047–1054.

Lo Ten Foe, J., Rooimans, M. A., Bosnoyan–Collins, L., Alon, N., Wijker, M., Parker, L., Lightfoot, J., Carreau, M., Callen, D. F., Savoia, A., Cheng, N. C., van Berkel, C. G. M., Strunk, M. H. P., Gille, J. J. P., Pals, G., Kruyt, F. A. E., Pronk, J. C., Arwert, F., Buchwald, M. and Joenje, H. (1996) Expression cloning of a cDNA for the major Fanconi anemia gene, *FAA. Nature Genetics*, **14**, 320–3.

Moustacchi, E., Guillouf, C., Fraser, D., Rosselli, F., Diatloff–Zito, C. and Papadopoulo, D. (1990) Fanconi's anemia: genetic and molecular aspects of the defect. *Nouvelle Revue Francaise d'Hematologie*, **32**, 387–9.

Parker, L., dos Santos, C. and Buchwald, M. (1998) A mutation (delta 327) in the Fanconi anemia group C gene generates a novel transcript lacking the first two coding exons. *Human Mutation Supplement*, **1**, S275–S277.

Poll, E. H., Arwert, F., Joenje, H. and Eriksson, A. W. (1982) Cytogenetic toxicity of antitumor platinum compounds in Fanconi's anemia. *Human Genetics*, **61**, 228–30.

Pronk, J. C., Gibson, R. A., Savoia, A., Wijker, M., Morgan, N. V., Melchionda, S., Ford, D., Temtamy, S., Ortega, J. J., Jansen, S. et al. (1995) Localisation of the Fanconi anaemia complementation group A gene to chromosome 16q24.3. *Nature Genetics*, **11**, 338–40.

Rathbun, R. K., Faulkner, G. R., Ostroski, M. H., Christianson, T. A., Grant-Hughes, Jones, G., Cahn, R., Maziarz, R., Royle, G., Keeble, W. C., Heinrich, M., Grompe, M., Tower, P. A. and Bagby, G. C. (1997) Inactivation of the Fanconi anemia group C gene augments interferon-induced apoptotic responses in hemopoietic cells. *Blood*, **90**, 974–85.

Rosselli, F., Ridet, A., Soussi, T., Duchaud, E., Alapetite, C. and Moustacchi, E. (1995) p53-dependent pathway of radio-induced apoptosis is altered in Fanconi anemia. *Oncogene*, **10**, 9–17.

Sasaki, M. S. and Tonomura, A. (1973) A high susceptibility of Fanconi's anemia to chromosome breakage by DNA cross-linking agents. *Cancer Research*, **33**, 1829–36.

Savitsky, K., Bar–Shira, A., Gilad, S., Rotman, G., Ziv, Y., Vanagaite, L., Tagle, D. A., Smith, S., Uziel, T., Sfez, S. et al. (1995) A single ataxia telangiectasia gene with a product similar to PI-3 kinase [see comments]. *Science*, **268**, 1749–53.

Savoia, A., Centra, M., Ianzano, L., de Cillis, G. P., Zelante, L. and Buchwald, M. (1995) Characterization of the 5' region of the Fanconi anaemia group C (FACC) gene. *Human Molecular Genetics*, **4**, 1321–6.

Savoia, A., Zatterale, A., Del Principe, D. and Joenje, H. (1996) Fanconi anaemia in Italy: high prevalence of complementation group A in two geographic clusters. *Human Genetics*, **97**, 599–603.

Schroeder, T. M., Anschutz, F. and Knopp, A. (1964) Spontaneous chromosome aberrations in familial panmyelopathy. [In German.] *Humangenetik*, **1**, 194–6.

Schroeder, T. M., Tilgen, D., Kruger, J. and Vogel, F. (1976) Formal genetics of Fanconi's anemia. *Human Genetics*, **32**, 257–88.

Segal, G. M., Magenis, R. E., Brown, M., Keeble, W., Smith, T. D., Heinrich, M. C. and Bagby, G. C. Jr. (1994) Repression of Fanconi anemia gene (FACC) expression inhibits growth of hemopoietic progenitor cells. *Journal of Clinical Investigation*, **94**, 846–52.

Stavropoulos, D. J., Sood, S., Tomkins, D. J. and Buchwald, M. (1996) Correction of the spontaneous and DEB-induced chromosomal aberrations in Fanconi anemia cells of the FA(C) complementation group by the FACC gene. *Cytogenetics and Cell Genetics*, **72**, 194–6.

Strathdee, C. A., Duncan, A. M. and Buchwald, M. (1992*a*) Evidence for at least four Fanconi anaemia genes including FACC on chromosome 9. *Nature Genetics*, **1**, 196–8.

Strathdee, C. A., Gavish, H., Shannon, W. R. and Buchwald, M. (1992*b*) Cloning of cDNAs for Fanconi's anaemia by functional complementation. *Nature*, **358**, 434.

The Fanconi Anaemia Breast Cancer Consortium (1996) Positional cloning of the Fanconi anaemia group A gene. *Nature Genetics*, **14**, 324–8.

Thompson, L. H. (1991) Properties and applications of human DNA repair genes. *Mutation Research*, **247**, 213–19.

Verlander, P. C., Lin, J. D., Udono, M. U., Zhang, Q., Gibson, R. A., Mathew, C. G. and Auerbach, A. D. (1994) Mutation analysis of the Fanconi anemia gene FACC. *American Journal of Human Genetics*, **54**, 595–601.

Verlander, P. C., Kaporis, A., Liu, Q., Zhang, Q., Seligsohn, U. and Auerbach, A. D. (1995) Carrier frequency of the IVS4 + 4 A→T mutation of the Fanconi anemia gene FAC in the Ashkenazi Jewish population. *Blood*, **86**, 4034–8.

Wevrick, R., Clarke, C. A. and Buchwald, M. (1993) Cloning and analysis of the murine Fanconi anemia group C cDNA. *Human Molecular Genetics*, **2**, 655–62.

Whitney, M. A., Saito, H., Jakobs, P. M., Gibson, R. A., Moses, R. E. and Grompe, M. (1993) A common mutation in the FACC gene causes Fanconi anaemia in Ashkenazi Jews. *Nature Genetics*, **4**, 202–5.

Whitney, M. A., Thayer, M., Reifsteck, C., Olson, S., Smith, L., Jakobs, P. M., Leach, R., Naylor, S., Joenje, H. and Grompe, M. (1995) Microcell mediated chromosome transfer maps the Fanconi anaemia group D gene to chromosome 3p. *Nature Genetics*, **11**, 341–3.

Whitney, M. A., Royle, G., Low, M. J., Kelly, M. A., Axthelm, M. K., Reifsteck, C., Olson, S., Braun, R. E., Heinrich, M. C., Rathbun, R. K., Bagby, G. C. and Grompe, M. (1996) Germ cell defects and hemopoietic hypersensitivity to gamma-interferon in mice with a targeted disruption of the Fanconi anemia C gene. *Blood*, **88**, 49–58.

Wong, J. C. Y. and Buchwald, M. (1997) Cloning of the bovine and rat Fanconi anemia group C cDNA. *Mammalian Genome*, **8**, 522–5.

Yamashita, T., Barber, D. L., Zhu, Y., Wu, N. and D'Andrea, A. D. (1994) The Fanconi anemia polypeptide FACC is localized to the cytoplasm. *Proceedings of the National Academy of Sciences of the USA*, **91**, 6712–16.

Yamashita, T., Wu, N., Kupfer, G., Corless, C., Joenje, H., Grompe, M. and D'Andrea, A. D. (1996) Clinical variability of Fanconi anemia (type C) results from expression of an amino terminal truncated Fanconi anemia complementation group C polypeptide with partial activity. *Blood*, **87**, 4424–32.

Youssoufian, H. (1994) Localization of Fanconi anemia C protein to the cytoplasm of mammalian cells. *Proceedings of the National Academy of Sciences of the USA*, **91**, 7975–9.

Youssoufian, H. (1996) Cytoplasmic localization of FAC is essential for the correction of a prerepair defect in Fanconi anemia group C cells. *Journal of Clinical Investigtion*, **97**, 2003–10.

Youssoufian, H., Auerbach, A. D., Verlander, P. C., Steimle, V. and Mach, B. (1995) Identification of cytosolic proteins that bind to the Fanconi anemia complementation group C polypeptide in vitro. Evidence for a multimeric complex. *Journal of Biological Chemistry*, **270**, 9876–82.

Youssoufian, H., Li, Y., Martin, M. E. and Buchwald, M. (1996) Induction of Fanconi anemia cellular phenotype in human 293 cells by overexpression of a mutant FAC allele. *Journal of Clinical Investigation*, **97**, 957–62.

Zakrzewski, S. and Sperling, K. (1980) Genetic heterogeneity of Fanconi's anemia demonstrated by somatic cell hybrids. *Human Genetics*, **56**, 81–4.

19

Treatment of Fanconi's anemia

Eliane Gluckman, Gérard Socié, Philippe Guardiola

for the European Blood and Marrow Transplant Group (EBMT) and European Fanconi's Anemia Registry (EUFAR)

Hôpital Saint-Louis, Paris

Introduction

Fanconi's anemia (FA) was originally described as an autosomal recessive disorder, characterized by progressive pancytopenia, diverse congenital abnormalities, and increased predisposition to malignancy (Auerbach et al., 1989). FA cells show a high level of chromosomal breakage, both spontaneously and induced by crosslinking agents such as mitomycin C, nitrogen mustard, diepoxybutane or photoactivated psoralens (Auerbach and Wolman, 1976; Berger et al., 1980). At least eight genetic complementation groups (A–H) have been described (Joenje et al., 1995). Genes for groups A, C, D, and G have been localized to chromosomes 16q24.3, 9q22.3, 3p, and 9p13, respectively, but the complementary deoxyribonucleic acid (cDNA) has been cloned and sequenced only for groups C (*FANC*), A (*FANCA*) and G (*FANG*) (de Winter et al., 1998; Fanconi Anaemia/Breast Cancer Consortium, 1996; Lo Ten Foe et al., 1996; Strathdee et al., 1992*a,b*; Whitney et al., 1995).

FA is a heterogeneous disorder that varies in both the genotype and phenotype (Gillio et al., 1997). Bone marrow failure is the most frequent hematological abnormality, occurring typically around 5 years of age, but aplasia can occur in older patients. Clonal abnormalities, including a high frequency of monosomy 7 and duplications involving 11q, can be observed on marrow cytogenetic analysis, as a sign of transformation to myelodysplastic syndrome or acute myeloblastic leukemia (Auerbach and Allen, 1991; Butturini et al., 1994). Bone marrow studies, including clonogeneic assays and long-term marrow cultures, show that the hemopoietic stem-cell pool gets smaller without gross defects in its microenvironment (Stark et al., 1993*a*). The persistence of normal hemopoietic stem cells in FA has never been demonstrated. Although the molecular expression of the c-*kit* proto-oncogene and Kit ligand in long-term marrow culture is normal (Stark et al., 1993b), there is evidence of a subtle defect in the microenvironment, consisting of dysregulation of cytokines such as interleukin-6, tumor necrosis factor and granulocyte/macrophage colony-stimulating factor (GM-CSF), which may contribute to marrow failure (Rosselli et al., 1994). It has been shown recently that inactivation of the *FANCC* gene augments interferon-γ-induced apoptotic responses in hemopoietic cells (Rathbun et al., 1997). The *FANCC* gene interferes with cell cycle progression, and the binding of FANCC to cdc2 is required for normal G_2/M progression (Kipfer et al., 1997). Without treatment survival is poor, death occurring during the second decade of life from aplastic anemia, leukemia or cancer. Treatment with androgens, steroids or hemopoietic growth factors can improve the situation transiently (Guinan et al., 1994). Allogeneic hemopoietic stem-cell transplantation is currently the only treatment that can restore normal hemopoiesis.

HLA-identical sibling bone marrow transplants

Cyclophosphamide (Cy), used to condition patients with idiopathic aplastic anemia at the total dose of 200mg/kg, has proven to be too toxic for FA patients, leading to a high rate of transplant-related mortality (Gluckman et al., 1980). Radiosensitivity studies, both in vitro and in vivo, have shown a delayed and an abnormal reaction in the form of radiation-induced skin lesions and a failure to repair DNA following fractionated irradiation (Dutreix and Gluckman, 1983). These findings agree with in vitro data showing an increased number of chromosome breaks and cell death when cells are incubated with alkylating agents, and that DNA fails to repair after irradiation. For this reason, the conditioning regimen for bone marrow transplantation (BMT) was modified by our team in 1980; it includes Cy 20mg/kg given intravenously over 4 days and a 5 Gy thoracoabdominal irradiation (TAI), followed by cyclosporin (CsA) alone to prevent graft-versus-host disease (GVHD) (Gluckman, 1989; Gluckman et al., 1983).

In our center from October 1981 to April 1996, 50 patients with FA were transplanted with bone marrow (46 patients) or cord blood (four patients) from an HLA-identical sibling donor, with a median follow-up time of 57 months. The median age at transplant was 11 years (range 4–26). All patients received Cy at a total dose of 20mg/kg except four patients with myelodysplastic changes in the bone marrow, who received 40 mg/kg Cy. All received 5 Gy TAI for conditioning and CsA to prevent GVHD.

The 5-year probability of disease-free survival was $74.4 \pm 6\%$ (Figure 19.1). In a univariate analysis, a small number of transfusions before BMT and the absence of acute or chronic GVHD were associated with improved survival. In the Cox's model, the number of transfusions before transplant was the only factor associated with survival with a relative risk of 7 (2.5–20, $P = 0.0003$). All patients without chronic GVHD survived. All but three patients had engraftment; when

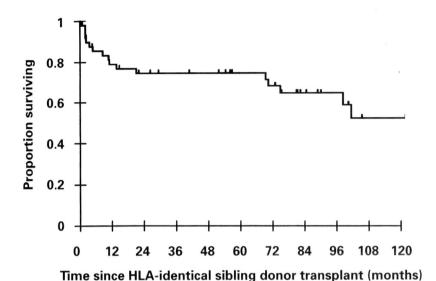

Figure 19.1. Survival of 50 patients with Fanconi's anemia who received a bone marrow transplant from a sibling donor.

assessing hemopoietic chimerism, all engrafted patients were of the donor type with no residual host cells, confirming that the decrease of immunosuppression prior to transplant is able to induce short- and long-term tolerance (Socié et al., 1993). Early complications included hemorrhagic cystitis in four cases, interstitial pneumonitis in four cases, and veno-occlusive disease of the liver in one case. Acute GVHD greater than or equal to grade II was observed in 26 cases (26%), with ten patients having grade III–IV. Chronic GVHD did not occur in 19 cases, was limited in 18 and extensive in two cases. Late complications included six epidermoid carcinoma of the tongue, appearing at a median time of 8 years after BMT; none of the patients developed myelodysplasia or acute leukemia. Hypothyroidism was observed in four cases, cataracts in four cases, two patients had a growth hormone deficiency and were treated, six boys had a normal puberty and one girl menstruated normally and spontaneously. One patient had vaginal stenosis which required surgery, three had esophageal stenosis, one femoral head osteonecrosis, one bronchiolitis and one hemolytic and uremic syndrome. The early causes of death observed in 11 patients were acute GVHD with infection in four cases, chronic GVHD in three cases, rejection in one case and other causes in three cases. After 2 years, eight patients died, four from epidermoid carcinoma of the tongue, one from liver adenocarcinoma, one from encephalitis, one from acquired immune deficiency syndrome (AIDS) and one from hepatitis B cirrhosis.

For 154 patients recorded by the European Blood and Bone Marrow Transplant (EBMT) Registry between 1972 and 1996, the 5-year survival was $66 \pm 4\%$ and the

10-year survival $50 \pm 9\%$. Most of the patients had received the low-dose Cy and TAI protocol. The median follow-up was 2.8 years (range 1 month to 21 years). Chronic extensive GVHD was also a highly significant factor affecting survival ($P = 0.009$, RR$= 3.35$, standard error 0.5). Reports from the International Bone Marrow Transplant Registry (IBMTR) (Gluckman et al., 1995) and from individual centers have confirmed that regimens including low-dose Cy give a better survival than regimens using >100 mg/kg Cy (Hows et al., 1989; Kohli-Kumar et al., 1994). The IBMTR study analyzed the results of allogeneic BMT in 151 patients transplanted with an HLA-identical sibling and in 48 patients transplanted with an alternative related or unrelated donor. FA was documented by cytogenetics in all the cases. The 2-year probability of survival was 66% after HLA-identical sibling transplants and 29% after alternative donor transplants. Being younger, having higher pretransplant platelets counts, use of antithymocyte globulin and use of low-dose Cy plus limited field irradiation and CsA for GVHD prophylaxis were associated with improved survival. These results show that early transplant and decreasing the dose of Cy reduce the toxicity and improve survival.

However, some centers have reported that Cy doses in the order of 100 mg/kg to 140 mg/kg with or without ATG but without irradiation give long-term survival rates greater than 50% (Flowers et al., 1992; Zanis-Neto et al., 1995). These results should be tempered because of the small size of the series and because the overall toxicity was reported as high. These results raise the hypothesis that the sensitivity to alkylating agents may vary according to the type of genetic mutation, which is reflected in vivo by phenotype heterogeneity and by variation in the number of chromosome breaks. Some mutations may be more severe than others. Cases of spontaneous mosaicism have been observed, which could restore a higher resistance rate to conventional doses of chemotherapy (Lo Ten Foe et al., 1997).

The observation of secondary tumors (ST) after transplant is of major concern. The probability of developing malignant tumors is very high in this population because of the addition of several risk factors, including the method of conditioning with or without irradiation, environmental exposure and chromosome instability that is characteristic of the disease. All ST were observed in males at an interval of 6–11 years after transplant. They were mostly head and neck squamous carcinoma.(Deeg et al., 1996; Socié et al., 1991). A joint analysis between the Seattle group and the Paris group has shown that the relative risk of ST is 42% and that irradiation is not the only risk factor, as the Seattle group never used irradiation in the conditioning regimen. In a multivariate analysis, the factors associated with a high risk of developing ST are acute GVHD (RR$= 7.7$) and increasing age (RR$= 1.3$). The fact that only solid tumors and no lymphomyeloproliferative malignancies are observed posttransplant is consistent with the fact that transplantation provides patients with a normal hemopoietic system, but does not affect the congenital defect in other tissues.

The good results of allogeneic BMT with an HLA-identical sibling raises several questions about the optimal date of BMT and the best conditioning regimen.

Concerning the date of transplant, there is general agreement to use BMT with an HLA-identical sibling, as first-line therapy, without trying androgens or steroids which have secondary effects. When blood counts show the criteria of severe aplastic anemia (hemoglobin <8g/100ml, polymorphonuclear cells <500/mm^3 or platelets <20,000/mm^3), transfusions are necessary; therefore, this limit seems a suitable indicator of BMT. During this waiting period, it is very important to perform bone marrow aspiration and cytogenetic analyses regularly for detecting clonal abnormalities or leukemic transformation, as BMT performed late after a long period of aplasia or during leukemic transformation gives poor results.

The problem of the best conditioning regimen is more difficult to solve for several reasons. First, the number of patients is too small for a prospective randomized multicenter study. Second, currently there is no in vitro test for predicting the sensitivity of a given patient to the conditioning regimen. There is no information about the sensitivity of cell subsets to alkylating agents. The sensitivity of leukemic cells seems to be increased, as some remissions have been obtained after low-dose chemotherapy or after conditioning with low-dose Cy without any attempt to induce remission, but these cases are rare and most of the patients treated for acute leukemia do not tolerate standard-dose chemotherapy and have a very poor prognosis. It is possible that the genetic diagnosis, which will be performed in the future, will delineate criteria for disease severity (Gillio et al., 1997). For this reason, it is highly important to report all the new cases in Registries and perform gene mutation studies, as is performed in EUFAR. Third, it will be very difficult to prove any further improvement when most survival curves show more than 75% long-term survival. Furthermore, omitting irradiation from the conditioning regimen does not seem to diminish the risk of secondary tumors, which are also related to the genetic defect and to the environment, as shown by the observation of different phenotypic expression of the disease in homozygous twins.(Lo Ten Foe et al., 1997). A proposal of our current protocol is shown in Table 19.1.

Alternative donor transplants

The development of large international registries including more than four million donors has enabled physicians to find bone marrow donors for patients without HLA-identical siblings. In FA, the results of mismatched family transplants or transplants performed with HLA-'identical' unrelated donors have been disappointing. In our retrospective series of 18 patients transplanted with a nonT-depleted unrelated BMT, only two are alive. Deaths were attributed to multivisceral failure (six patients), acute GVHD (five patients), rejection (two patients), infection (one patient), and interstitial pneumonitis (two patients). Of

Table 19.1. Proposed protocol for matched related
bone marrow transplantation in Fanconi's anemia

I – Objective		
Absence of irradiation for prevention of secondary tumor		
II – Conditioning		
Myleran	1.5 mg/kg per day	
	days –8, –7, –6, –5	
	Total dose 6 mg/kg	
Cyclophosphamide	10 mg/kg per day	
	days –5, –4, –3, –2	
	Total dose 40 mg/kg	
III – Prevention of GVHD		
Cyclosporin A	3 mg/kg starting day –1 for at	
	least 6 months	
Methotrexate	5 mg/m²	
	days +1, +3, +6	

Note:
GVHD = graft-versus-host disease.

41 patients with alternative donors reported to the IBMTR, 2-year survival was 29%; the probability of rejection was 24%; the probability of grade II–IV GVHD was 51%; of chronic GVHD 46% and of IP 25%. The number of patients was too small to analyze risk factors (Gluckman et al., 1995).

The European Blood and Marrow Transplantation (EBMT) Working Party on Aplastic Anemia has recently analyzed the outcome of allogeneic BMT using alternative donors for FA. Patients receiving grafts from HLA-pheno-identical related donors were excluded from this analysis ($n=16$) as their outcome was similar to that reported for patients transplanted with a geno-identical sibling ($P=0.6$). Seventy-six patients reported by 18 centers were analyzed, the median age at transplant was 10 years (range 4–31). The median time from diagnosis to transplant was 42 months (range 2–303). The donor was an unrelated HLA-'matched' donor in 53 cases defined by serology for class I and low-resolution DRB1 typing, a mismatched unrelated donor for at least one antigen in seven cases and an HLA-mismatched family donor in the last 16. For conditioning, low-dose Cy either 20 mg/kg ($n=22$) or 40 mg/kg ($n=34$) was used combined with TAI ($n=35$) or total-body irradiation ($n=29$). Nine patients did not receive irradiation. Antithymocyte globulin or antiT monoclonal antibody was given prior to transplant in 39 cases. GVHD prevention consisted of CsA alone ($n=12$) or associated with corticosteroids (methylprednisolone) ($n=16$) or CsA+methylpredisolone+methotrexate (MTX) ($n=16$) or CsA+ATG or monoclonal antibody with or without MTX ($n=26$). Three patients only did not receive CsA. Bone

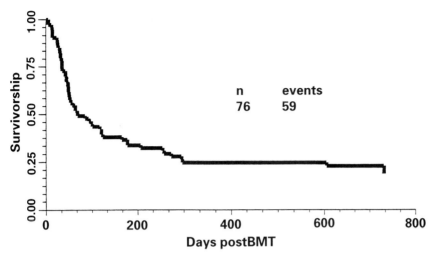

Figure 19.2. Survival of patients with Fanconi's anemia who received a bone marrow transplant from an unrelated or a mismatched related donor.

marrow T-cell depletion was performed in 20 cases (CD34+ selection in 9 cases and other methods in 11 cases). The median number of nucleated cells infused was 3.6×10^8/kg (range 0.2–22.5).

With a median follow-up of 32 months (range 1–166), the 2-year survival was $23 \pm 5\%$ (Figure 19.2). Engraftment was complete in 58 cases, 11 patients had a primary graft failure including four patients who died before day 21. Acute grade II–IV GVHD was observed in 38 of 69 patients at risk, and 23 patients developed grade III–IV acute GVHD. Among 28 patients surviving more than 90 days, two had limited and seven extensive chronic GVHD. Main causes of death were infections and GVHD. In univariate analysis, factors associated with survival were donor gender (male $38 \pm 9\%$ versus female $13 \pm 5\%$, $P = 0.003$) and T-cell depletion: with T-cell depletion survival was $47 \pm 11\%$ whereas it was $16 \pm 5\%$ without T-cell depletion, $P = 0.03$ (Figure 19.3). Patients receiving a graft from an HLA-'matched' unrelated donor had a significantly better outcome than those transplanted with an HLA-mismatched related one (2-year event-free survival $30 \pm 7\%$ versus $6 \pm 6\%$, $P = 0.04$). When separately analyzing patients transplanted with an HLA-'identical' unrelated donor in a Cox's model donor, gender (RR = 2.2, $P = 0.04$) and T-cell depletion (RR = 2.7, $P = 0.03$) remained significant factors affecting survival. Survival was not modified by using a higher dose of Cy (20 versus 40 mg/kg) or ATG or monoclonal antibody.

GVHD was associated with the recipient's gender: female patients were more likely to have GVHD than males ($P = 0.03$). Being younger ($P = 0.02$) and T-cell depletion ($P = 0.027$) were associated with diminution of GVHD.

These results show that the outcome of unrelated BMT is improving. This is probably due to several factors, including better selection of the patients, improved techniques of HLA matching by high-resolution molecular techniques and modifications of the transplant procedure. To overcome GVHD, T-cell

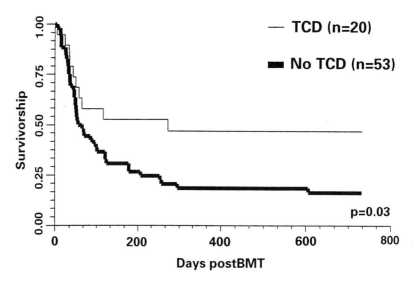

Figure 19.3. Impact of T-cell depletion of the graft on survival of patients with Fanconi's anemia who received a bone marrow transplant from an unrelated or a mismatched related donor.

depletion can be used either by positive selection of bone marrow CD34+ cells on columns or magnetic beads, or by T-cell depletion with elutriation or lysis with monoclonal antibodies. This approach is likely to increase the frequency of rejection. As the intensification of the conditioning regimen will certainly increase the risk of toxicity, agents not yet tested, such as busulphan or thiotepa, may be worth testing in vitro and in vivo. It is also possible to increase the number of stem cells infused by adding to the bone-marrow-derived CD34+ cells G-CSF-mobilized peripheral blood CD34+ cells. The add-back of lymphocytes after transplant may also improve engraftment in patients without GVHD.

In our center, we currently use a modified conditioning regimen with a higher dose of Cy (total dose 40 mg/kg), associated with 4.5 Gy total-body irradiation and ATG (six doses) from day –6 followed by a CD34+-selected unrelated bone marrow transplant (Table 19.2). This new protocol has markedly improved our results with nine out of 11 patients alive with good engraftment and minimal GVHD. One patient rejected and one died of aspergillosis associated with acute GVHD. More patients and longer follow-up are required to evaluate this new encouraging strategy.

New strategies

Cord blood transplant

The first successful HLA-identical cord blood transplant was performed on a FA patient. The donor was known, before birth, to be HLA identical to the patient and not affected by FA. His cord blood was collected at birth and transplanted,

Table 19.2. Proposed protocol for unrelated bone marrow
transplantation in Fanconi's anemia

I – Conditioning	
Cyclophosphamide	1.0 mg/kg per day
	days –6, –5, –4, –3
	Total dose 40 mg/kg
ATG	12 mg/kg
	days –6 to –1 (6 doses)
Total body irradiation	Single dose 4.5 Gy
	dose rate 26 cGy/min per day

II – Prevention of GVHD

T-cell depletion by CD34+ cell selection Isolex Baxter

Cyclosporin A 3 mg/kg per day –1 to day 30 then orally for 1 year

Prednisone 1 mg/kg on day –6 slowly taper after day 20

after thawing, to his HLA-identical brother who had severe aplastic anemia
caused by FA. The patient received before transplant low-dose CY and TAI and,
after transplant, CsA to prevent GVHD. This patient's hematology and immunology were completely reconstituted with a complete donor chimerism, with a
follow-up of more than 9 years. Since this first successful transplant, the number
of cases of cord blood transplants has been increasing worldwide, including more
than 700 patients, adults and children with various hematological diseases.
Simultaneously, cord blood banks have developed, mostly in the USA and in
Europe, for unrelated matched or mismatched cord blood transplants. Eurocord
has collected 16 patients transplanted with cord blood for FA (Gluckman et al.,
1997): eight received HLA-identical sibling cord blood, five are currently alive and
three died early. Eight patients received a partially 'matched' unrelated cord
blood transplant; only one is currently alive, the others died early after transplant.
It seems that one of the advantages of using cord blood, instead of bone marrow,
is a reduced severity of GVHD, because of the relative immaturity of the
newborn's immune system.

Gene therapy

Autologous transplant has been discussed but seems of limited value in FA, where
the few CD34+ cells isolated from G-CSF-mobilized hemopoietic stem cells from
the blood do not grow in long-term culture and are unlikely to give short- or long-
term engraftment. Collection of cord blood at birth or of peripheral-blood CD34+
stem cells can be performed at an early phase of the disease for gene transfer. The
recent localization of *FANCA*, *FANCC* and *FANCG* genes and the demonstration in

vitro that transfected cells have a selective growth advantage over FA cells have increased the interest in designing gene therapy protocols (Liu et al., 1994). Several questions remain unsolved, including the integration site of the gene in primitive hemopoietic stem cells, the level of integration required for the correction of the disease, the long-term expression of the transfected gene, the selective growth advantage of transfected cells, and the function of the FA genes' protein (Segal et al., 1994; Walsh et al., 1994; Yamashita et al., 1994). On the other hand, prenatal diagnosis and early recognition of the disease as well as detection of the heterozygous state are very likely to diminish the incidence of the disease.

Conclusion

FA is a hereditary disorder characterized by chromosomal breaks increased by crosslinking agents. BMT is the treatment of choice when an HLA-identical sibling donor has been identified. Results have improved since it was realized that in vitro sensitivity to alkylating agents explains the in vivo toxicity of high-dose cyclophosphamide used for conditioning. The reduction of the dose of cyclophosphamide to 20mg/kg with 5 Gy TAI/TLI has given rise to 75% long-term survival. In the long term, most patients are completely cured of the bone marrow disease but there is concern about the observed increased frequency of secondary tumors, all of which were head and neck secondary carcinoma. The results of mismatched family transplants or unrelated matched transplant are improving with the use of total-body irradiation and T-cell depletion. New approaches are being explored, including cord blood transplant and gene therapy.

References

Auerbach, A. D. and Allen, R. G. (1991) Leukemia and preleukemia in Fanconi anemia patients. *Cancer Genetics and Cytogenetics*, **51**, 1–12.

Auerbach, A. D. and Wolman, S. R. (1976) Susceptibility of Fanconi anaemia fibroblasts to chromosome damage by carcinogens. *Nature*, **261**, 494–6.

Auerbach., A. D., Rogatko, A. and Schroeder-Kurth, T. M. (1989) International Fanconi anemia registry: relation of clinical symptoms to diepoxybutane sensitivity. *Blood*, **73**, 391–6.

Berger, R., Bernheim, A. and Gluckman, E. (1980) In vitro effect of cyclophosphamide metabolites on chromosomes of Fanconi's anaemia patients. *British Journal of Haematology*, **45**, 565–8.

Butturini, A., Gale, R. P., Verlander, P. C., Adler-Brecher, B., Gillio, A. P. and Auerbach, A. D. (1994) Hematological abnormalities in Fanconi anemia: an international Fanconi anemia registry study. *Blood*, **84**, 1650–5.

De Winter, J. P., Waisfisz, Q., Rooimans, M. A., van Barkel, C. G. M., Bosnoyam–Collins, L.,

Alon, N., Carreau, M., Bender, O., Demuth, J., Schindler, D., Pronk, J. C., Arwert, F., Hoehn, H., Digwal, M., Buhwald, M. and Joenje, H. (1998) The Fanconi anemia group G gene *FANCG* is identical with *XRCC9*. *Nature Genetics*, **20**, 281–3.

Deeg, H. J., Socié, G., Schoch, G., Henry-Amar, M., Flowers, M., Witherspoon, R. P., Devergie, A., Sullivan, K. M., Gluckman, E. and Storb, R. (1996) Malignancies after marrow transplantation for aplastic anemia and Fanconi anemia: a joint Seattle and Paris analysis of results in 700 patients. *Blood*, **87**, 386–92.

Dutreix, J. and Gluckman, E. (1983) Skin test of radiosensitivity. Application to Fanconi anemia. *Journal of European Radiotherapy*, **4**, 3–8.

Fanconi Anaemia/Breast Cancer Consortium (1996) Positional cloning of the Fanconi anaemia group A gene. *Nature Genetics*, **14**, 324–8.

Flowers, M. E. D., Doney, K.C., Storb, R. et al. (1992) Marrow transplantation for Fanconi anemia with or without leukemic transformation: an update of the Seattle experience. *Bone Marrow Transplantation*, **9**,167–73.

Gillio, A. P., Verlander, P. C., Batish, S. D., Giampetro, P. F. and Auerbach, A. D. (1997) Phenotypic consequences of mutations in the Fanconi anemia FAC gene: an international Fanconi anemia registry study. *Blood*, **90**, 105–10.

Gluckman, E. (1989) Bone marrow transplantation for Fanconi anemia. *Baillière's Clinical Haematology*, **2**, 153–62.

Gluckman, E., Devergie, A., Schaison, G. et al. (1980) Bone marrow transplantation in Fanconi anemia. *British Journal of Haematology*, **45**, 557–64.

Gluckman, E., Devergie, A. and Dutreix, J. (1983) Radiosensitivity in Fanconi anemia: application to the conditioning for bone marrow transplantation. *British Journal of Haematology*, **54**, 431–40.

Gluckman, E., Auerbach, A. D. and Horowitz, M. (1995) Bone marrow transplants in Fanconi anemia from the International bone marrow transplant registry. *Blood*, **86**, 2856–62.

Gluckman, E., Rocha, V., Boyer-Chammard, A., Locatelli, F., Arcese, W., Pasquini, R., Ortega, J., Souillet, G., Ferreira, E., Laporte, J. P., Fernandez, M., Chastang, C. for EUROCORD Transplant Group and European Blood and Marrow Transplant Group (EBMT) (1997) Clinical outcome in recipients of cord blood transplant from related and unrelated donors. *New England Journal of Medicine*, **337**, 373–81.

Guinan, E. C., Lopez, K. D., Huhn, R. D., Felser, J. M. and Nathan, D. G. (1994) Evaluation of granulocyte-macrophage colony-stimulating factor for treatment of cytopenia in children with Fanconi anemia. *Journal of Pediatrics*, **124**, 144–50.

Hows, J. M., Chapple, M., Marsch, J. C. W., Durrant, S., Vin, J. L. and Swirsky, D. (1989) Bone marrow transplantation for Fanconi anemia: the Hammersmith experience 1977–1989. *Bone Marrow Transplantation*, **4**, 629–34.

Joenje, H., Ten Foe, J. R. L., Oostra, A. B., Van Berkel, C. G. N., Rooimans, M. A., Schroeder-Kurth, T., Wegner, R. D., Gille, J. J. P., Buchwald, M. and Arwert, F. (1995) Classification of Fanconi anemia patients by complementation analysis: evidence for a fifth genetic subtype. *Blood*, **86**, 2156–60.

Kipfer, G. M., Yashimata, T., Naf, D., Suliman, A., Asano, S. and D'Andrea, A. D. (1997) The Fanconi anemia polypeptide, FAC, binds to the cycline-dependent kinase, cdc2. *Blood*, **90**, 1047–54.

Kohli-Kumar, M., Morris, C., Delaat, C., Sambrano, J., Masterson, M., Mueller, R., Shahidi,

N. T., Yanik, G., Desantes, K., Friedman, D. J., Auerbach, A. D. and Harris, R. E. (1994) Bone marrow transplantation in Fanconi anemia using matched sibling donors. *Blood*, **84**, 2050–4.

Liu, J. M., Buchwald, M., Walsh, C. E. and Young, N. S. (1994) Fanconi anemia and novel strategies for therapy. *Blood*, **84**, 3995–4007.

Lo Ten Foe, J. R., Rooimans, M. A., Bosnoyan-Collins, L., Alon, N., Wijker, M., Parker, L., Lightfoot, J., Carreau, M., Callen, D. F., Savoia, A., Cheng, N. C., Van Berkel, C. G. M., Strunk, M. H. P., Gille, J. J. P., Pals, G., Kruyt Fae, Pronk, J. C., Arwert, F., Buchwald, M. and Joenje, H. (1996) Expression cloning of a cDNAs for the major Fanconi anaemia gene FAA. *Nature Genetics*, **14**, 320–4.

Lo Ten Foe, J. R., Kwee, M. L., Rooimans, M. A., Oostra, A. B., Veerman, A. J. P., Van Weel, M., Pauli, R. M., Shahidi, N. T., Dokal, I., Roberts, I., Alatay, C., Gluckman, E., Gibson, R. A., Mathew, C. G., Arwert, F. and Joenje, H. (1997) Somatic mosaicism in Fanconi anaemia: molecular basis and clinical significance. *European Journal of Human Genetics*, **5**, 137–48.

Rathbun, R. K., Faulkner, G. R., Ostroski, M. H., Christianson, H. G., Hughes, G., Jones, S. G., Cahn, R., Maziarz, R., Royle, G., Keeble, W., Heinrich, M. C., Grompe, M., Tower, P. A. and Bagby, G. C. (1997) Inactivation of the Fanconi Anemia group C gene augments interferon γ induced apoptotic responses in hemopoietic cells. *Blood*, **90**, 974–85.

Rosselli, F., Sanceau, J., Gluckman, E., Wiettzerbin, J. and Moustacchi, E. (1994) Abnormal lymphokine production a novel feature of the genetic disease Fanconi anemia: II in-vitro and in-vivo spontaneous overproduction of tumor necrosis factor alpha. *Blood*, **83**, 1216–25.

Segal, G. M., Magenis, R. E., Brown, M., Keeble, W., Smith, T. D., Heinrich, M. C. and Bagby, G. C. (1994) Repression of Fanconi anemia gene (FACC) expression inhibits growth of hemopoietic progenitor cells. *Journal of Clinical Investigations*, **94**, 846–52

Socié, G., Henry-Amar, M., Cosset, J. M., Devergie, A., Girinsky, T. and Gluckman, E. (1991) Increased incidence of solid malignant tumors after bone marrow transplantation for severe aplastic anemia. *Blood*, **78**, 277–9.

Socié, G., Gluckman, E., Raynal, B. et al. (1993) Bone marrow transplantation for Fanconi anemia using low dose cyclophosphamide/thoraco abdominal irradiation as conditioning regimen: chimerism study by the polymerase chain reaction. *Blood*, **82**, 2249–56.

Stark, R., Thierry, D., Richard, P. and Gluckman, E. (1993*a*) Long-term bone marrow culture in Fanconi's anaemia. *British Journal of Haematology*, **83**, 554–9.

Stark, R., Andre, C., Thierry, D., Cherel, M., Galibert, F. and Gluckman, E. (1993*b*) The expression of cytokines and cytosine receptor genes in long-term bone marrow culture in congenital and acquired bone marrow hypoplasias. *British Journal of Haematology*, **83**, 560–6.

Strathdee, C. A., Duncan, A. M. V. and Buchwald, M. (1992*a*) Evidence for at least four Fanconi anaemia genes including FACC on chromosome nine. *Nature Genetics*, **1**, 196–8.

Strathdee, C. A., Gavish, H., Shannon, W. R. and Buchwald, M. (1992*b*) Cloning of cDNAs for Fanconi's anaemia by functional complementation. *Nature*, **356**, 763–7.

Walsh, C. E., Nienhuis, A. W., Samulski, R. J., Brown, M. G., Miller, J. M., Young, N. S. and Liu, J. M. (1994) Phenotypic correction of Fanconi anemia in human hemopoietic cells with a recombinant adeno-associated virus vector. *Journal of Clinical Investigations*, **94**, 1440–8.

Whitney, M., Thayer, M., Reifsteck, C., Olson, S., Smith, L., Jakobs, P. M., Leach, R., Naylor,

S., Joenje, H. and Grompe, M. (1995) Microcell mediated chromosome transfer maps the Fanconi anaemia group D gene to chromosome 3p. *Nature Genetics*, **11**, 341–3.

Yamashita, T., Barber, D. L., Zhu, Y., Wu, N. and D'Andrea, A. D. (1994) The Fanconi anemia polypeptide FACC is localized to the cytoplasm. *Proceedings of the National Academy of Sciences of the USA*, **91**, 6712–16.

Zanis-Neto, J., Ribeiro, R. C., Meideros, C., Andrade, R. J., Ogasawara, V., Hush, M., Magdalena, N., Friedrich, M. L., Bitencourt, M. A., Bonfim, C. and Pasquini, A. R. (1995) Bone marrow transplantation for patients with Fanconi anemia: a study of 24 cases from a single institution. *Bone Marrow Transplantation*, **15**, 293–8.

20

Genetic correction of Fanconi's anemia

Johnson M. Liu

National Institutes of Health, Bethesda

Introduction

Fanconi's anemia (FA) is a genetic syndrome that leads to bone marrow failure, congenital anomalies, and a predisposition to cancer in affected individuals (Fanconi, 1927, 1967). FA's clinical features and genetic basis, as well as the conventional approaches to treating FA patients, are detailed in Chapters 17–19. The purpose of this review is to summarize both the rationale and the progress of gene therapy strategies aimed at correcting the hemopoietic defect of FA, usually manifesting as aplastic bone marrow failure.

FA is thought to affect the hemopoietic stem cell (HSC), as evidenced by profoundly diminished numbers of platelets, erythrocytes, and granulocytes in patients. As a stem-cell disorder, the hemopoietic consequences of FA can be effectively treated by complete replacement of the patient's stem cells with those from a histocompatible donor (Gluckman et al., 1989, 1995; Kohli–Kumar et al., 1993). Pretreatment with chemotherapy and irradiation is required to destroy the diseased marrow as well as to suppress the patient's immune system so that it cannot reject the transplanted stem cells. Historically, this has been difficult to accomplish in FA patients since they are particularly sensitive to these toxic agents. Doses of therapy typically required to eliminate a patient's immune system cannot routinely be given, and, at this time, an individual patient's sensitivity to the chemotherapy and irradiation cannot be predicted. Even with the lower doses of therapy given today, some patients are inordinately sensitive and will die as a result of organ failure. Moreover, FA patients appear to have more difficulties with graft-versus-host disease. For these reasons, allogeneic stem-cell transplantation is currently limited to patients with an unaffected matched sibling donor. Stem-cell transplantation from alternative donors, while successful in selected cases, is associated with a high risk of graft failure and must be carefully considered in terms of risk and benefit for each individual. For FA patients lacking an appropriate donor, experimental therapies should be considered.

Gene transfer is as yet unproven as a therapeutic modality (Liu et al., 1995*b*). Although some encouraging results have been reported for adenosine deaminase deficiency (Bordignon et al., 1995; Kohn et al., 1995), the concept of gene augmentation has been difficult to realize, in part because of low transfection efficiency. The hemopoietic stem cell has been targeted for genetic manipulation because of its potential for continuous production of blood elements (Dunbar, 1995). However, despite intensive efforts at altering the conditions of transduction, human HSC marking using currently available vectors has been disappointingly inefficient (Dunbar et al., 1995). Application of gene transfer to FA highlights many of the considerations and technical difficulties relevant to gene therapy of other hematological disorders. The new information obtained from these studies on the molecular function of FA genes and on the nature of the FA hemopoietic defect should ultimately prove useful for devising effective new treatment strategies. Perhaps equally as important, they may also guide future research efforts in the general application of gene therapy to other, more common, hematological diseases.

FANCC and FANCA

To briefly review, FA can be divided into at least eight groups according to somatic cell hybridization studies and complementation analysis. The genes for two groups, FA-C and FA-A, have been identified and are called *FANCC* (Strathdee et al., 1992) and *FANCA* (Fanconi Anaemia/Breast Cancer Consortium, 1996; Lo Ten Foe et al., 1996), respectively. Since the two genes are not homologous with each other and yet mutations in either gene lead to FA, the FANCC and FANCA proteins may either function in a common pathway (for example, as members of an enzymatic cascade), may physically associate, or may interact in some functional manner. Recently, Kupfer et al. (1997) reported that FANCC and FANCA proteins interact to form a nuclear complex. If reproducible, this finding suggests that FA proteins may be directly involved in a nuclear pathway.

There is now mounting evidence that at least one important function of the wild-type FANCC protein is in the modulation of apoptosis or programmed cell death. One series of experiments suggests that lymphoblastoid cell lines and peripheral blood lymphocytes from *FANCC*-mutant patients seem to be resistant to apoptosis induced by various stimuli (Ridet et al., 1997), whereas other investigators have found that overexpression of the wild-type FANCC protein also protects hemopoietic cells from undergoing apoptosis (Cumming et al., 1996). One possible explanation for these contradictory findings is that FANCC (and possibly other FA proteins) may act at a decision fork between apoptotic and nonapoptotic (necrotic) cell death. One prediction from this hypothesis is that overexpression of the FANCC protein may promote cell survival through suppression of apoptotic pathways. While none of these experiments has yielded definitive conclusions, they point out mechanisms which may be involved following transduction and complementation with the FA genes.

Hemopoietic defect in FA

The pathophysiological abnormalities leading to bone marrow failure in patients with FA are not well understood. Some hypotheses include qualitative or quantitative defects in stem cells or defects in the auxiliary cells of the hemopoietic microenvironment, resulting in reduced or even absent colony formation [as measured by myeloid (Daneshbod–Skibba et al., 1980) and erythroid (Alter et al., 1991) progenitor assays]. These clonogeneic assays do not necessarily provide information regarding stem cells, but reflect the hemopoietic defect at the progenitor level.

With respect to the auxiliary or stromal cells, the FA mutation does not seem to consistently abrogate the formation of an adherent layer (Stark et al., 1993), although the layer may be slower than normal to develop. The capacity of FA fibroblasts to produce stem-cell factor (SCF) and macrophage colony-stimulating factor (M-CSF) is normal, but the interleukin-1- (IL-1-) induced expression of granulocyte colony-stimulating factor (G-CSF), granulocyte/macrophage colony-stimulating factor (GM-CSF), and interleukin-6 (IL-6) varies between individuals, ranging from blunted responses to hypersensitive ones (Bagby et al., 1993). This variability may reflect the heterogeneity of the disorder but does not seem to be a direct effect of the FA mutation. By implication, the FA defect is not a primary disorder of stromal function but a disorder affecting the hemopoietic stem cell.

Assessment of human HSC reserve is technically difficult. HSC are classically defined by their ability to reconstitute multilineage hemopoiesis after transplantation into marrow-ablated animals. Enrichment of these rare cells is now based upon identifying cells with unique surface antigens such as the CD34 molecule. No direct assay to identify and quantitate true stem cells exists, although the long-term culture-initiating cell (LTC-IC) assay has been touted as a surrogate. The LTC-IC is defined as a primitive hemopoietic cell capable of producing clonogeneic progenitor cells after 5 weeks of long-term bone marrow culture (Eaves et al., 1991; Sutherland et al., 1989). Several investigators have examined FA hemopoiesis in long-term culture (Butturini and Gale, 1994; Stark et al., 1993). Secondary colonies were reported to develop from the nonadherent population of cells (Butturini and Gale, 1994). As yet, however, no studies have systematically assessed LTC-IC (from the adherent population) from FA patients.

FA gene transduction and hemopoiesis

Recombinant vectors to transfer foreign genes have been engineered from both deoxyribonucleic acid (DNA) and ribonucleic acid (RNA) viruses (Liu et al., 1995*a*). Currently, murine retroviruses are still the best-characterized vectors adapted to stable integration of foreign genetic material, a process referred to as transduction. Retroviruses are single-stranded RNA viruses that bind to a specific surface receptor for entry into cells. Once inside the cell, the viral RNA is converted into double-stranded DNA by the enzyme reverse transcriptase, before integration into the host cell genome as provirus. Recombinant retroviral vectors currently in use for human gene therapy are derived from the Moloney murine leukemia virus (MoMLV). These recombinant vectors contain the gene of interest flanked by the long terminal repeats (LTRs); the LTRs contain the promoter, polyadenylation signals and the sequences required for viral replication and integration. The utility of retroviruses as vectors for gene therapy has been greatly enhanced by the ability to engineer packaging cell lines that secrete retroviral virion particles. These cell lines are designed to express a helper genome encoding viral proteins. A separate vector genome that contains the gene to be transferred (along with cis elements necessary for RNA encapsidation, replication and integration) is then stably introduced into these cell lines to generate a 'producer' packaging line. The main advantage of using retroviral vectors is their ability to integrate into the host cell genome and confer long-term expression of the transgene. The major limitation of retroviral vectors is that the target cell must be actively replicating in order for the vector to integrate into the host chromosome.

Adeno-associated viruses (AAV) are single-stranded DNA parvoviruses (Liu et al., 1995*a*). The viral genome consists of *rep* genes encoding regulatory proteins and *cap* genes which encode the capsid proteins. The genome is flanked by inverted terminal repeats (ITR) that function as viral origins of replication and are necessary for encapsidation and integration of viral DNA into the cellular genome. In the absence of a helper virus such as adenovirus, AAV causes a latent infection characterized by the integration of viral DNA into the cellular genome. Recombinant AAV vector production involves cotransfection of a permissive cell line (such as the 293 line) with a recombinant plasmid containing the gene to be transferred (with a promoter and polyadenylation signal) flanked by the AAV ITRs and a helper plasmid carrying the *rep* and *cap* genes but lacking the AAV ITRs. The 293 cells are coinfected with adenovirus to generate AAV virion particles. These particles are released with cell lysis and are contaminated with helper adenovirus. Subsequent heating to destroy adenovirus is followed by purification and concentration of heat-stable recombinant AAV particles.

We have used both recombinant retroviral and AAV vectors to transfer copies of the normal *FANCC* complementary DNA (cDNA) to cells from patients with *FANCC* mutations (Walsh et al., 1994*a*,*b*, 1995). Phenotypic correction was demonstrated following viral transduction by resistance to mitomycin-C-(MMC-) induced cell death and insusceptibility to induced chromosomal aberrations. Next, we demonstrated that CD34-enriched hemopoietic progenitors isolated from FA patients exhibit the same hypersensitivity to MMC characteristic of cultured FA cells. Gene transduction of *FANCC* progenitor cells using a viral vector containing the *FANCC* cDNA significantly improved colony formation in clonogeneic assays in the absence, as well as in the presence, of low concentrations of MMC (Walsh et al., 1994*a,b*). We have recently extended our transduction studies to include the newly identified *FANCA* cDNA (Fu et al., 1997). We first engineered a recombinant retroviral vector containing the normal *FANCA* cDNA. Transduction with this vector also appeared to improve the viability of hemopoietic progenitor colonies from patients with *FANCA* mutations. These experiments imply that both FANCC and FANCA proteins are involved in the maintenance of hemopoietic progenitor cell viability, perhaps by countering programmed cell death. As yet unclear is whether the *FANCC* and *FANCA* genes exert a function on true hemopoietic stem cells and whether it might be possible to expand progenitor cell (measured as LTC-IC) numbers following gene transfer.

Hemopoietic stem cell targets and rationale for gene therapy

Theoretically, HSC represent an ideal target for gene therapy since they can be harvested from bone marrow (BM), peripheral blood (PB), or umbilical cord blood and transduced ex vivo (Lu et al., 1996). Replication (self-renewal) of stem cells and repopulation with progeny blood cells should result in the continuous maintenance of the transgene in blood cells of the patient. In practice, many technical obstacles limit gene transfer to HSC (Dunbar, 1996; Liu et al., 1995*b*). First, as discussed, no direct assay to identify and quantitate true stem cells exists. For example, no direct correlation exists between transduction of LTC-IC and HSC. Second, true HSC may be predominantly quiescent (in the G_0 phase of the cell cycle), making them unsusceptible to proviral integration and transduction. Third, since chromosomal integration is necessary for delivery of the transgene to progeny cells, adenoviral and other nonDNA-integrating delivery systems will result in only transient expression. Gene-marking studies have been conducted as part of autologous BM or PB stem-cell transplantation protocols for the treatment of malignancies (Brenner et al., 1993*a,b*). For the most part, these studies have confirmed that transfer of genes to HSC is very inefficient (Dunbar et al., 1995).

It has been possible to model HSC gene therapy with computer simulation studies in which the contribution of labeled (genetically marked) progenitor cells to hemopoiesis is assessed under various circumstances (Abkowitz et al., 1997).

For this purpose, HSC are assumed to undergo either replication (self-renewal), differentiation, or apoptosis, and these parameters are assigned probabilities. These studies have confirmed that gene transfer experiments that render an HSC either a proliferative (replication rate) or survival (antiapoptosis) advantage can significantly increase the number of marked cells. However, transplantation of small numbers of HSC led to dramatic variation in terms of the contribution of marked clones to hemopoiesis, whereas variability was minimized when large numbers of HSC were transplanted (Abkowitz et al., 1997). These predictions highlight the difficulties in devising effective HSC gene therapy, since the large numbers of HSC needed for successful transplantation may be inefficiently transduced. This problem is magnified in FA, in one sense, as the number of HSC may be lower than that of a normal individual. On the other hand, if FA gene transfer confers a survival advantage to the corrected HSC, corrected clones may eventually dominate hemopoiesis.

Recent observations have suggested that, within the hypoplastic FA bone marrow microenvironment, the mutant cell may be at a selective disadvantage relative to the wild-type. Perhaps the clearest example is that, rarely, FA patients may develop spontaneous reversion of the cellular phenotype as manifested by the presence of two subpopulations of lymphocytes, one of which retains sensitivity to DNA cross-linking agents (MMC) while the other has acquired resistance to these agents (Lo Ten Foe et al., 1997). These cases of phenotypic reversion were found to be caused by intragenic recombination events generating a wild-type allele at the disease locus. In one of the patients described, the degree of reversion was sufficient to allow replacement of the majority of the mutant cells, implying that a single revertant stem cell gradually gained clonal dominance over the mutant cell.

NIH experimental trial of *FANCC* gene therapy

Based upon our preclinical data (Walsh et al., 1995) as well as safety studies of animals (Liu et al., 1995*a*), we recently initiated an experimental trial of gene therapy for group-C FA patients. This ongoing study is meant to test two hypotheses:

1. Given the known inefficiency of retroviral vectors in transducing human hemopoietic stem cells, can that efficiency be improved by multiple cycles of gene therapy in a nonmyeloablated host?

2. Can *FANCC* gene-complemented stem and progenitor cells outcompete defective mutant cells in vivo and selectively repopulate patient bone marrow?

Our trial used mobilized PB progenitor cells based on previous experimental data indicating that retrovirally marked CD34-enriched PB cells can contribute to long-term engraftment after autologous transplantation (Dunbar et al., 1995). PB progenitor cells were collected by apheresis following mobilization with G-CSF. G-CSF-mobilized cell populations may not be quiescent (Lemoli et al., 1997) and may therefore be more susceptible to retroviral gene transduction, a process that requires cell division. Because of the inefficiency of retroviral transduction of hemopoietic stem cells, we designed our study to include four cycles of mobilization, collection, transduction, and infusion, in an attempt to increase the number of gene-corrected cells. Ex vivo transduction conditions were based on our pilot studies comparing gene transfer into FA-C progenitors cultured with either autologous stromal cells or the hemopoietic growth factors SCF, IL-3, and IL-6. The addition of the exogenous growth factors was found to be necessary for efficient progenitor transduction (Walsh et al., 1995). Because of the hypoplastic state of the FA host bone marrow, ablative chemotherapy was not included prior to cell infusion.

Three FA patients, each bearing a different *FANCC* mutation (exon 1, exon 14, intron 4), have thus far participated in this trial. The *FANCC* transgene was demonstrated in transduced CD34-enriched progenitor cells. Following infusion, *FANCC* was also present transiently in PB cells. Function of the normal *FANCC* transgene was suggested by a marked increase in hemopoietic colonies following successive transduction cycles in all patients. Transient improvement in BM cellularity coincided with this expansion of hemopoietic progenitors. Apparently, transduction of the normal *FANCC* gene into hemopoietic cells from patients with *FANCC* mutations was able to improve the pathological process affecting FA hemopoiesis. However, despite the in vitro selective advantage resulting from *FANCC* gene transfer, we did not observe long-term hemopoietic reconstitution with gene-corrected clones.

Lessons from the NIH trial

Genetic manipulation of true human HSC continues to be an elusive goal. Although our small trial was able to confirm that relatively long-lived hemopoietic progenitors can be genetically altered, the number of PB mononuclear cells marked by the *FANCC* transgene was only 1/1000, remaining relatively constant following an initial tenfold increase. Despite the apparent growth advantage of corrected cells in vitro, we were unable to confirm selective amplification of the transfected clone in vivo.

The three patients who participated in our experimental trial differed greatly in the clinical and molecular features of their disease. The major *FANCC* mutations described thus far (Verlander et al., 1994), affecting exon 1, exon 14, and intron 4, were represented in our patient group. Clonal karyotypic abnormalities (Alter et al., 1993) were present in 100% of the BM cells of two of our patients. Despite progenitor mobilization patterns that were near-normal, transduction of a long-lived hemopoietic progenitor was not achieved in either of these two individuals. The observed differences in outcome may reflect differences in the biological manifestations of FA in individual patients. They also suggest that gene therapy may be more suitable for patients who have not developed clonal hemopoiesis with a dominant karyotypically abnormal precursor cell.

For FA, a number of conclusions can be drawn from our pilot study. First, our work suggests that gene complementation has at least transient positive effects on FA hemopoiesis as measured by progenitor growth and marrow cellularity, suggesting that collection of hemopoietic stem cells in FA patients prior to the outgrowth of dysplastic clones may be desirable. Those stem cells might then be transduced and reinfused at a later point should leukemia develop. Second, amplification of the transduced clone may require additional selective pressure, perhaps from the use of DNA cross-linking agents to select for resistant (transduced) clones or to purge dysplastic cells. In addition, a suicide gene could be included with the FA vector, so that dysplastic clones that had been inadvertently transfected could be eliminated.

Conclusion

Currently, stem cell transplantation is the only treatment proven to cure the marrow and blood abnormalities associated with FA (Gluckman et al., 1995). Clearly, young patients with a brother or sister who has an identical human leukocyte antigen (HLA) type should be treated by stem cell transplantation (either from bone marrow or umbilical cord blood) at the earliest stages of BM failure in preference to other therapies. However, most patients do not have an HLA-identical donor and are dependent upon finding a suitably matched nonsibling relative or unrelated donor. To date, the largest single-institution experience with mismatched related or unrelated donor stem cell transplantation for FA has been at the University of Minnesota (Dr. John Wagner, personal communication). All 23 of their patients were treated with cyclophosphamide (40 mg/kg) and total-body irradiation (400–450 cGy in a single dose) followed by stem cell transplantation using marrow or umbilical cord blood from related (nonsibling) or unrelated donors. The overall probability of marrow and white blood cell recovery was 64% (i.e., 36% failed to engraft with donor cells). At this time, graft failure clearly remains the single most important complication limiting the successful use of alternative donor transplantation. One important, unanswered question is whether autologous BM cells transduced with the *FANCC* transgene can be used to reconstitute FA-C patients who have developed graft failure following allogeneic stem cell transplantation from an unrelated donor. We have recently begun a trial to examine this issue. In theory, additional selective pressure for *FANCC* gene-modified cells may exist because the recipient will have received immune suppression and chemotherapy.

As alluded to above, one of the fundamental problems with current gene therapy protocols is the low efficiency of transduction to multipotential HSC. Two important hindrances suggested by computer modeling studies (Abkowitz et al., 1996, 1997) are the need to transduce large numbers of HSC and, second, the infrequency of stem cell replication (once every 3 weeks). If HSC do not replicate often, they may be unsusceptible to viral transduction. Future efforts to address these problems may include the use of ex vivo expansion (Emerson, 1996). The stroma plays an important role in supporting the growth of HSC through cell–cell interaction and production of the various hemopoietic cytokines. Previous studies have examined whether autologous or allogeneic stroma has the capacity to expand the hemopoietic culture of primitive progenitor and stem cells. Various combinations of cytokines have also been tested for the ability to expand the growth of LTC-IC (Zandstra et al., 1997). Recently, investigators used a stroma-free culture system with a combination of the FLT3 ligand and thrombopoietin to expand hemopoietic progenitors belonging to all lineages (Piacibello et al., 1997). In particular, there was prolonged maintenance and expansion of LTC-IC and blast cell colony-forming units for up to 6 months, suggesting extensive self-renewal with limited differentiation. If reproducible, these protocols may enable both the expansion and the replication of primitive progenitors. It may be possible to combine expansion protocols with FA gene transduction with the aim of targeting larger numbers of cycling progenitors and HSC.

With the recent identification of the major FA gene, *FANCA*, transduction strategies should become applicable for a larger number of patients within the context of carefully designed research trials. As the field of hemopoietic-cell gene transfer continues to evolve, with both minor alterations in transduction conditions (to include newer and more potent cytokines) as well as radical improvements in vector development and HSC growth, persistent expression of the FA genes in HSC may become feasible. Such studies should help define the role of gene transfer directed at HSC and lead to a better understanding of the complex pathophysiological processes underlying FA.

References

Abkowitz, J. L., Catlin, S. N. and Guttorp, P. (1996) Evidence that hemopoiesis may be a stochastic in vivo. *Nature Medicine*, **2**, 190–7.

Abkowitz, J. L., Catlin, S. N. and Guttorp, P. (1997) Strategies for hemopoietic stem cell gene therapy: insights from computer simulation studies. *Blood*, **89**, 3192–8.

Alter, B. P., Knobloch, M. E. and Weinberg, R. S. (1991) Erythropoiesis in Fanconi's anemia. *Blood*, **78**, 602–8.

Alter, B. P., Scalise, A., McCombs, J. and Najfeld, V. (1993) Clonal chromosomal abnormalities in Fanconi's anemia: what do they really mean? *British Journal of Haematology*, **85**, 627–30.

Bagby, G. C., Segal, G. M., Auerbach, A. D., Onega, T., Keeble, W. and Heinrich, M. C. (1993) Constitutive and induced expression of hemopoietic growth factor genes by fibroblasts from children with Fanconi anemia. *Experimental Hematology*, **21**, 1419–26.

Bordignon, C., Notarangelo, L. D., Nobili, N., Ferrari, G., Casorati, G., Panina, P., Mazzolari, E., Maggioni, D., Rossi, C., Servida, P., Ugazio, A. G. and Mavilio, F. (1995) Gene therapy in peripheral blood lymphocytes and bone marrow for ADA-immunodeficient patients. *Science*, **270**, 470–5.

Brenner, M. K., Rill, D. R., Holladay, M. S., Heslop, H. E., Moen, R. C., Buschle, M., Krance, R. A., Santana, V. M., Anderson, W. F. and Ihle, J. N. (1993*a*) Gene marking to determine whether autologous marrow infusion restores long-term haemopoiesis in cancer patients. *Lancet*, **342**, 1134–7.

Brenner, M. K., Rill, D. R., Moen, R. C., Krance, R. A., Mirro, J. Jr., Anderson, W. F. and Ihle, J. N. (1993*b*) Gene marking to trace origin of relapse after autologous bone-marrow transplantation. *Lancet*, **341**, 85–6.

Butturini, A. and Gale, R. P. (1994) Long-term bone marrow culture in persons with Fanconi anemia and bone marrow failure. *Blood*, **83**, 336–9.

Cumming, R. C., Liu, J. M., Youssoufian, H. and Buchwald, M. (1996) Suppression of apoptosis in hemopoietic factor-dependent progenitor cell lines by expression of the FAC gene. *Blood*, **88**, 4558–67.

Daneshbod–Skibba, G., Martin, J. and Shahidi, N. T. (1980) Myeloid and erythroid colony growth in non-anaemic patients with Fanconi's anaemia. *British Journal of Haematology*, **44**, 33–8.

Dunbar, C. E. (1996) Gene transfer to hemopoietic stem cells: implications for gene therapy of human disease. *Annual Reviews in Medicine*, **47**, 11–20.

Dunbar, C. E., Cottler, F., O'Shaughnessy, J. A., Doren, S., Carter, C., Berenson, R., Brown, S., Moen, R. C., Greenblatt, J., Stewart, F. M., Leitman, S., Wilson, W. H., Cowan, K., Young, N. S. and Nienhuis, A. W. (1995) Retrovirally-marked CD34-enriched peripheral blood and bone marrow cells contribute to long-term engraftment after autologous transplantation. *Blood*, **85**, 3048–57.

Eaves, C. J., Sutherland, H. J., Cashman, J. D., Otsuka, T., Lansdorp, P. M., Humphries, R. K., Eaves, A. C. and Hogge, D. E. (1991) Regulation of primitive human hemopoietic cells in long-term marrow culture. *Seminars in Hematology*, **28**, 126–31.

Emerson, S. G. (1996) Ex vivo expansion of hemopoietic precursors, progenitors, and stem cells: the next generation of cellular therapeutics. *Blood*, **87**, 3082–8.

Fanconi Anaemia/Breast Cancer Consortium (1996) Positional cloning of the Fanconi anaemia group A gene. *Nature Genetics*, **14**, 324–8.

Fanconi, G. (1927) Familiäre infantile periziosaartige Anämie (perniziöses Blutbild und Konstitution). *Jahrbuch Kinder*, **117**, 257.

Fanconi, G. (1967) Familial constitutional panmyelopathy, Fanconi's anemia (FA) I. Clinical aspects. *Seminars in Hematology*, **4**, 233.

Fu, K–L., Lo Ten Foe, J. R., Joenje, H., Rao, K. W., Liu, J. M. and Walsh, C. E. (1997) Functional correction of Fanconi anemia group A hemopoietic cells by retroviral gene transfer. *Blood*, **90**, 3296–303.

Gluckman, E., Broxmeyer, H. E., Auerbach, A. D., Friedman, H. S., Douglas, G. W., Devergie, A., Esperou, H., Thierry, D., Socié, G., Lehn, P., Cooper, S., English, D., Kurtzberg, J., Bard, J. and Boyse, E. A. (1989) Hemopoietic reconstitution in a patient with Fanconi's anemia by means of umbilical-cord blood from an HLA-identical sibling. *New England Journal of Medicine*, **321**, 1174–8.

Gluckman, E., Auerbach, A. D., Horowitz, M. M., Sobocinski, K. A., Ash, R. C., Bortin, M. M., Butturini, A., Camitta, B. M., Champlin, R. E., Friedrich, W., Good, R. A., Gordon–Smith, E. C., Harris, R. E., Klein, J. P., Ortega, J. J., Pasquini, R., Ramsay, N. K. C., Speck, B., Vowels, M. R., Zhang, M.–J. and Gale, R. P. (1995) Bone marrow transplantation for Fanconi anemia. *Blood*, **86**, 2856–62.

Kohli–Kumar, M., Shahidi, N. T., Broxmeyer, H. E., Masterson, M., Delaat, C., Sambrano, J., Morris, C., Auerbach, A. D. and Harris, R. E. (1993) Haemopoietic stem/progenitor cell transplant in Fanconi anaemia using HLA-matched sibling umbilical cord blood cells. *British Journal of Haematology*, **85**, 419–22.

Kohn, D. B., Weinberg, K. I., Nolta, J. A., Heiss, L. N., Lenarsky, C., Crooks, G. M., Hanley, M. E., Annett, G., Brooks, J. S., El–Khoureiy, A., Lawrence, K., Wells, S., Moen, R. C., Bastian, J., Williams–Herman, D. E., Elder, M., Wara, D., Bowen, T., Hershfield, M. S., Mullen, C. A., Blaese, R. M. and Parkman, R. (1995) Engraftment of gene-modified umbilical cord blood cells in neonates with adenosine deaminase deficiency. *Nature Medicine*, **1**, 1017–23.

Kupfer, G. M., Naf, D., Suliman, A., Pulsipher, M. and D'Andrea, A. D. (1997) The Fanconi anaemia proteins, FAA and FAC, interact to form a nuclear complex. *Nature Genetics*, **17**, 487–90.

Lemoli, R. M., Tafuri, A., Fortuna, A., Petrucci, M. T., Ricciardi, M. R., Catani, L., Rondelli, D., Fogli, M., Leopardi, G., Ariola, C. and Tura, S. (1997) Cycling status of CD34+ cells mobilized into peripheral blood of healthy donors by recombinant human granulocyte colony-stimulating factor. *Blood*, **89**, 1189–96.

Liu, J., Kim, K. and Walsh, C. E. (1995*a*) Retroviral-mediated transduction of the Fanconi anemia C complementing (FACC) gene in two murine transplantation models. *Blood Cells Molecules Diseases*, **21**, 56–63.

Liu, J. M., Walsh, C. E. and Nienhuis, A. W. (1995*b*) Gene therapy for hematologic disorders. In *Hematology: basic principles and practice*, ed. R. Hoffman, E. J. Benz, S. J. Shattil, B. Furie, H. J. Cohen and L. E. Silberstein, p. 427. New York: Churchill Livingstone.

Lo Ten Foe, J. R., Rooimans, M. A., Bosnoyan–Collins, L., Alon, N., Wijker, M., Parker, L., Lightfoot, J., Carreau, M., Callen, D. F., Savoia, A., Cheng, N. C., van Berkel, C. G. M., Strunk, M. H. P., Gille, J. J. P., Pals, G., Kruyt, F. A. E., Pronk, J. C., Arwert, F., Buchwald, M. and Joenje, H. (1996) Expression cloning of a cDNA for the major Fanconi anaemia gene, FAA. *Nature Genetics*, **14**, 320–3.

Lo Ten Foe, J. R., Kwee, M. L., Rooimans, M. A., Oostra, A. B., Veerman, A. J., van Weel, M., Pauli, R. M., Shahidi, N. T., Dokal, I., Roberts, I., Altay, C., Gluckman, E., Gibson, R. A., Mathew, C. G., Arwert, F. and Joenje, H. (1997) Somatic mosaicism in Fanconi anaemia: molecular basis and clinical significance. *European Journal of Human Genetics*, **5**, 137–48.

Lu, L., Shen, R–N. and Broxmeyer, H. E. (1996) Stem cells from bone marrow, umbilical cord blood and peripheral blood for clinical application: current status and future application. *Critical Reviews in Oncology/Hematology*, **22**, 61–78.

Piacibello, W., Sanavio, F., Garetto, L., Severino, A., Bergandi, D., Ferrario, J., Fagioli, F., Berger, M. and Aglietta, M. (1997) Extensive amplification and self-renewal of human primitive hemopoietic stem cells from cord blood. *Blood*, **89**, 2644–53.

Ridet, A., Guillouf, C., Duchaud, E., Cundari, E., Fiore, M., Moustacchi, E. and Rosselli, F. (1997) Deregulated apoptosis is a hallmark of the Fanconi anemia syndrome. *Cancer Research*, **57**, 1722–30.

Stark, R., Thierry, D., Richard, P. and Gluckman, E. (1993) Long-term bone marrow culture in Fanconi's anaemia. *British Journal of Haematology*, **83**, 554–9.

Strathdee, C. A., Gavish, H., Shannon, W. R. and Buchwald, M. (1992) Cloning of cDNAs for Fanconi's anaemia by functional complementation. *Nature*, **356**, 763–7.

Sutherland, H. J., Eaves, C. J., Eaves, A. C., Dragowska, W. and Lansdorp, P. M. (1989) Characterization and partial purification of human marrow cells capable of initiating long-term hemopoiesis in vitro. *Blood*, **74**, 1563–70.

Verlander, P. C., Lin, J. D., Udono, M. U., Zhang, Q., Gibson, R. A., Mathew, C. G. and Auerbach, A. D. (1994) Mutation analysis of the Fanconi anemia gene FACC. *American Journal of Human Genetics*, **54**, 595–601.

Walsh, C. E., Grompe, M., Vanin, E., Buchwald, M., Young, N. S., Nienhuis, A. W. and Liu, J. M. (1994*a*) A functionally active retrovirus vector for gene therapy in Fanconi anemia group C. *Blood*, **84**, 453–9.

Walsh, C. E., Nienhuis, A. W., Samulski, R. J., Brown, M. G., Miller, J. L., Young, N. S. and Liu, J. M. (1994*b*) Phenotypic correction of Fanconi anemia in human hemopoietic cells with a recombinant adeno-associated virus vector. *Journal of Clinical Investigation*, **94**, 1440–8.

Walsh, C. E., Mann, M. M., Emmons, R. V. B., Wang, S. and Liu, J. L. (1995) Transduction of CD-34-enriched human peripheral andumblical cord blood progenitors using a retroviral vector with the Fanconi anemia group C gene. *Journal of Investigative Medicine*, **43**, 379–85.

Zandstra, P. W., Conneally, E., Petzer, A. L., Piret, J. M. and Eaves, C. J. (1997) Cytokine manipulation of primitive human hemopoietic cell self-renewal. *Proceedings of the National Academy of Sciences USA*, **94**, 4698–703.

Index

Note: Aplastic anemia is referred to as 'AA' and severe aplastic anemia as 'SAA'. Page numbers in *italics* refer to figures and tables.